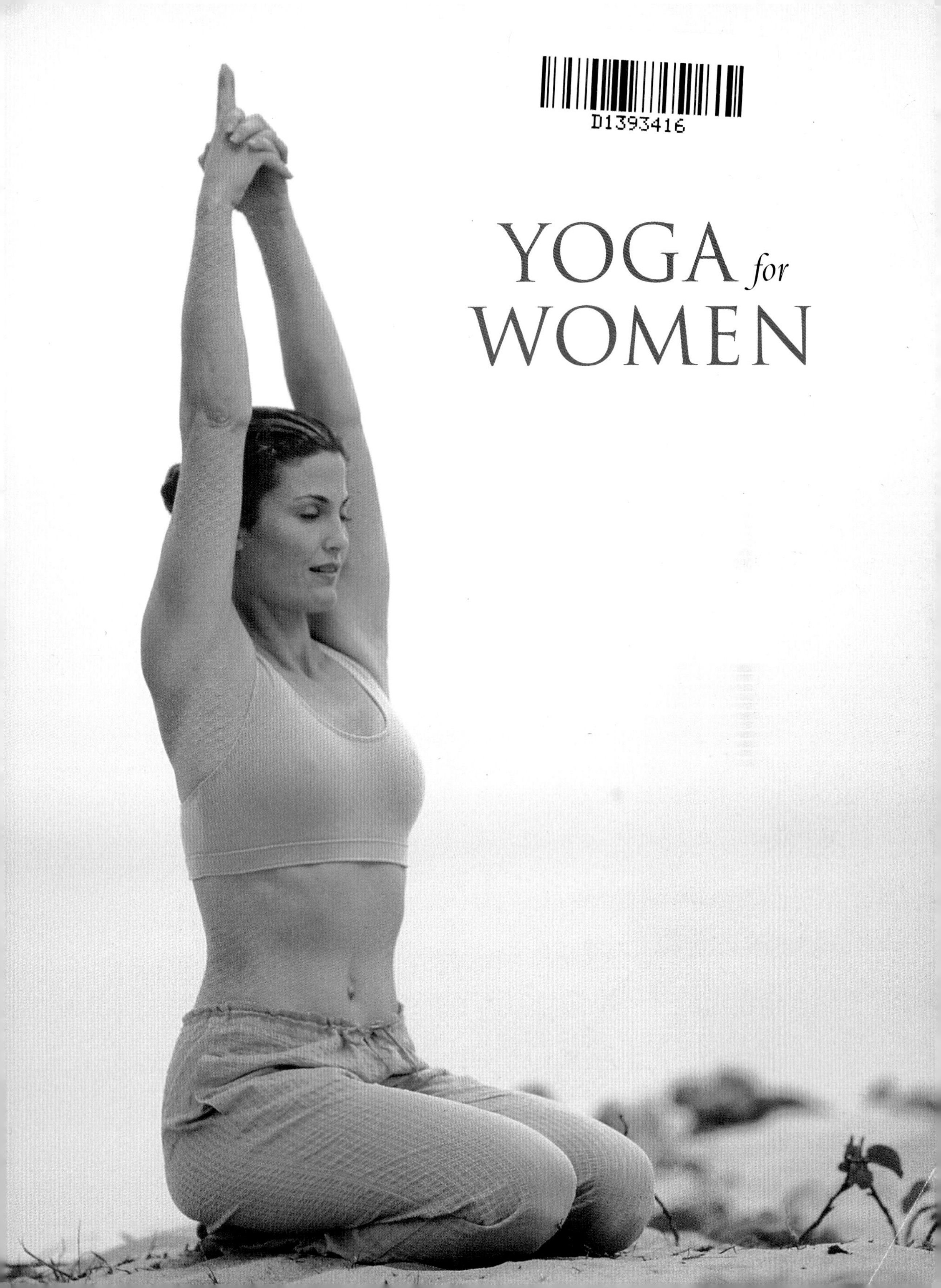
D1393416
YOGA for
WOMEN

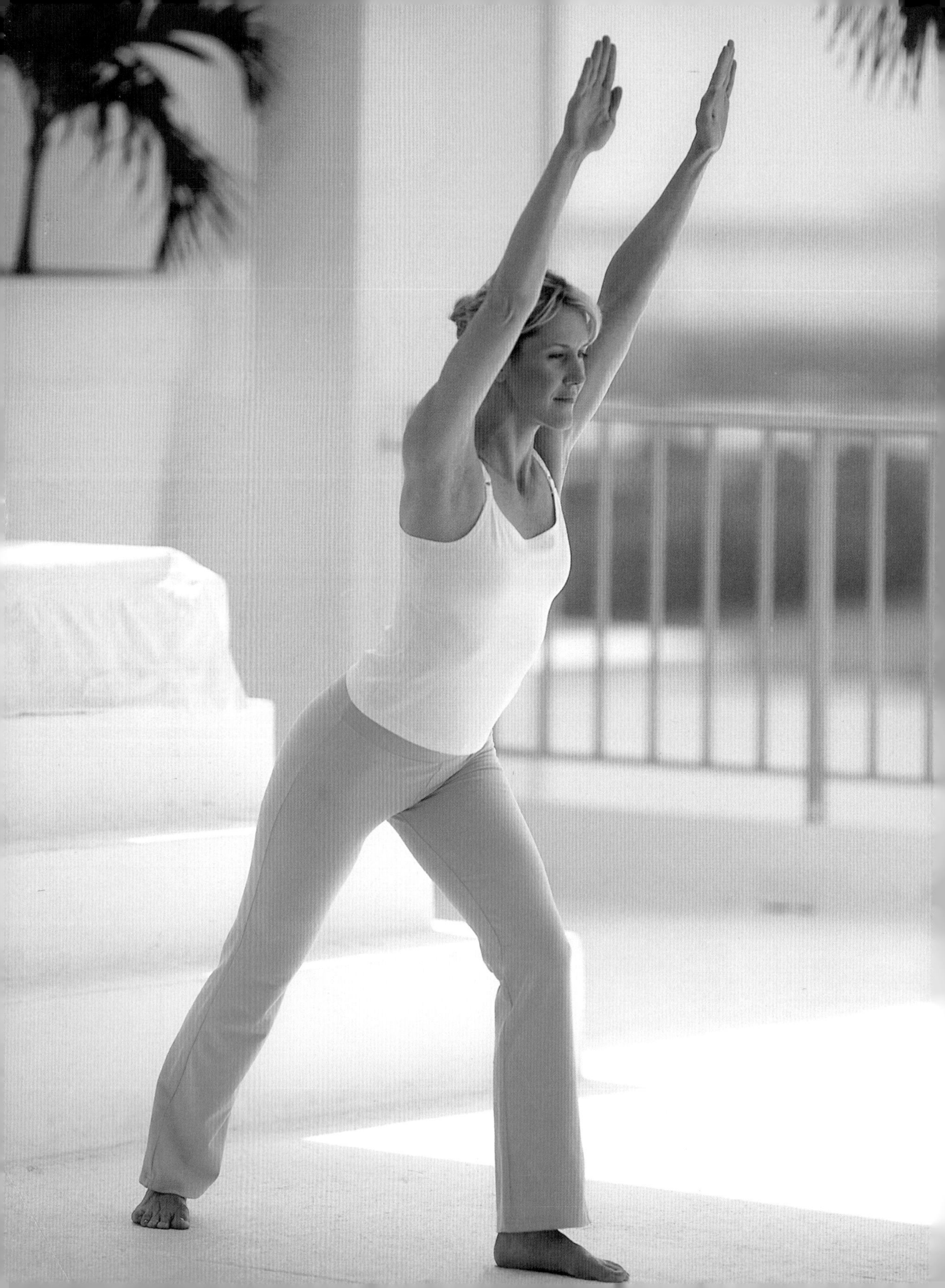

YOGA *for* WOMEN

SHAKTA KAUR KHALSA

Photography by Russell Sadur

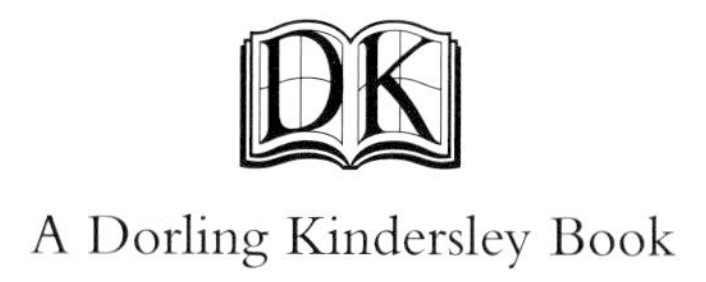

A Dorling Kindersley Book

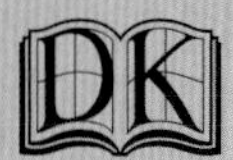

London, New York, Munich,
Melbourne, and Delhi

Dedicated with love and gratitude to Yogi Bhajan, my spiritual teacher and Master of Kundalini Yoga, and to my mother, Grace Meyers, for her unfailing love and support.

Project Editor Susannah Steel
Art Editor Claire Legemah
Managing Editor Gillian Roberts
Senior Art Editor Karen Sawyer
Art Director Carole Ash
Category Publisher Mary-Clare Jerram
DTP Designer Sonia Charbonnier
Production Controller Joanna Bull

First published in Great Britain in 2002
by Dorling Kindersley Limited
80 Strand, London WC2R 0RL
A Penguin Company

This paperback edition published 2004

A CIP catalogue record for this book
is available from The British Library

ISBN 1 4053 0704 8

Colour reproduced in Great Britain by
Media Development and Printing, Ltd.
Printed in China by
C&C Offset Printing Co., Ltd.

Discover more at
www.dk.com

NOTE TO READERS
Always consult your GP before beginning any exercise programme. Nothing in this book is to be construed as medical advice. Benefits attributed to the practice of yoga come from the ancient yogic traditions. Results will vary with each individual.

This book is intended as a complement to instruction from trained yoga teachers. Personal guidance from a trained teacher and the experience of group yoga classes are of equal importance as the guidance of this book. See *Resources* to locate qualified instructors in your area.

Whenever possible, the information presented in this book has been verified for authenticity through the official organizations and yogic traditions that are represented within these pages. Additionally, this book has been granted the the seal of approval for authenticity of information from the Kundalini Research Institute (KRI).

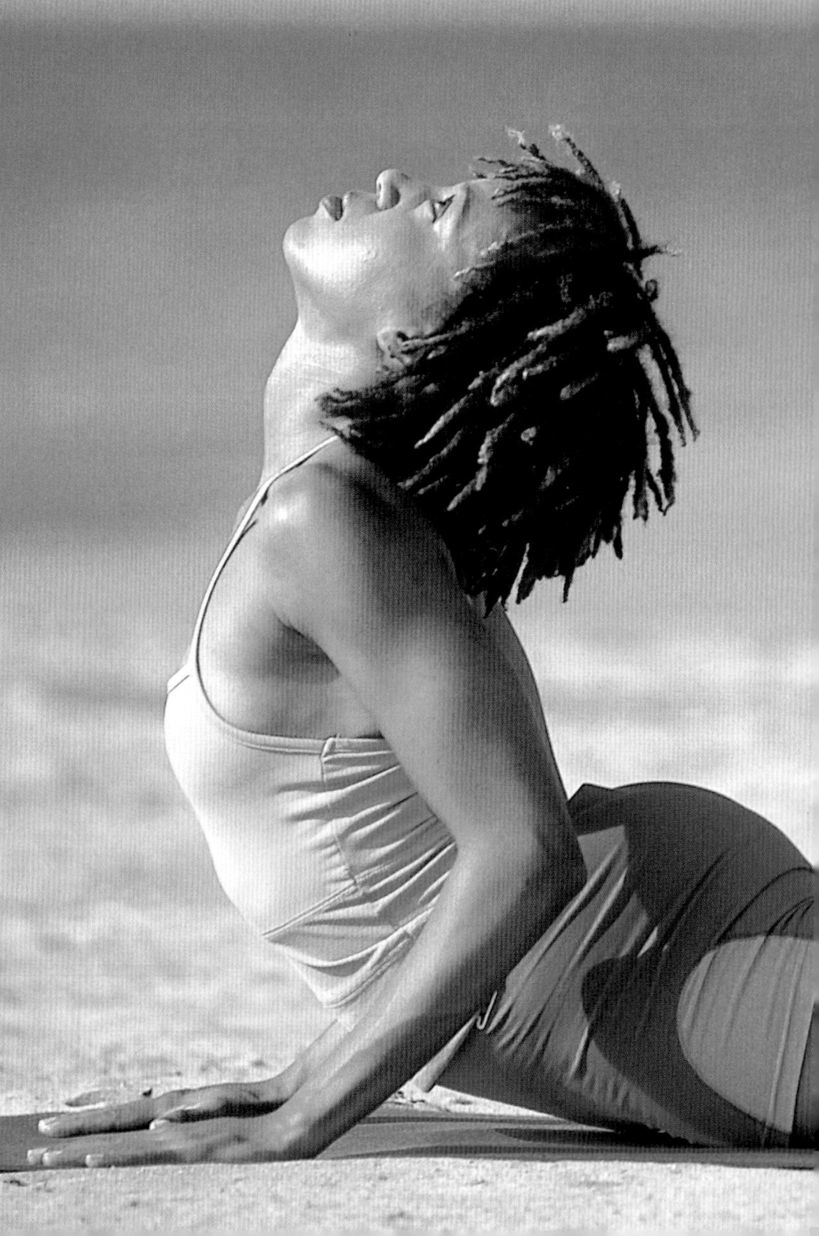

CONTENTS

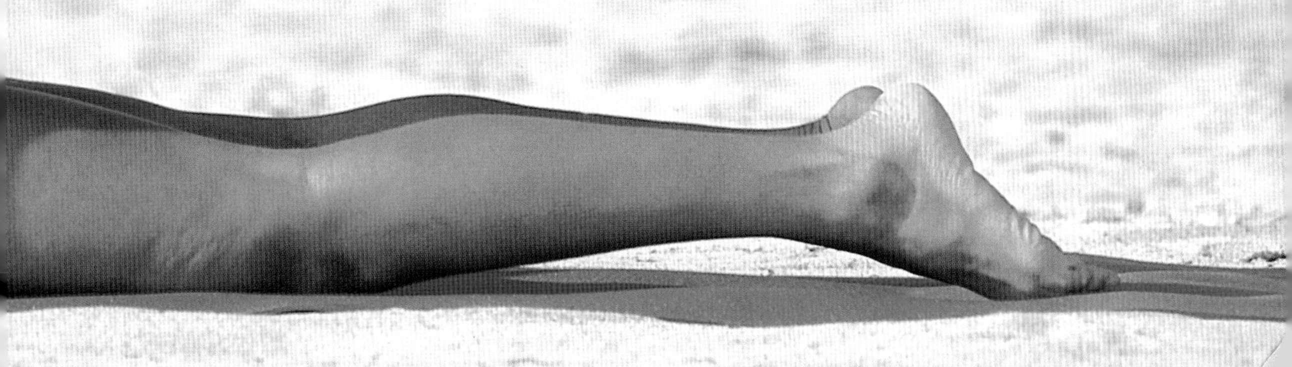

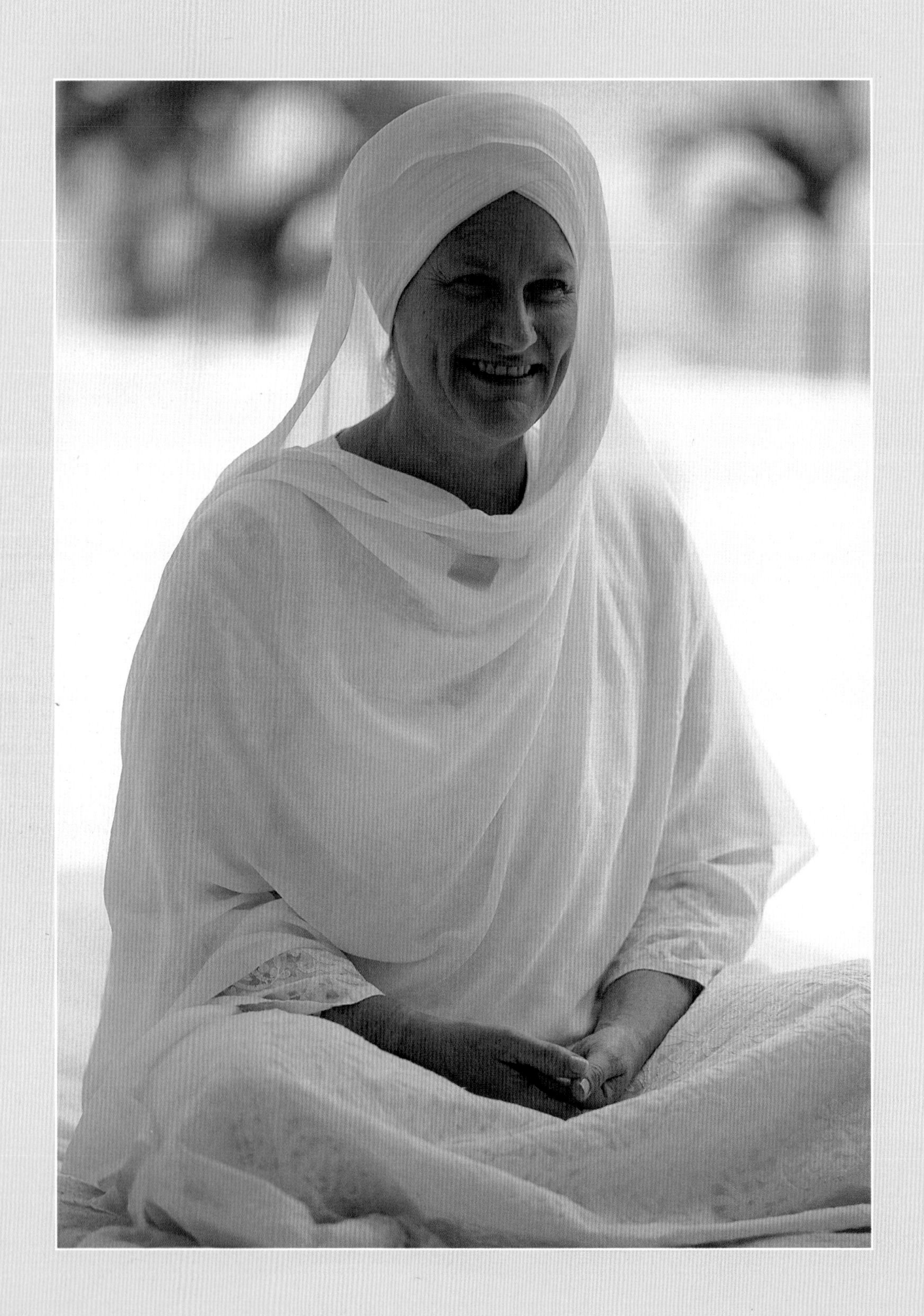

A NOTE FROM THE AUTHOR

I adore teaching women yoga. Yoga and women go together like tea and toast. It's a cozy, homey fit. Women love to relax with other women. We love to share our experiences with each other, and after a yoga class there are often much inspired and somewhat intimate conversations around. Someone is sure to say, "Wow, I needed that class!"

Just on the other side of yoga's relaxing coziness is its dynamic, transformational power. During the many years that I've been practising yoga, I have grown in ways that I never would have imagined possible. I am not the same person I was – literally. I believe the atoms and molecules in my body are different than they were before I began a life of daily yoga practice. Life is so much easier, not because it doesn't present challenges, but because I can handle the challenges now. My ability to move on from life's crises I attribute to the consistent, honest work – and joy – of a daily yoga practice.

The key word is "daily". Don't let this intimidate you. Start out by thinking of it as a "steady" practice, 10 or 15 minutes a day, an hour every few days or so. You will begin to feel taller, straighter, fitter. You will become more aware of the rhythm of your breath, and deepen your breathing in order to relax yourself. You may experience a new and positive outlook that becomes more permanent. Emotions even out. Little things, and even big things, no longer hold the same power over you that they used to. Over time, past hurts – mental and emotional scars – heal and fade, as though from another dim lifetime. You begin to find the strength and confidence to live your dreams, and beyond!

Such is the healing and transformational power of the yoga that is held within these pages. And now, if you are ready, let's begin.

INTRODUCING WOMEN'S YOGA

Within the pages of this book you will find a practical manual for nurturing the many facets of you as a woman. Yoga – as you may know – is an ancient art and science that brings health and wellbeing to your body, mind, and spirit. Yoga accomplishes this through a practice of movements, held postures, breathing exercises, and mental focus. People who practise yoga say that they feel more relaxed, accomplish more with less stress, and feel in touch with their inner being, their sense of authentic self.

WHY YOGA FOR WOMEN?

Yoga is good for everyone – men, women, and children. Why, then, a yoga book just for women? We women have well-defined needs, issues, and stages of life. Just think, for a moment, how a woman's outlook and physical health are affected by her hormones, which control menstrual cycle, pregnancy, and menopause. Yoga balances these hormones efficiently and effectively through the many stages of a woman's life. But yoga is not just for the bodily changes that women undergo. It is for balancing emotions. For reducing the impact of diseases such as breast cancer and osteoporosis. And for the feminine need to have a cosy, relaxed way of life, supported by a spiritual outlook.

About 85 per cent of those who practise yoga are women, and we are attracted to it for many reasons – to find relaxation, gain energy, and to remain flexible physically

MEDICAL CONDITIONS

Practise yoga gently and slowly, and include the use of recommended props – or avoid certain poses altogether – if you have one of the following medical conditions:

- *Heart conditions and asthma. Avoid breathing exercises and aerobic or strenuous poses.*
- *Spinal conditions and osteoporosis. Avoid strenuous backbends, inverted poses, spinal twists, and balancing poses.*
- *High-risk pregnancy and complications after the birth. Check with your GP before starting yoga.*
- *Balancing problems and neurological diseases. Avoid poses that require balancing, especially on one foot or on the hands.*

Remember, yoga is non-competitive so practise only to your capacity. Some restrictions may apply, depending on your physical abilities. If a pose causes discomfort, stop and go on to another pose, or do the easy-does-it version if one is provided. Always consult your GP with concerns you may have about any poses or exercises before doing them.

and mentally, nurturing the spirit and developing inner strength and higher awareness. Generally, women exhibit more physical and mental flexibility than men. To be able to carry and birth babies, we have been designed with flexible bodies. We have an innate capacity to do many things at once – take care of a sick child, cook, talk on the telephone, and perhaps three other things all at the same time. We have a natural mental flexibility that allows us to "go with the flow". These star qualities shine brightly with a practice of yoga and meditation that can be enhanced by beautiful, inspiring music designed especially for use with this book *(see* Music Resources, *p.224)*. And through yoga, we experience the balanced interplay of vitality and relaxation – the ability to be alert yet peaceful, relaxed and energized, all at the same time.

As women, we also have needs. I have found from my years of practice and teaching that yoga goes directly to the heart of women's needs. We need to feel loved. Yoga develops self-love. We need to feel secure. Yoga lets a woman know her security lies within. We need to feel fulfilled. Yoga develops self-awareness and self-fulfillment. When a woman knows she is complete in herself, all her relationships enjoy the benefit of that knowledge. Just with her presence she uplifts her partner, her children, her parents, her co-workers, her friends, and even those she meets in passing.

I believe that you will find *Yoga for Women* to be a treasure house filled with the best gems and jewels that women's yoga has to offer.

REMEDIES & MORE

In this book you will find healing remedies and recipes based on the ancient science of yoga. These include:

✻ *Self-massage of the lymphatic system in the upper chest and armpit areas to stimulate blood and energy circulation and help prevent stagnation (a factor in the formation of cysts).*

✻ *A tasty recipe for Golden Milk made with turmeric, an Indian spice that is known to keep joints lubricated.*

✻ *Special drinks for a woman in the first few days after giving birth, which will give her energy, be easy on the sensitive digestive system, and optimize the nutritional content of her breast milk, providing the richest nourishment for her new baby.*

✻ *An ancient recipe for a wonderfully luxurious "yogurt bath" that cleans your skin down to the pores and keeps you feeling and looking both young and relaxed.*

Additionally, throughout the book are scattered inspiring stories by women whose lives were changed through yoga. You may have your own story to tell as you develop your lifelong relationship with a wonderful best friend... yoga.

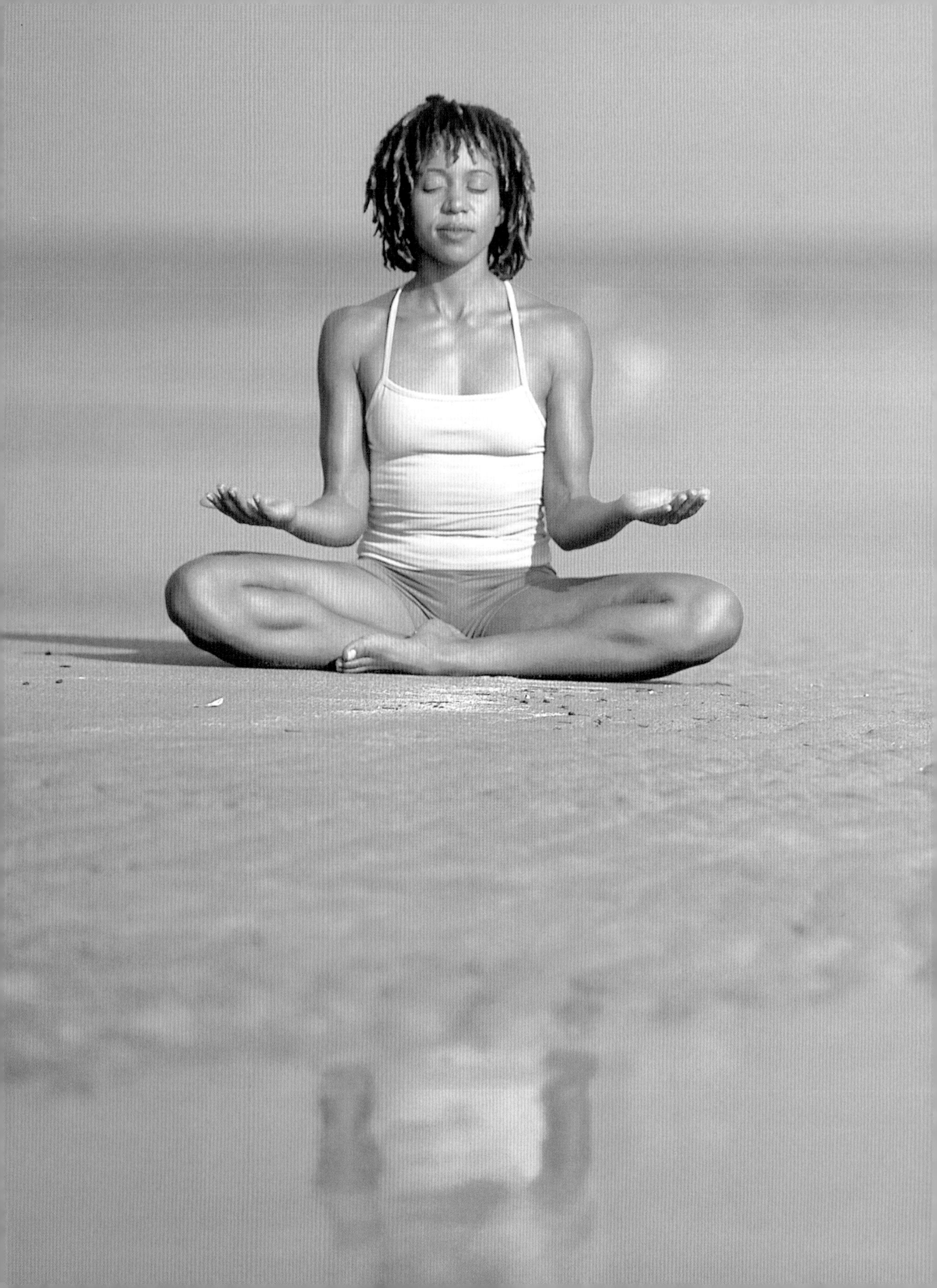

BEGINNINGS

The genius of yoga is that it is a self-perpetuating system. I have found that in practising yoga I feel inspired and empowered to want to do more yoga. It is as if yoga says to me, "You take the first step, and let me do the rest." Of course, experience is everything. So set yourself in a quiet space and get ready to begin your yoga journey.

Here, at the beginning, is always a good place to start. In this part of the book you will come to understand the big picture of yoga and begin to glean many of the finer points that make yoga the wonderful, transforming practice that it is.

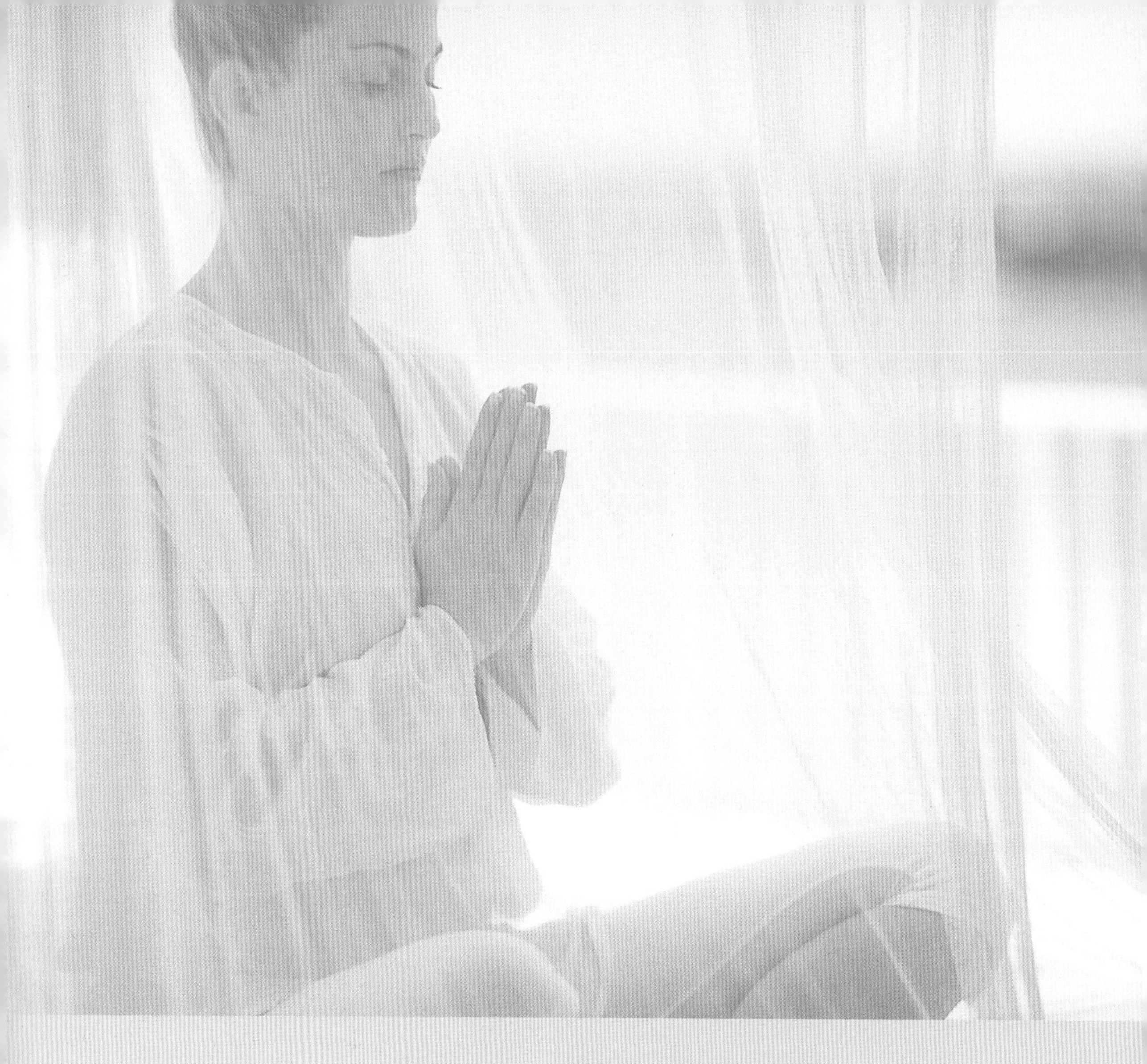

THE BASICS

Yoga is older than recorded time. It may well be tens of thousands of years old. Yoga's beauty lies in the realization that a practice of yoga is as relevant to our lives in the 21st century as it was all those many centuries ago – maybe even more so, given the stresses and uncertainties of our fast-paced, modern lives. If I were to name one thing that has been the greatest blessing in my life, I would say it is my daily yoga practice and meditation. I like to practise in the quiet early morning hours, finishing up just as the light creeps across the sky and the birds begin their morning call. Throughout the day when things get rough, I sometimes remember how I felt early that morning and can recapture that peaceful clarity.

So well-known is the idea of yoga that it hardly needs explanation. But what, in essence, does yoga mean? Being an inquisitive sort of person, I always enjoy delving into the origin of a word in order to glimpse its essential meaning. The word "yoga" comes from the Sanskrit word *yug*, which means "to yoke", or bind together. And what does yoga bind together? All the various parts of ourselves, often thought of as body, mind, and spirit. Yoga is an instrument of wholeness. And by the way, did you know that the word "whole" is the origin of the words health, heal, and holy? Amazing, isn't it, how even an ordinary dictionary can be a source of enlightenment.

The main focus of this book is instructional, working with asana (postures and exercises), pranayama (breathing techniques), and the practice of meditation. These are the tools of yoga – tools to pick up and use to change ourselves for the better, to drop self-defeating patterns and to live to our deepest and highest idea of who we are. As you move deeper into your practice, still more elements of yoga come in to play *(see* Yoga Sutras, *right).*

UNDERSTANDING THE YOGA IN THIS BOOK

Although Kundalini Yoga has been the primary style of yoga I've practised and taught for many years, I also very much enjoy my practice of Hatha Yoga. My vision in shaping this book is to create an artful, harmonious blend of Hatha and Kundalini Yoga. The idea is to take the best of both worlds, although in reality Hatha and Kundalini are both from the same world of yoga, using many of the

YOGA SUTRAS

The science of yoga was known and practised but not clearly documented until around 200AD, when a physician-sage called Patanjali systematized and codified the science of yoga into what became known as the Yoga Sutras:

* ***Yama*** *encourages moderation and restraint.*
* ***Niyama*** *gives the ground rules for self-discipline and inner awareness.*
* ***Asana,*** *or yoga postures, keep the body healthy and the mind calm, creating an atmosphere in which the life energy can flow more easily.*
* ***Pranayama*** *focuses on experiencing the link between the breath, mind, and body.*
* ***Pratyahara*** *is the process of becoming aware of, and learning to control, thought patterns.*
* ***Dharana*** *is when the mind, once withdrawn into itself, is fixed in one-pointed inner concentration.*
* ***Dhyana*** *is meditation without focus on an object, founded in a deep, inner space of awareness.*
* ***Samadhi*** *is the ecstatic state of being, in which the meditator becomes one with the object of meditation.*

same postures and following the same yogic teachings. But for those of you who may be new to yoga in general, or to Hatha and Kundalini Yoga specifically, I have included some background and basics about each yoga style here.

ABOUT HATHA YOGA

The word "Hatha" comes from two Sanskrit words, *Ha,* meaning sun, and *Tha*, meaning moon. Hatha Yoga blends the sun/male/active energy with the moon/female/receptive energy that is in each of us.

Hatha Yoga practice consists of held and moving postures, called asanas. There are a wide variety of asanas (over 200), each one with its own distinct form dictated by stretching, counter-stretching, and resistance. The alignment of the muscular and skeletal structures is a major focus of the asanas. Adding a conscious breathing pattern to the postures helps circulate energy and blood, and brings balance to the sympathetic and parasympathetic nervous systems, which govern the function of just about every other system in the body. In other words, asana practice is the key to the body, which is the key to the mind, which is the key to the spirit.

There are a wide variety of Hatha Yoga styles and traditions. Most of the Hatha Yoga included in this book is general, with some influence from the Viniyoga tradition. *Vini* can be translated from its original Sanskrit word to mean individual. It can also mean step-by-step and gradual. With Viniyoga, the pace is relaxed and poses are adjusted to meet individual needs.

DIFFERENT YOGA STYLES

The plethora of different styles of yoga is enough to make your head spin. Try to think of them as rays of light emanating from the same sun, and since they are from the same source, they are all related. It is only natural, though, that distinct differences between the various schools of yoga have developed over time, and thankfully so – there's something for everyone when it comes to yoga.

UNSEEN ENERGY CENTRES

According to the science of yoga, the body is made up of centres of energy called chakras that are not visible to most of us. Those who can see chakras say that these fields of energy are like fluid whirlpools of light, each with its own colour, which are constantly moving and changing in complex patterns. Chakras function as intake organs for energy from the universal life force (prana) that is all around us. There are eight chakras (see side bar, opposite).

ABOUT KUNDALINI YOGA

Kundalini comes from the word *kundal*, which means "lock of hair from the beloved". The uncoiling of this "hair" is the awakening of the kundalini, the creative potential that already exists in every human. The easiest way to understand kundalini is to realize that there is the universal spirit, sometimes referred to as God, that uncoils him/her/itself. This uncoiling process is known as kundalini. What is uncoiling and awakening is you, nothing more and nothing less. It is an innate capacity that most people simply are not utilizing. Yoga is the science of the Self, and kundalini is the awakening of the Self. It is that simple.

The main aim of Hatha Yoga is to bring about a balanced flow of energy through the body's energy centres, called chakras *(see side bar, right)*. But, besides the energy that is already flowing within our bodies, there is a vast reservoir of untapped energy stored (according to yogic tradition) under the fourth vertebra of the spinal column. This latent energy is activated through Kundalini Yoga.

This untapped energy is stimulated through the proper practice of Kundalini Yoga as given by my teacher, Yogi Bhajan. As you maintain a steady yoga practice over a period of time, the energy gradually rises up the central column of the spine, balancing the body's chakras and activating the secretion of the pineal gland, which is located in the centre of the skull. Although some functions of the pineal gland are yet to be properly understood, in yogic science it is considered the very key to life, both physical and spiritual.

CHAKRAS

* ***The first chakra*** *at the base of the spine is our "root", grounding us on the earth, and relates to primal needs.*

* ***The second chakra*** *is located beside the reproductive organs and relates to sexual energy and creativity.*

* ***The third chakra*** *is at the navel and relates to stamina, willpower, and wellbeing.*

* ***The fourth chakra*** *is at the centre of the chest, the heart centre, and relates to personal and universal feelings of love.*

* ***The fifth chakra*** *is at the throat, and relates to the ability to speak truth.*

* ***The sixth chakra*** *is at the centre of the forehead where the eyebrows meet, known as the "brow point", and relates to the power of intuition and visionary qualities.*

* ***The seventh chakra*** *is located at the top of the head at the crown, and relates to all-expansive merger with universal spirit.*

* ***The eighth chakra*** *is sometimes considered to be the aura, or electromagnetic energy field surrounding the entire body, as well as interpenetrating each of the seven chakras in the body.*

TIPS FOR YOUR YOGA PRACTICE

* *It is best to practise yoga barefoot on a non-slip mat with a blanket, rug, or sheepskin for extra padding.*
* *Warm up with exercises in* Warming up to Yoga (pp.30–41) *before practising a yoga set.*
* *Let your eyes have a soft focus or be closed. Turn your attention inwards.*
* *Move slowly into the pose to avoid injury and to increase your inner awareness. If the instructions are to move quickly, build up to a fast pace, as much as you are able.*
* *Discomfort is fine, pain is not. Stretch as far as is comfortable. Work on the edge of the stretch, but stop if you experience any pain.*
* *Breathe, breathe, breathe! Unless instructed otherwise, inhale and exhale through the nose, not the mouth.*
* *Hold the poses for the minimum time if you are new to yoga, eventually working up to the maximum time.*
* *To conclude an exercise or posture, inhale and pause the breath briefly, then exhale and relax the posture.*

Kundalini Yoga, which includes many of the same postures found in Hatha Yoga, provides a good challenge yet is very doable; the positive effects can be experienced in a matter of minutes. It consists of both held postures and active exercises, often coordinated with strong breathing patterns.

MENTAL FOCUS DURING YOGA

During yoga practice, hold your mind in the present moment by keeping your attention focused on each breath that you take: you can hear it, feel it, even visualize the breath. As you inhale, see prana, or life energy, entering your body and mind. See and feel it as sparkling light, vital and fresh, bringing all possibilities to you. Then as you exhale, release the apana, the used-up energy, old thoughts and feelings, tensions, discomfort, and anything you are ready to let go of to make way for new beginnings on the next inbreath.

As well as listening, feeling, and visualizing your breath moving in and out, you can also imagine hearing a sound on your breath. One sound that is often used in yoga is *Om*. Another is *Sat Nam* (rhymes with "but mum"). *Sat* is heard on the inhalation, and *Nam* on the exhalation. This means "Truth is my/our essence". You can also use affirmations in your own language that speak to you, for example, "I am, I am".

RELAXATION AND MEDITATION

Following the natural flow of a routine of yoga, a period of deep relaxation and then meditation gives the perfect energy balance to the body and mind. A meditative mind and a relaxed mind go together: your relaxation practice will enhance your meditation, and the practice of meditation will teach you to relax. The yogic teachings say that there are different "processing" times needed to create certain desired effects during meditation. Although some meditations are given for a specific amount of time and should not exceed that amount, most meditations are done for 11 minutes, which adjusts your pituitary, or master gland, and your nervous system, and also changes your outlook for the better. After 31 minutes of meditation, your entire mind and all the chakras are positively affected. After a 62-minute meditation, your subconscious mind is positively transformed and integrated with your conscious mind.

Each chapter in this book is designed as a beautiful and effective dance of yoga and meditation, set to the tune of women's themes. As much as possible, leave time at the end of your practice for at least five minutes of meditation, and preferably 11 minutes.

Starting your day with yoga can make a very real difference to how well your day goes. Some women find an afternoon practice rejuvenates and relaxes them for the rest of the day. Many women, especially those with children, find that their favourite time to turn to yoga is in the evening when the house is quiet. However you can squeeze your yoga time into your busy life, I guarantee that the effort will be worth it.

RELAXING WITH YOGA

✻ *Twenty seconds to a minute of relaxation between postures allows the energy to circulate throughout your body and mind.*

✻ *Follow your practice with a deep relaxation on your back for a minimum of 10 minutes, more if possible.*

✻ *The optimal time for meditation is after your yoga practice, usually after a period of relaxation.*

✻ *Above all, enjoy. A little smiling goes a long way!*

YOGIC CYCLES OF TIME

The yogic teachings talk of specific cycles of time that help to change old habits and develop new ones. For a really special experience, choose a specific yoga set or meditation in this book and commit to a programme of practice for one of the following times:

✻ ***40 days*** *will change an old habit into a more positive one.*
✻ ***90 days*** *confirms the new habit in you.*
✻ ***120 days*** *allows the habit to become who you are*
✻ ***1,000 days*** *ensures that you have mastered the habit.*

BASIC POSTURES

Knowing how to sit is a very important component in yoga and meditation. Your sitting posture should provide a firm base for your spine to stack up straight. Why is this important? Think of a garden hose. When it is straight the water flow is strong, when it is curved or twisted the water flow is weak. In a similar way your spine conducts spinal fluid, which nourishes every nerve and carries messages to your brain. It also contains prana, the Sanskrit word for the life force energy that flows through all of your body's energy centres, enlivening your vital awareness and your sense of self.

Straightening your spine is a matter of paying attention to how well your vertebrae are lining up. You can help this process by slightly tightening your abdominal muscles to hold the pelvis in place while lifting your breastbone slightly, and subtly pulling your chin in towards your neck to straighten the cervical vertebrae. Keep your shoulders relaxed. Visualize your spine lengthening and straightening, and relax into the feeling.

YOUR YOGA SPACE

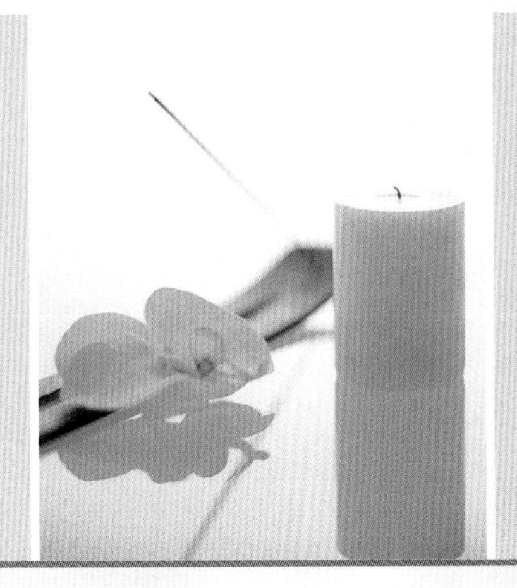

Think of your yoga space as your personal sanctuary, a place where you can drop everything and be in a haven of peace. You may like to decorate a low table or altar with objects such as a candle, meaningful photos or objects, and a vase of flowers.

If you don't have a particular place set up for yoga, just find a quiet spot where you will have room to move. Spread out a mat that will fit the length of your body, perhaps adding a blanket or sheepskin for padding. If you have a wooden floor, use a yoga mat that will not slip.

EASY POSE

Let's explore the most common sitting poses in yoga. The basic sitting posture is Easy pose. Besides being the most often-used meditation posture, it is the starting position for many yoga exercises.

Sit on the ground with your legs crossed at the ankles so that your body forms a triangular base. Straighten the spine, relax the shoulders, and rest your hands on your knees. To straighten the lower spine and allow the knees to relax down, place a firm pillow, bolster, or thick blanket under your buttocks.

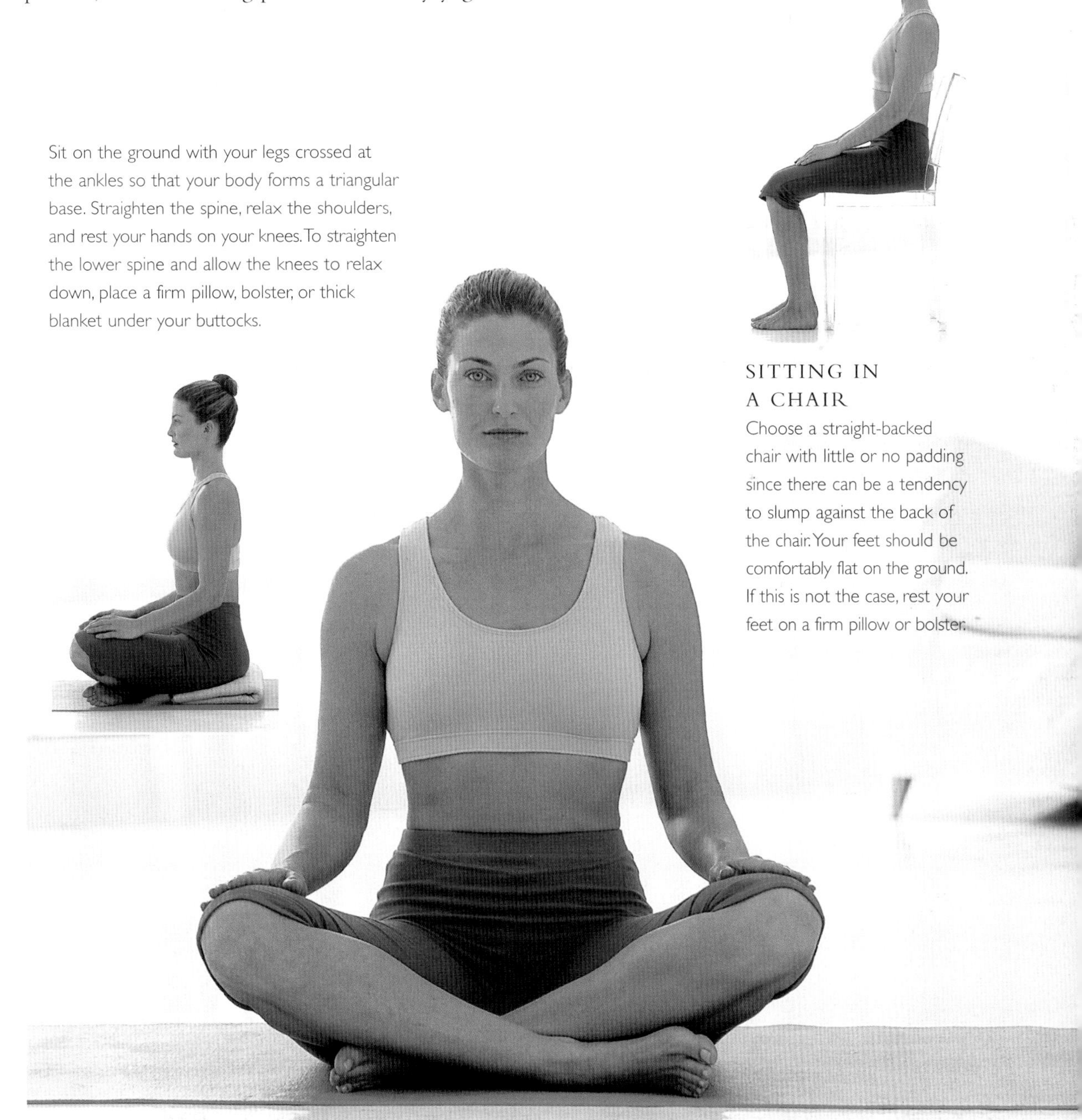

SITTING IN A CHAIR

Choose a straight-backed chair with little or no padding since there can be a tendency to slump against the back of the chair. Your feet should be comfortably flat on the ground. If this is not the case, rest your feet on a firm pillow or bolster.

ROCK POSE

This pose gains its name from the idea that whoever masters Rock pose can sit and "digest rocks" since the position is beneficial for the digestive system. Rock pose also encourages a straight spine and helps you to sit as steady as a rock.

ALMOND OIL

The almond is a wonderful nut. Its oil is excellent both internally and externally for the skin. Add 25ml (1fl oz) of raw almond oil (available from health food stores), to food or drink each day to help lower cholesterol, reduce body fat and hunger, cleanse the body of toxins, and keep the skin healthy and lustrous. Use instead of butter on food.

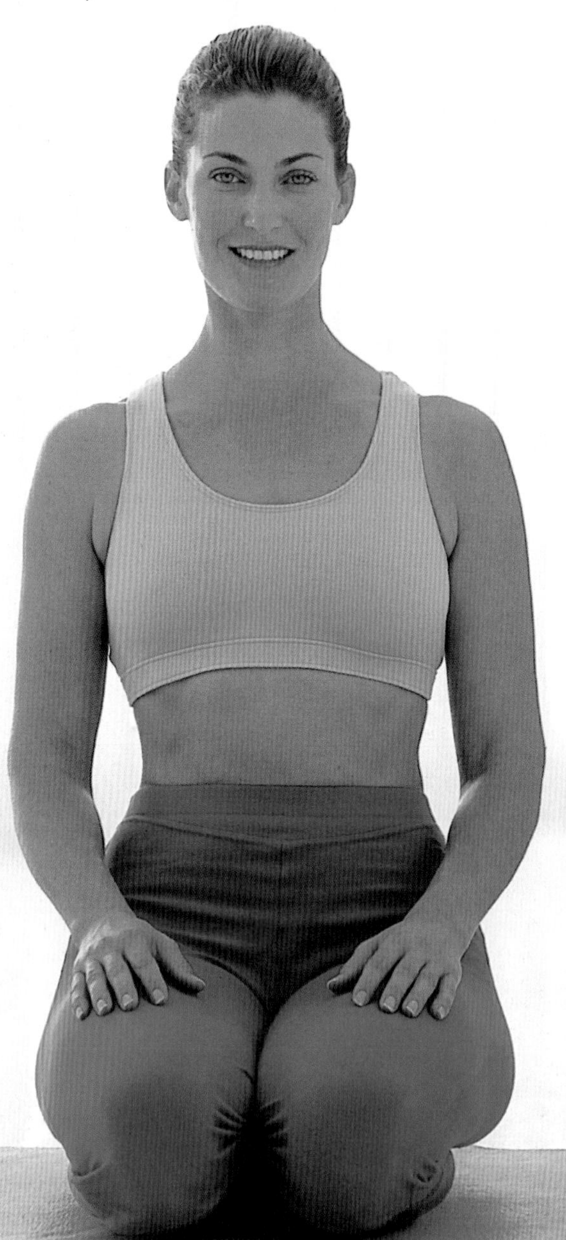

Sit on your heels with your feet relaxed under you. Straighten your spine. Place your hands on your thighs. To relieve excess pressure on the knees, sit with a rolled blanket or firm pillow between your buttocks and heels.

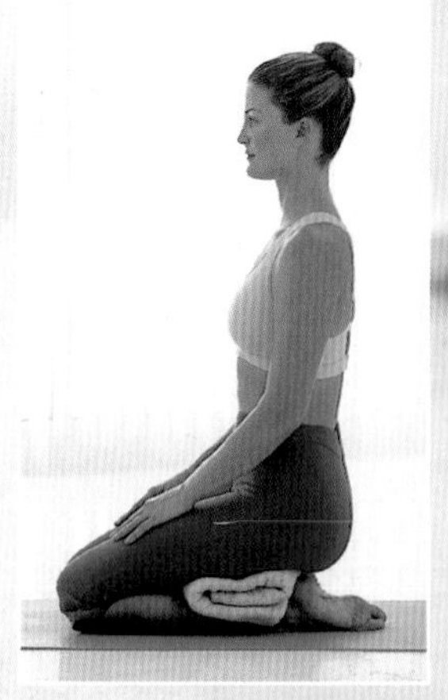

MUDRA

The hands form their own yoga positions, especially during meditative practices such as pranayama (breathing exercises), and sitting meditations. These hand positions, called mudras, are used to activate certain pressure points on the fingers. Each mudra is a technique for giving clear messages to the mind/body energy system.

The most common hand position is called Gyan ("gee-yawn") Mudra. This mudra activates the qualities of knowledge and wisdom (which is what *gyan* means in Sanskrit.) There are two forms: passive and active.

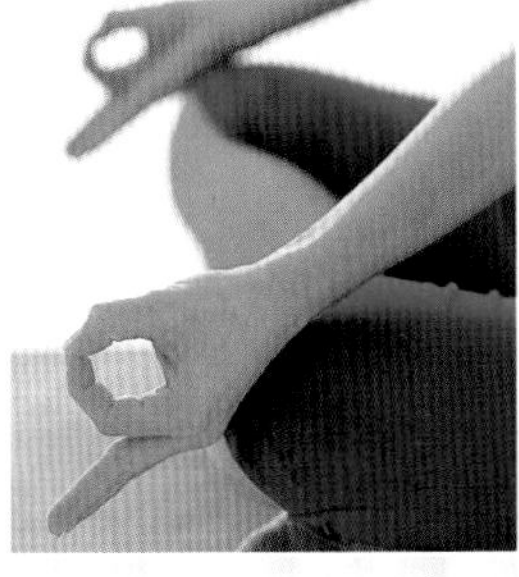

PASSIVE GYAN MUDRA
Put the tip of the thumb together with the tip of the index finger. This gives receptivity and calmness.

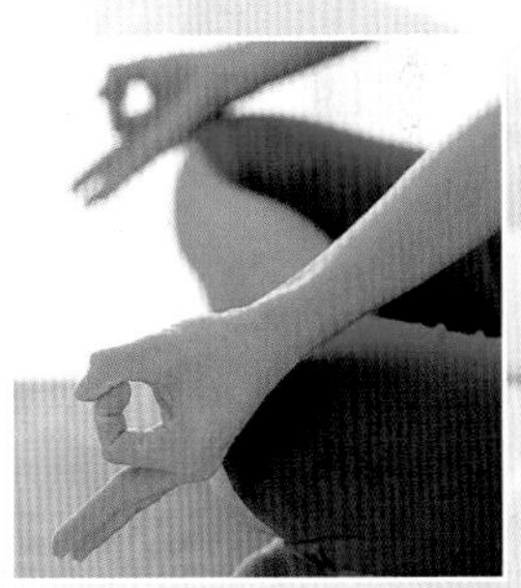

ACTIVE GYAN MUDRA
Curl the index finger under the thumb so that the fingernail is on the second joint of the thumb. This gives all the same qualities as passive Gyan Mudra, but with a more active, or projective energy.

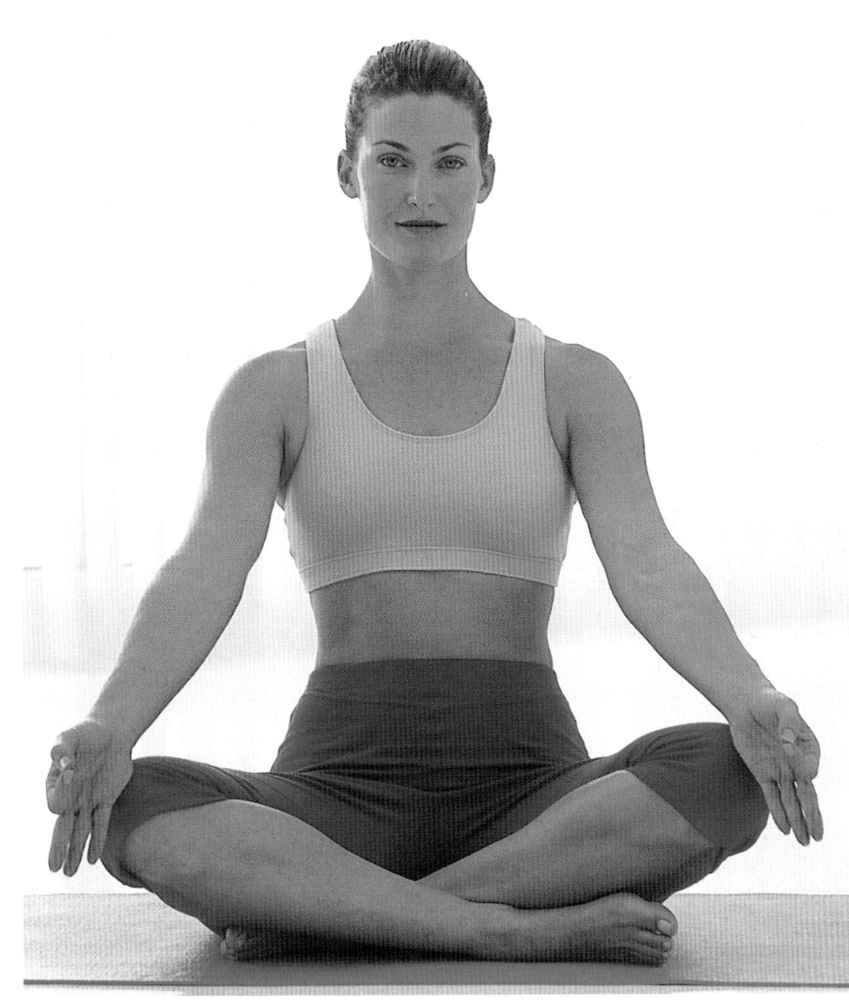

TUNING IN

In Kundalini Yoga there is a sound intonation, called a mantra, that is used to begin a yoga practice. Mantras (from Sanskrit, *man*, "mind", *tra*, "guiding") are ancient, time-tested sounds that have been used to calm, focus, and uplift the mind. According to yogic understanding, and validated by science, the basic nature of everything in the universe is composed of vibration – consisting of sound, light, and energy. When chanting a mantra, every cell begins to vibrate at a similar energy frequency in the same way that a note struck on a stringed instrument will automatically vibrate on a second instrument.

Before beginning each yoga practice, use this mantra as a centring technique to attune you to your inner guidance. *Ong Namo Guru Dev Namo* means "I call on the Universal Spirit, I call on the ever-present guidance." To chant the mantra, feel the navel come in towards the spine slightly on the long "o" sound of *Ong*. Then feel the "ng" at the point between your two eyebrows. *Namo* is pronounced "nah-moe". *Guru* is "gu-roo", making sure to roll the "r" sound. *Dev* sounds like "dave", and then finally *Namo* again.

The cosmic syllable Om *is considered to be the primal sound of which all things are created. It begins with the open "o" or "au" sound, then extends the "m" sound, creating a soothing hum in the throat and root of the nose. In Kundalini Yoga* Om *is changed slightly to* Ong, *which is considered to be the active form of* Om.

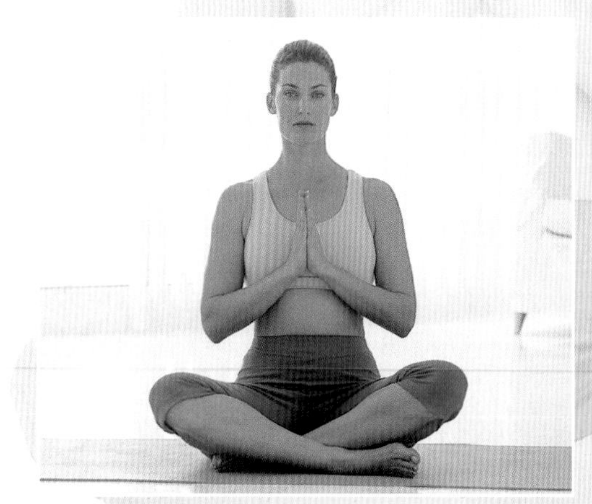

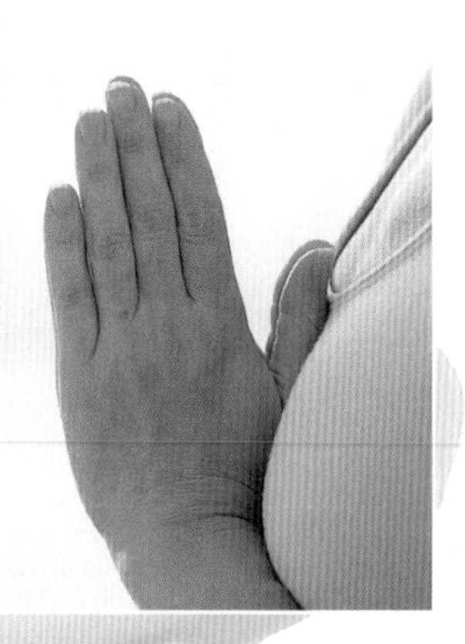

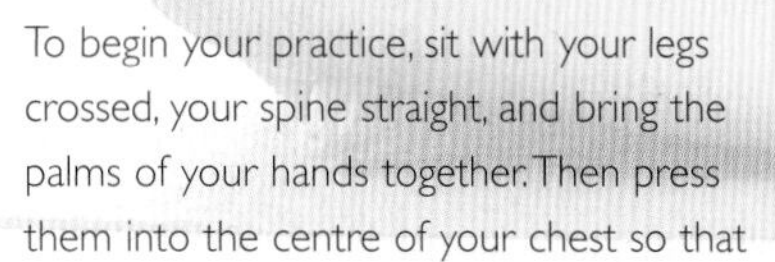

To begin your practice, sit with your legs crossed, your spine straight, and bring the palms of your hands together. Then press them into the centre of your chest so that your thumbs press against your sternum. This is called Prayer pose. Inhale deeply with your eyes closed and chant the mantra once. Repeat for a total of three repetitions.

DEEP BREATHING

To understand the mechanics of deep breathing, the most common breath used in yoga, take a look at a sleeping baby. Watch her abdomen rise effortlessly on the inhale and fall on the exhale. This is our natural, inborn way of breathing. Realize that you have known this way of breathing and it is preserved in your cell memory. If you have forgotten how, here is how to retrain yourself.

Taking long, slow, deep breaths calms you, relaxes your heart, relieves stress, clears your mind, and brings awareness of your inner being.

1

Lie on your back with your knees bent. Place one hand on your abdomen and the other on your upper chest. Exhale all of your breath out. Make a conscious effort to push the remaining breath out with your abdominal muscles, creating a vacuum for a deep breath to enter.

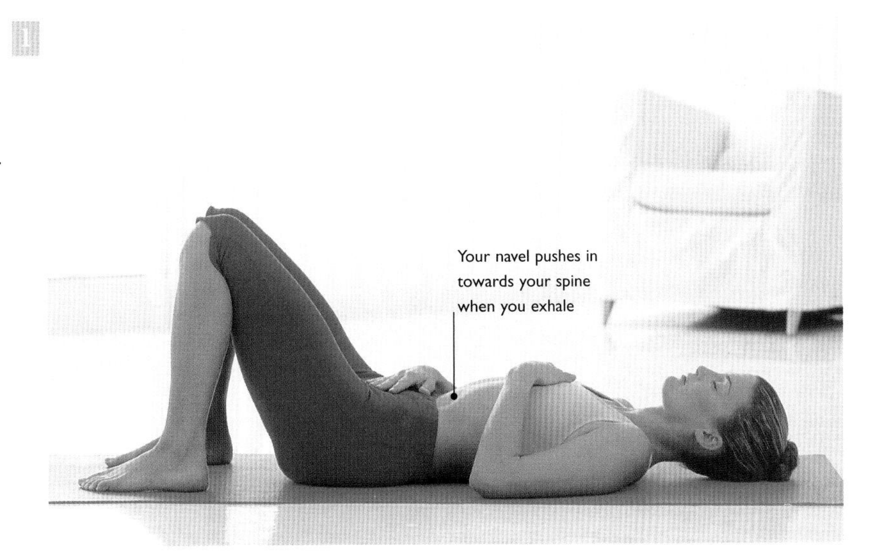

Your navel pushes in towards your spine when you exhale

2

As you begin to inhale, your abdominal muscles will relax and expand outwards to allow the diaphragm to drop. Pause the breath for 1–2 seconds at the end of your inhalation. As you exhale, your abdominals will naturally move inwards to press the diaphragm up against the lungs. Notice the breath leaving the upper chest first. Continue exhaling smoothly and completely, and feel the abdominals press slightly towards the spine. Pause the breath, then begin another deep inhalation.

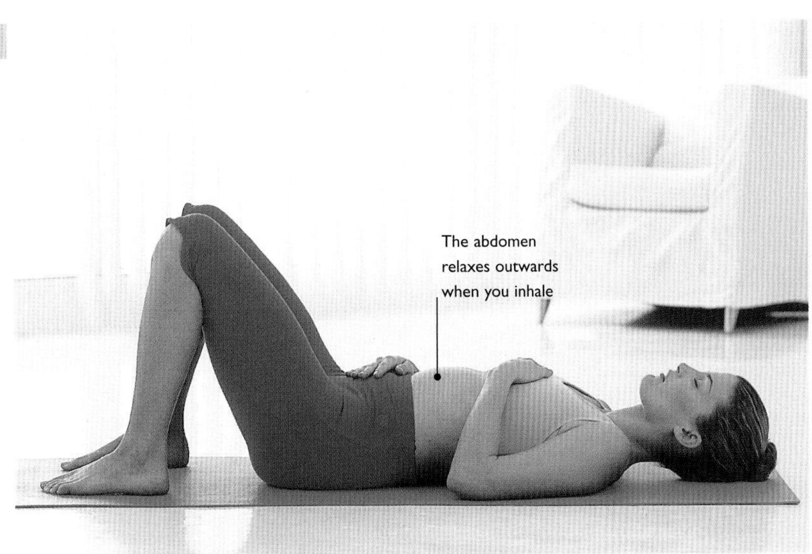

The abdomen relaxes outwards when you inhale

BREATH OF FIRE

Breath of Fire is actually like one long, continuous breath being pumped in and out, over and over. Because of the way it moves energy and blood circulation, there are a few cautions: during menstruation a "light" practice of Breath of Fire will help regulate it, but do not practise if there is discomfort or cramping. During pregnancy, except possibly for the first trimester, Breath of Fire should not be done. In cases of major health issues, check first with your GP.

Breath of Fire cleanses the blood, the mucous linings of the lungs, and body cells. It rejuvenates your mind and expands your lung capacity while strengthening all the nerves in the body.

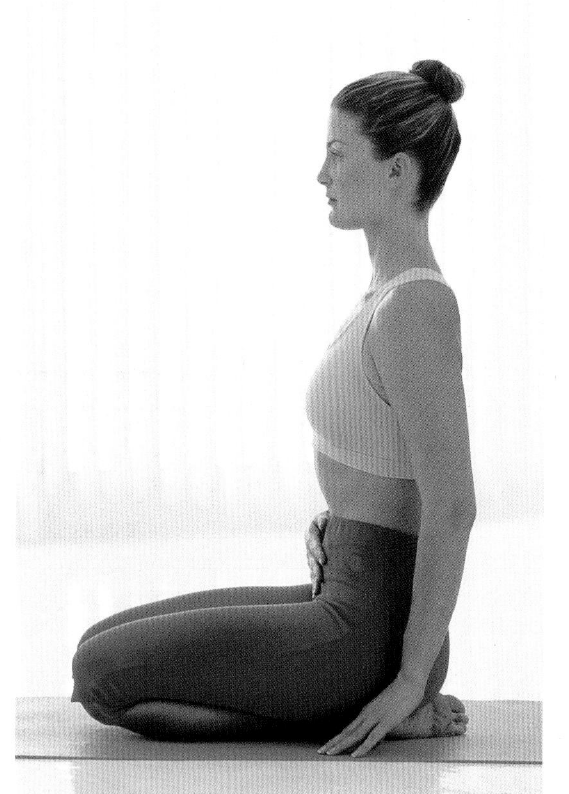

1 Sit in Easy pose, or on your heels in Rock pose. Straighten the spine and relax the shoulders. You may like to put one hand on the abdomen to monitor its movement. Inhale normally. Then exhale with force. Your navel will press back towards your spine and you may feel the slightly upward push of the diaphragm pressing the breath out of your lungs.

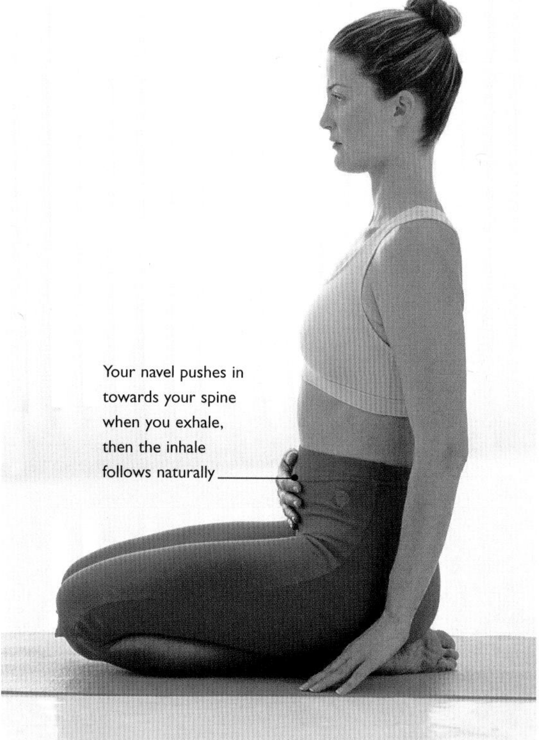

2 Let the breath enter naturally on the inhale, and press it out again on the exhale. Although the inhalation and exhalation are equal in length, it may be helpful to focus on the strong, quick exhalation. Start off slowly, at a rate of one exhale per two seconds, then as you get used to the movement, speed it up gradually so that you are exhaling at two per second or faster.

ROOT LOCK

Body Locks, or Bandhas ("bond" or "tie" in Sanskrit) are internal contractions of muscles that are used to strengthen those muscles, focus concentration, and move energy through the body, which translates into vitality and health. The most commonly used lock is called Root Lock. Women who practise pelvic floor exercises will recognize the vaginal squeeze as an integral part of Root Lock.

Exhale all your breath out. Contract and lift the pelvic floor muscles, which includes the anal muscles and the genitals. Try to keep the buttocks relaxed. Pull the navel in towards the spine. Hold for a few seconds. Then as you inhale relax the lock and focus your attention in an upwards motion from the base of the spine to the top of your head. Or you may focus at the brow point, the area between your eyebrows. Exhale again and repeat several times.

You can also contract Root Lock on the held inhalation and release it on the exhalation

Root Lock is great for certain times of a woman's life, as in the postnatal period when the internal muscles need firming and strengthening. Root Lock should not be practised during menstruation. In cases of major health issues, check with your GP before practising it.

CORPSE POSE

An essential part of yoga is the deep relaxation at the end of your practice. In fact, deep relaxation is actually a pose called Corpse pose. If you think this sounds morbid, think again. The idea is that you are "dead" to the world, to your bodily tensions, and the usual cacophony of mental noise. Corpse pose is the icing on the cake of yoga practice, held dear by long-time yoga practitioners and new ones alike. In deep relaxation you are "actively allowing" in the sense that you are consciously noticing tensions, thoughts, or feelings without giving them any extra attention. At the same time, you allow them to release. What this process does is bring you to an inner space of no resistance. In the openness of that space the transforming power of your yoga practice can have optimum effect.

Many people, upon learning yogic deep relaxation techniques, discover that they need to relearn what it feels like to relax deeply. As your yoga practice increases, you are more aware of tension in your body and mind, and so are able to consciously relax yourself immediately.

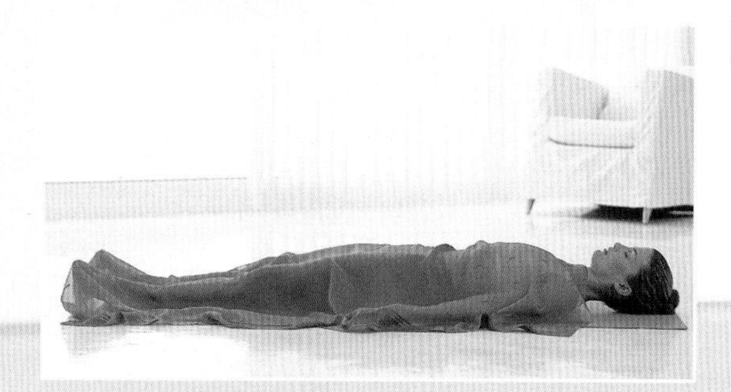

Corpse pose with shawl for added comfort.

1 Lie down on a comfortably padded mat. You may want to place a rolled blanket or bolster under your knees and/or neck and cover yourself with a light, natural fabric shawl to avoid a chill. If you are wearing glasses, take them off to relax the eyes. You may also like to have some beautifully uplifting music playing softly. If it is music with words, they should be elevating and divinely inspired. See Music Resources *(p.224)* for suggested relaxation music.

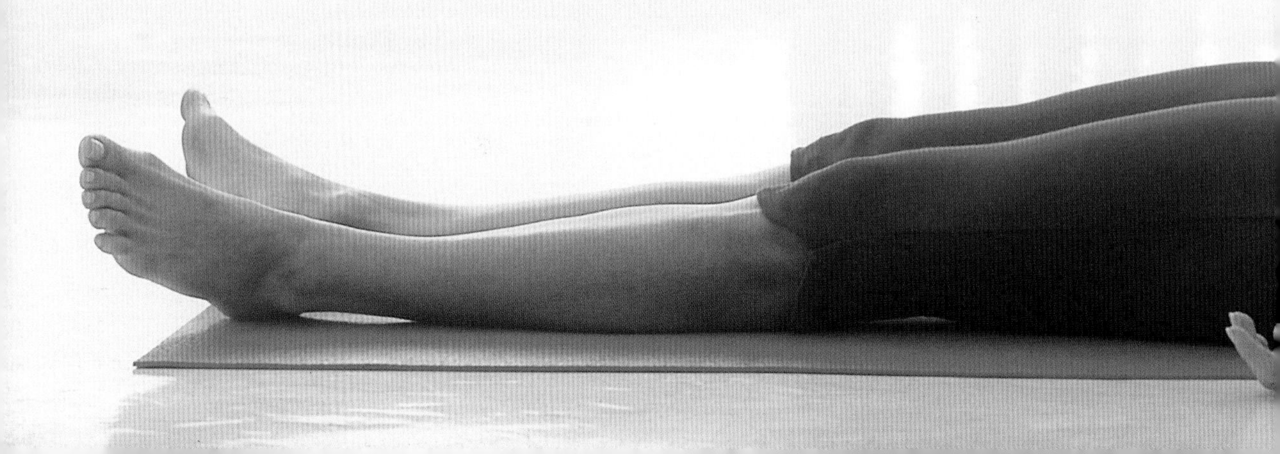

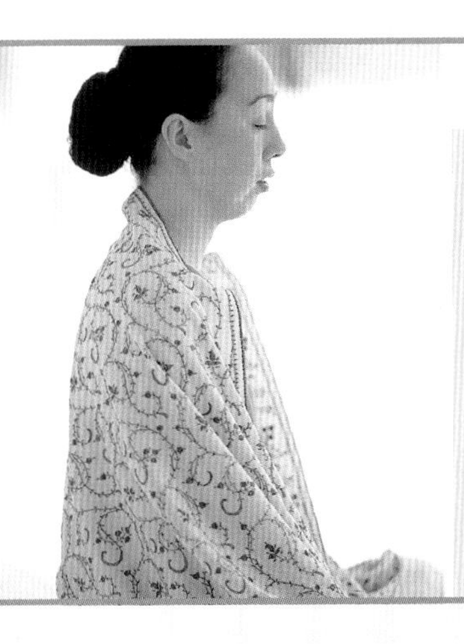

MEDITATION SHAWL

During yoga practice, heat builds in the body to the point that you may sweat lightly. This heat rises and cools off in the period of deep relaxation or meditation that often follows a yoga practice. Covering your body with a light cotton or wool shawl during a sitting meditation is just as important as during deep relaxation: the meditation shawl not only keeps the spine warm but allows for a subtle flow of energy through the entire spine, which empowers your meditation.

2 Close your eyes. Your arms are at your sides with the palms facing upwards, open and relaxed. Allow your body to feel as if it is sinking towards the ground. Consciously relax every part of your body, beginning with your feet and moving up your legs to your pelvis, torso, arms, and face, including your lips, jaw, and face muscles.

3 If your mind begins to wander, gently bring your attention back to the quiet inflow and outflow of your breath. You may like to imagine hearing a mantra or affirmation with each inhalation and exhalation. Continue to relax for at least 10 minutes, preferably longer. If you fall asleep it will be a self-healing sleep, so light that you may feel yourself almost dancing on the edge of awareness.

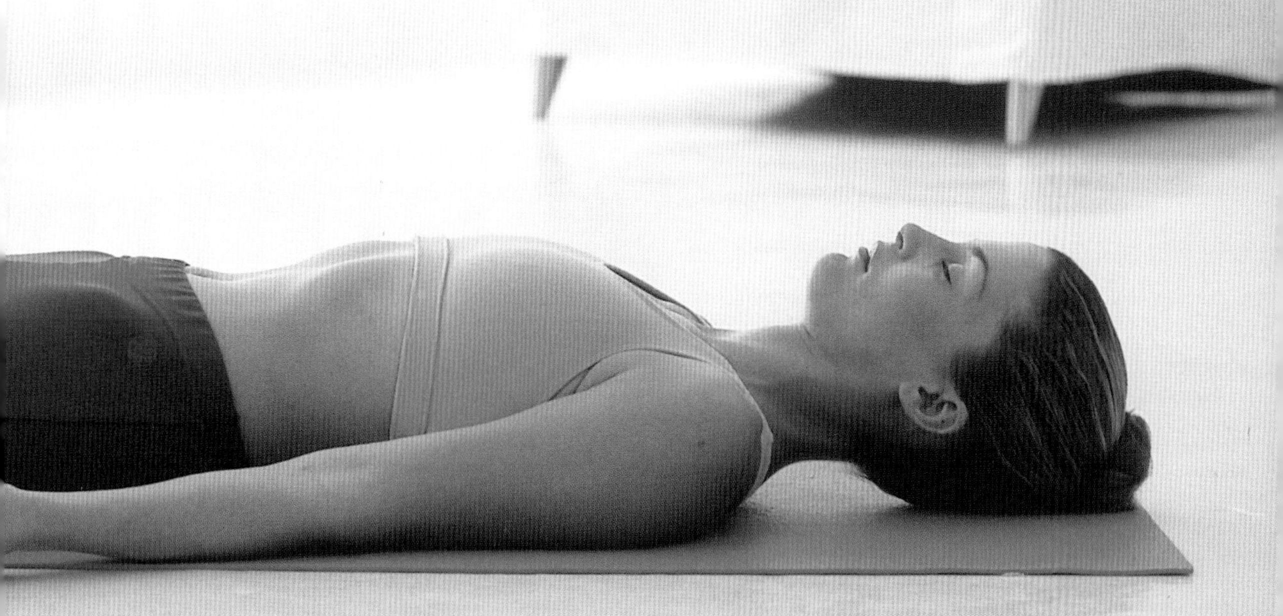

COMING BACK FROM DEEP RELAXATION

At the end of your relaxation time, when you come back to awareness of yourself, take a deep and conscious inhale and exhale. Do the following wake-up exercises for about 20 seconds each, using deep breathing.

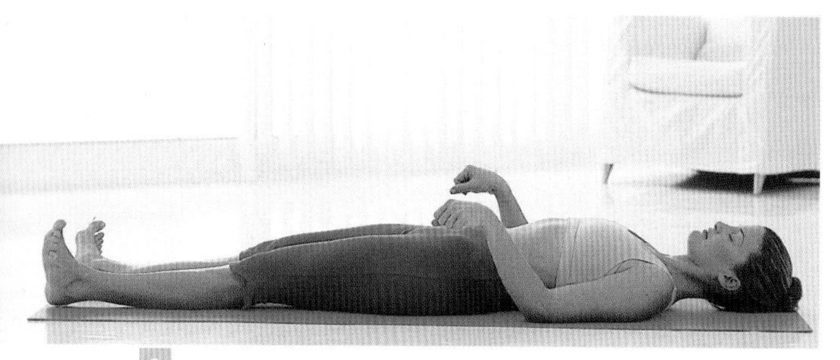

1 Roll your wrists and ankles in circles in both directions. This wakes up the extremities of the body.

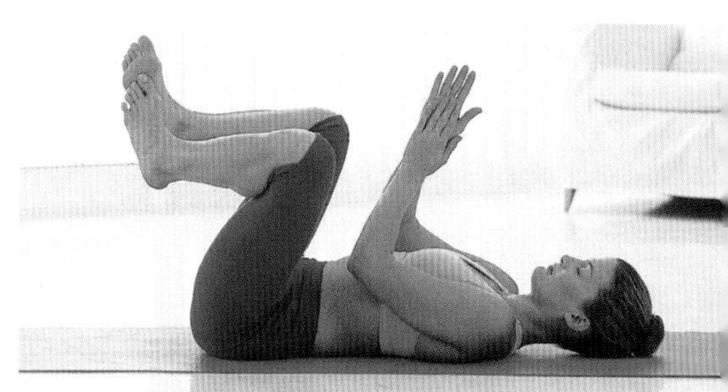

2 Lift your feet and rub the bare soles together. Rub your hands together at the same time. This wakes up the nerve endings in the feet and hands.

3 Begin a Cat Stretch: bring your arms out to the sides, lift one bent leg and bring it across the other in a diagonal stretch. Turn your head in the opposite direction from your bent leg. Breathe. Then switch sides. Do this a few times on each side to give the spine and body a good diagonal stretch.

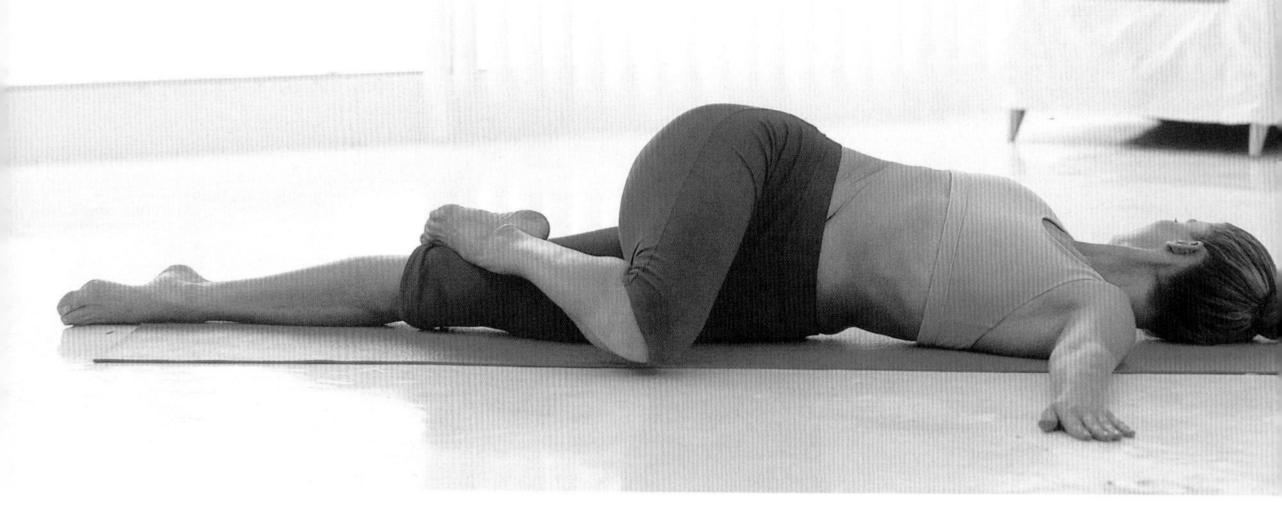

KATHY'S STORY (USA)

About four years ago, my heart led me to a yoga class for stress relief from a very demanding job. I immediately loved the challenge of the poses and the focus on my breath, but I rejected outright the meditation at the end as unnecessary for me and only went through the motions in class. But as time went on, I began to think, "Why not? I'll try it." Meditating made a subtle but very real difference. Whereas before I would leave my yoga class relaxed and feeling good physically, now I left with a peacefulness unlike anything I had felt before.

In the meantime, my job of almost 30 years began to lose its meaning, and I made the decision to leave without any plans for what to do next. Now there was no excuse not to indulge myself in my love of yoga, and a regular home practice emerged. I even toted my yoga mat abroad as I biked across Italy. Imagine doing Sun Salutations facing a breathtaking Italian countryside sunrise on a late May morning!

Indirectly, yoga also led me to my new vocation, Life Coaching. Yoga and meditation help prepare me for coaching sessions, and I also use them with my clients when appropriate.

Yoga keeps me in touch with who I am and why I am here, and helps me to live my life with the peace and harmony I once thought were possible to attain only from a weekly yoga class.

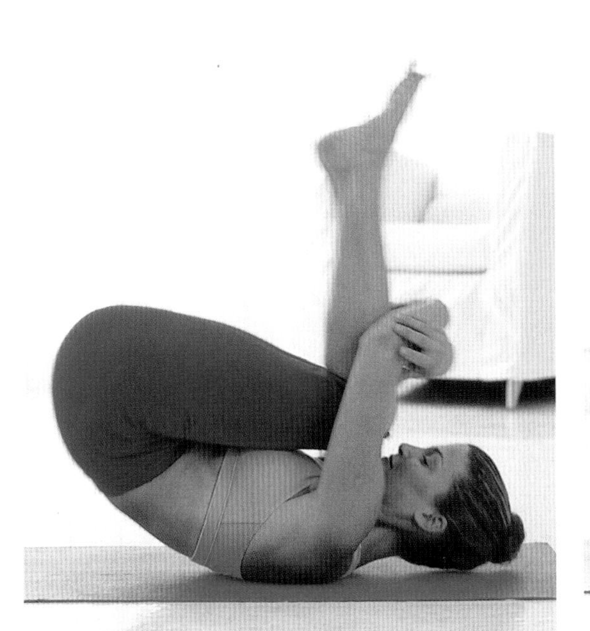

4 Draw your knees into your chest and wrap the arms around them. Tuck your head into your knees and begin rocking up and down on your spine 6–8 times. This wakes up the spine.

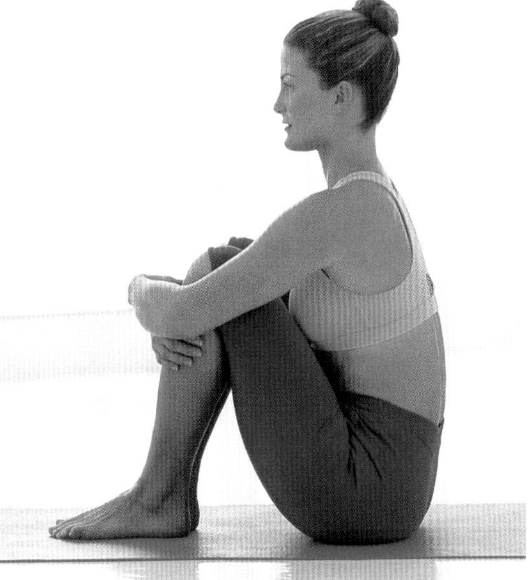

5 Sit up to end your practice or to meditate. These exercises bring your body and mind to consciousness gently and completely. Be sure to drink some spring water (room temperature) after relaxing or meditating to reground and rebalance the nervous system.

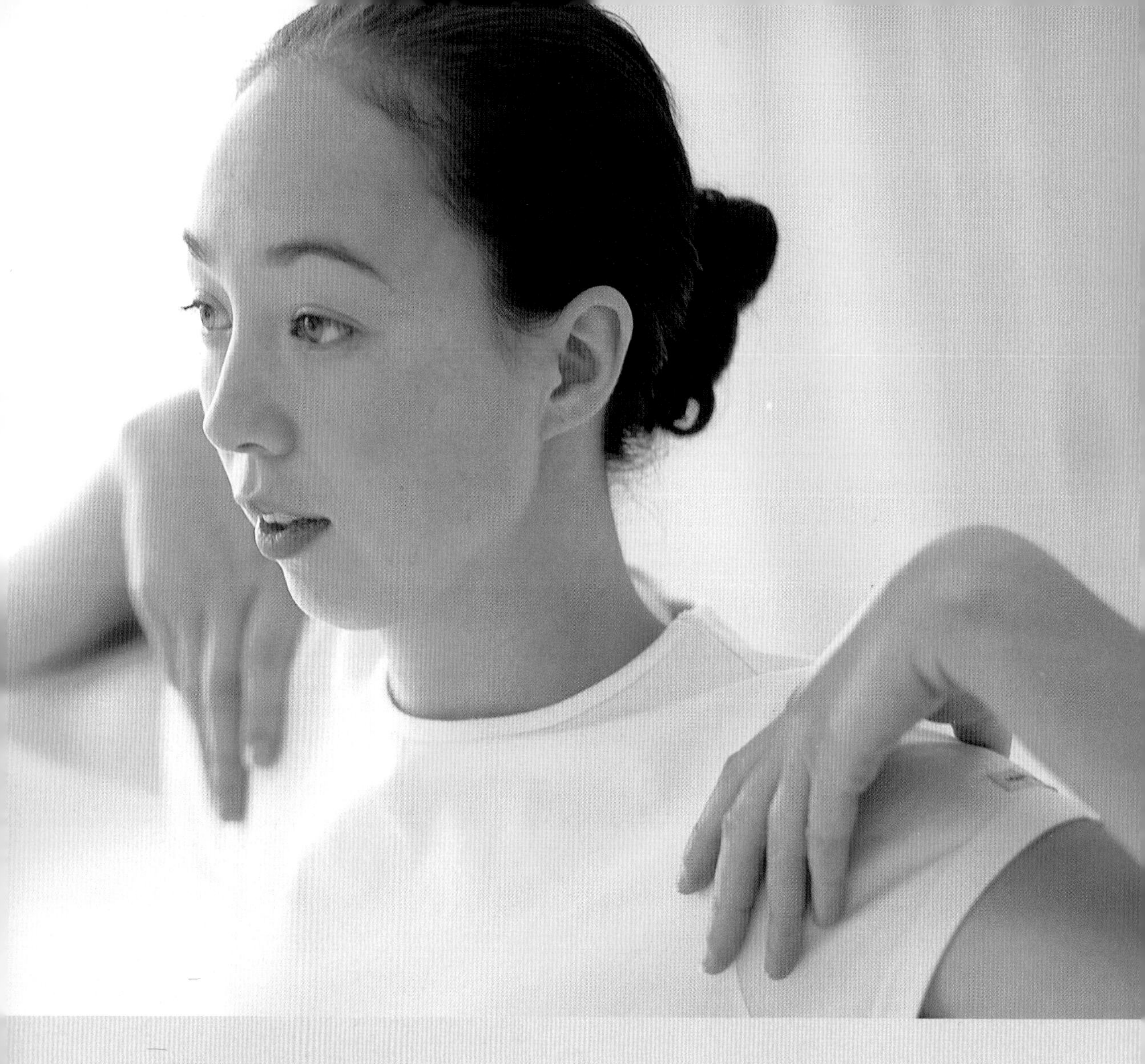

WARMING UP TO YOGA

As you leaf through this book you'll see a wide variety of yoga sets, or kriyas, and yoga poses. Many require some flexibility and should not be done "cold". As you choose different yoga sets, refer back to this chapter for essential warm-up poses and practise them for at least 10 minutes before you move on. Choose between the Spinal Warm-ups and Kneeling Sun Salutation, or do both for an especially satisfying experience. These exercises and poses loosen up your spine and back muscles, all the way from your tailbone to your neck. Rotating joints is key, as is stretching the nerves and muscles in the arms and legs. You will be able to accomplish all this in just 10–15 minutes.

SPINAL WARM-UPS

The following exercises prepare the body, and specifically the spine, for the rest of the yoga in this book. Although they need not all be done each time you practise yoga, the key point is to begin at the base of the spine and work your way upwards towards the neck.

Breathing consciously is an essential aspect of yoga. Breathe deeply to expand your lung capacity, energize your mind, and oxygenate your blood. Focus on each inflow and outflow of breath for a deeper experience of peace and clarity.

LOWER SPINE FLEX

In this exercise you are loosening the vertebrae of the lower spine. The spinal fluid and pranic life energy in the lower spine are also activated and begin to circulate upwards throughout the spine.

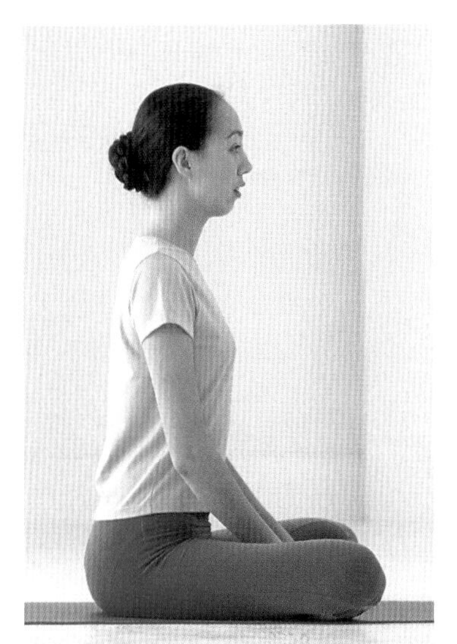

1 Start in Easy pose: sit on the ground with your legs crossed and tucked in. Straighten the spine by pressing the chest forwards slightly and lifting the rib cage. Relax the shoulders and slightly tuck the chin in.

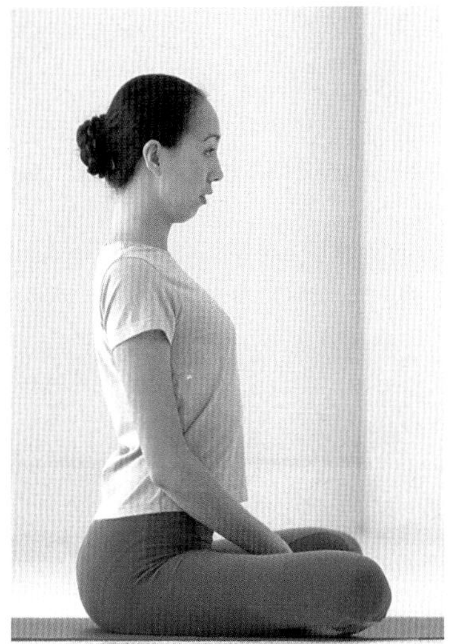

2 Now take hold of your outside ankles with both hands. Inhale and flex your spine forwards. The chest lifts and the shoulders drop back. Keep your head upright as you move your spine.

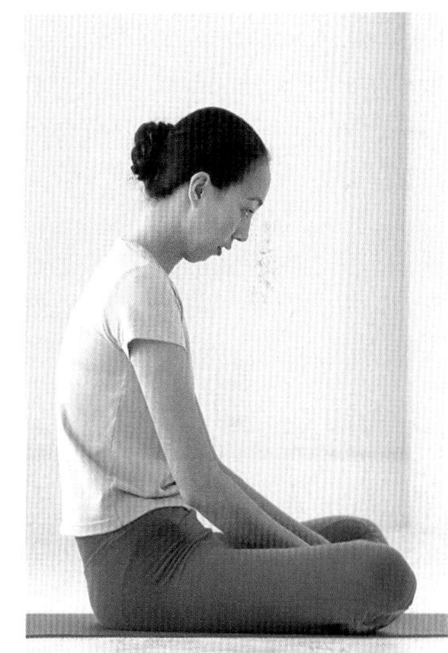

3 Exhale and round the back, slump the chest, and let the shoulders fall forwards. Continue in a rhythmic forwards and backwards manner. Feel your pelvis rock forwards and back as you flex, and each vertebra of your spine curl and uncurl. Pick up the pace for 1–2 minutes, then inhale deeply, hold, exhale, and relax your breath and the pose.

UPPER SPINE FLEX

The vertebrae of the mid-spine are flexed in this pose, and digestion is stimulated. Energy is circulated throughout the middle and upper back. The head moves in tandem with the spine in a fluid motion.

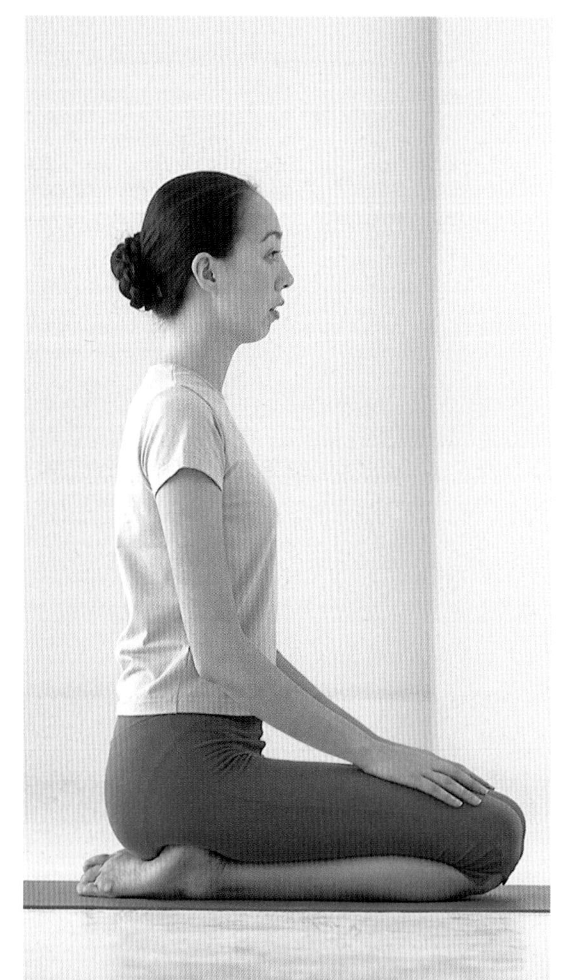

1 Sitting in Rock pose, grasp your knees with your hands and straighten your elbows. Inhale and stretch your body forwards. Your chest should be lifted, the shoulders back and relaxed, the chin slightly tucked in towards the neck.

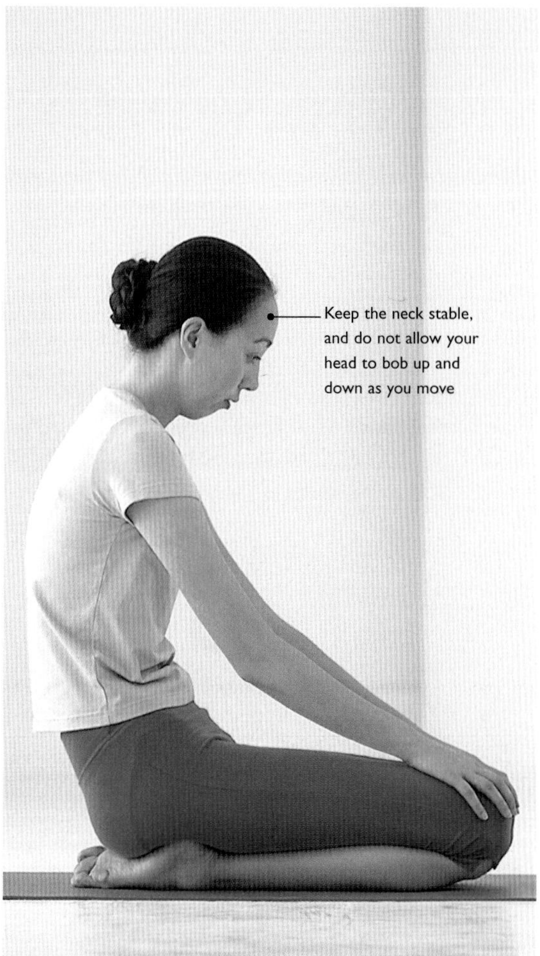

Keep the neck stable, and do not allow your head to bob up and down as you move

2 Exhale and slump the spine as far as possible, shoulders rounded forwards. Keep your elbows as straight as possible throughout the exercise. Focus your awareness on the areas from the mid-spine up through the shoulder blades. Feel each vertebra flexing. Begin slowly, and as you go pick up the pace for 1–2 minutes. Inhale deeply and stretch the chest out. Then exhale and relax the breath and the pose.

TWISTS

The entire spine is loosened and the vertebrae are adjusted. This active spinal twist massages all the organs of the body, improves digestion, and tones the lateral and abdominal muscles.

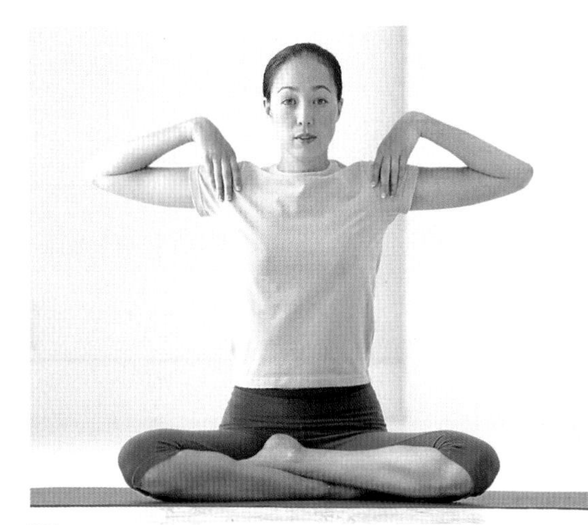

1 Sit in Easy pose *(p.19)*, stretch the spine up, chest out, and bring your hands up to grasp the shoulders with the fingers in the front and the thumbs in the back. Keep the upper arms parallel to the ground.

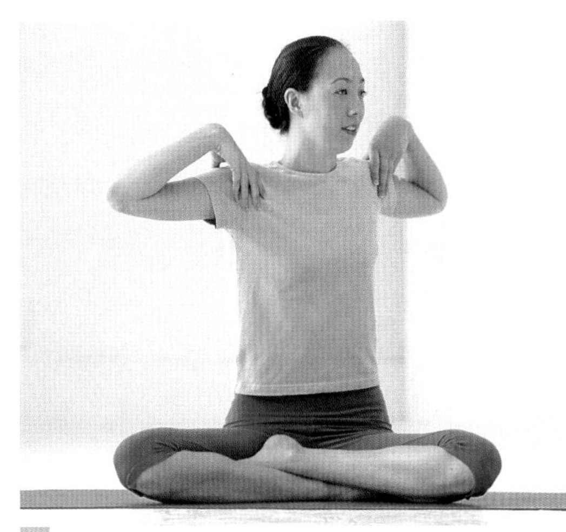

2 Twist as far as you can in each direction, swinging freely from side to side. Inhale to the left and exhale to the right. Breathe rhythmically and powerfully for 1–2 minutes.

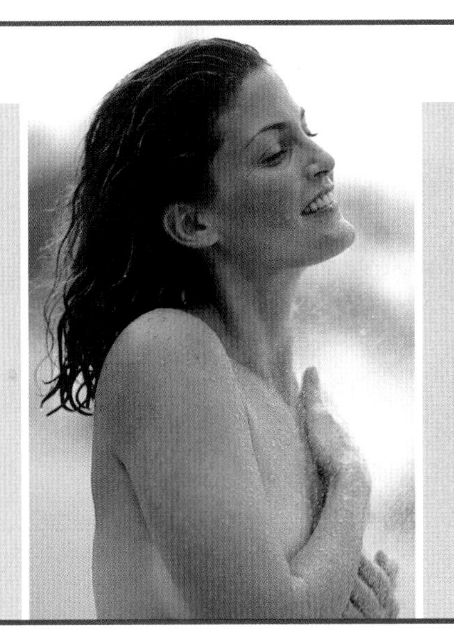

HYDROTHERAPY

A brief cold shower in the morning strengthens the nervous system and opens the capillaries, flushing impurities from the bloodstream. When the capillaries return to normal, the blood supply flushes and refreshes the organs and endocrine system. First massage your body with pure oil, preferably almond; this protective coating is driven into the pores of the skin while showering. Allow cold water to hit your feet, your body, and your face, but not the top of your head or thighs. Massage as you move in and out of the cold water. Breathe deeply or chant a mantra. Start at 30 seconds and work up to three minutes. Towel dry and rub the skin briskly. If you have circulatory problems or other conditions, seek medical advice first. Pregnant and menstruating women should take warm or tepid showers.

SHOULDER SHRUGS

Shoulder tension is common in the fast-paced lives most of us lead, and it often contributes to tension headaches as well. In this exercise, the tension in the shoulders is pressurized as you squeeze upwards, and then released as you drop the shoulders.

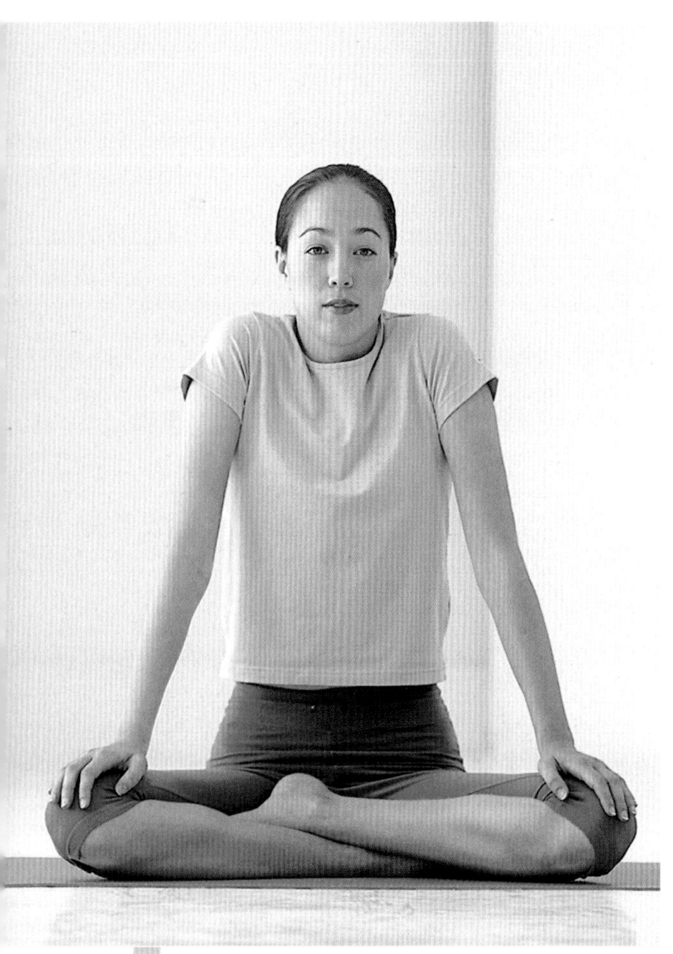

1 Sit in Easy pose. Straighten your spine and bring your neck and spinal vertebrae in line. Keep your hands relaxed on your knees. Inhale and lift your shoulders straight up.

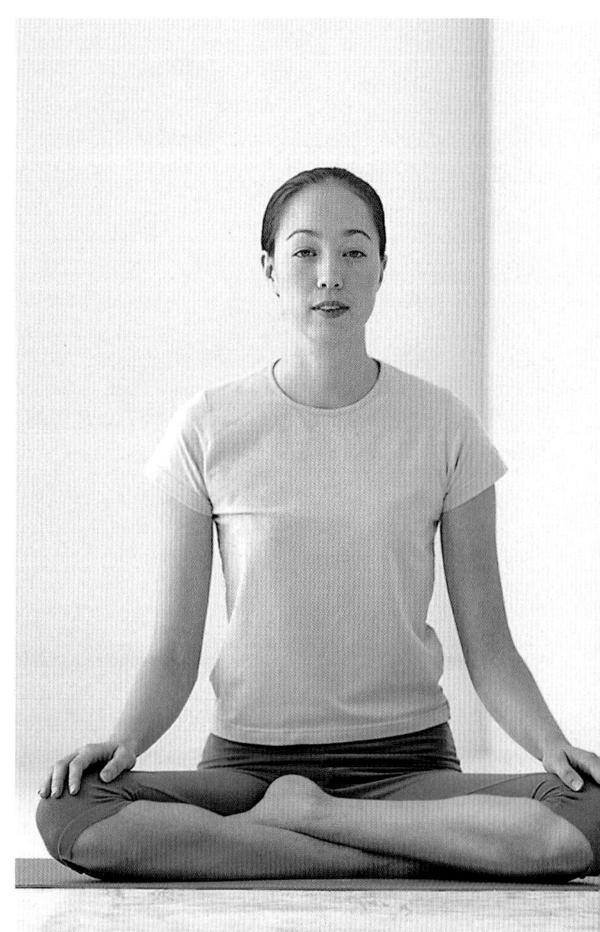

2 Exhale and let your shoulders drop down. Use a powerful breath and continue Shoulder Shrugs for 1–2 minutes. Then inhale deeply, stretch the shoulders up and hold for a few seconds, then exhale, relaxing down. Feel a warm energy circulating throughout the shoulder and neck area.

NECK ROLLS

In the previous exercises, spinal fluid and pranic life energy have been stimulated and circulated from the spine upwards. This exercise releases the tension in the neck, allowing the energy to flow into the head.

If you have reason to be cautious about neck movements, try Neck Turns: inhale and slowly turn your head to the left, bringing your chin towards or over your shoulder, then exhale and slowly turn your head toward the right shoulder. Repeat several times.

1 Keeping your jaw relaxed and your mouth slack, gently drop your head forwards, and as you inhale begin to rotate the head around to the left shoulder. Your chin will come over the left shoulder as you inhale and your head will slowly circle in a smooth, continuous motion.

2 As you exhale, your head will move over the right shoulder and back to the front. Move meditatively and slowly. After 3–4 circles, reverse the direction. Inhale to the right, and exhale as the head comes around to the left. Continue for 3–4 circles, then inhale and bring your head to the front. Exhale and relax.

Feel that the weight of your head is moving your neck around in a fluid circle

SPREAD STRETCH

This exercise increases flexibility. It stretches and strengthens the hips, lower spine, and lateral muscles from the upper chest to the pelvis. The sciatic nerve is strengthened as the leg muscles receive a beneficial stretch.

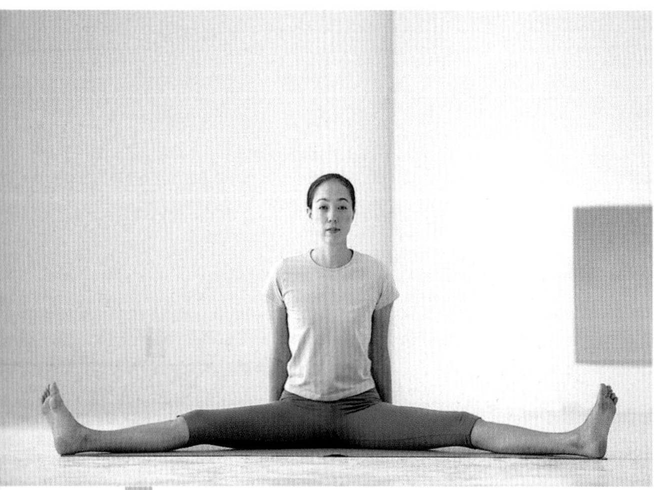

1 Spread the legs as far apart as is comfortable. Place your hands by your hips and lift your body slightly so that you are up on your buttocks and your lower spine is straight.

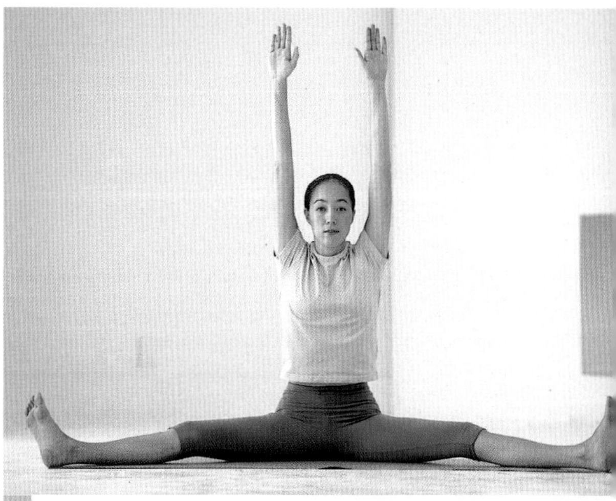

2 Inhale as you stretch your arms straight up overhead, lengthening the spine and lifting the rib cage.

Visualize lifting your chest and placing it on your thighs as you reach over

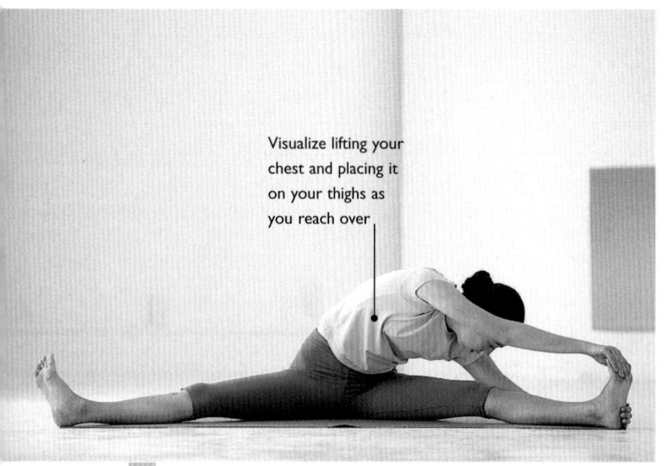

3 Exhale and reach for the outside of your left foot with your left hand, and the left toes with your right hand. If you cannot reach this far, reach your ankle or calf. Keep your chin parallel to the ground. Inhale and lift up to the centre.

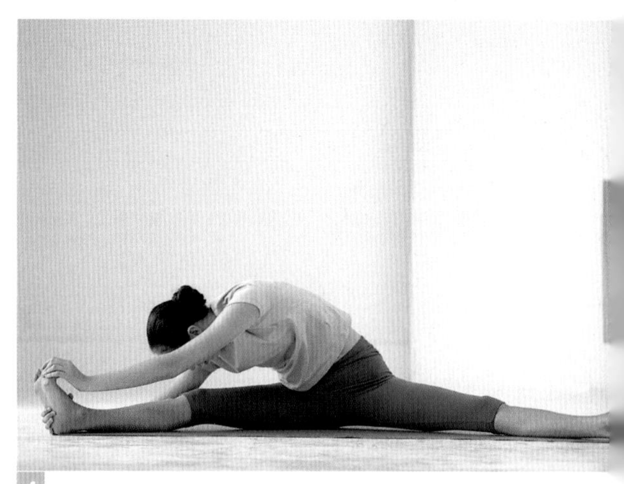

4 Exhale and stretch over the right leg in the same manner as for the left leg. Then inhale up to the centre again, and continue the stretching pattern for 1–2 minutes.

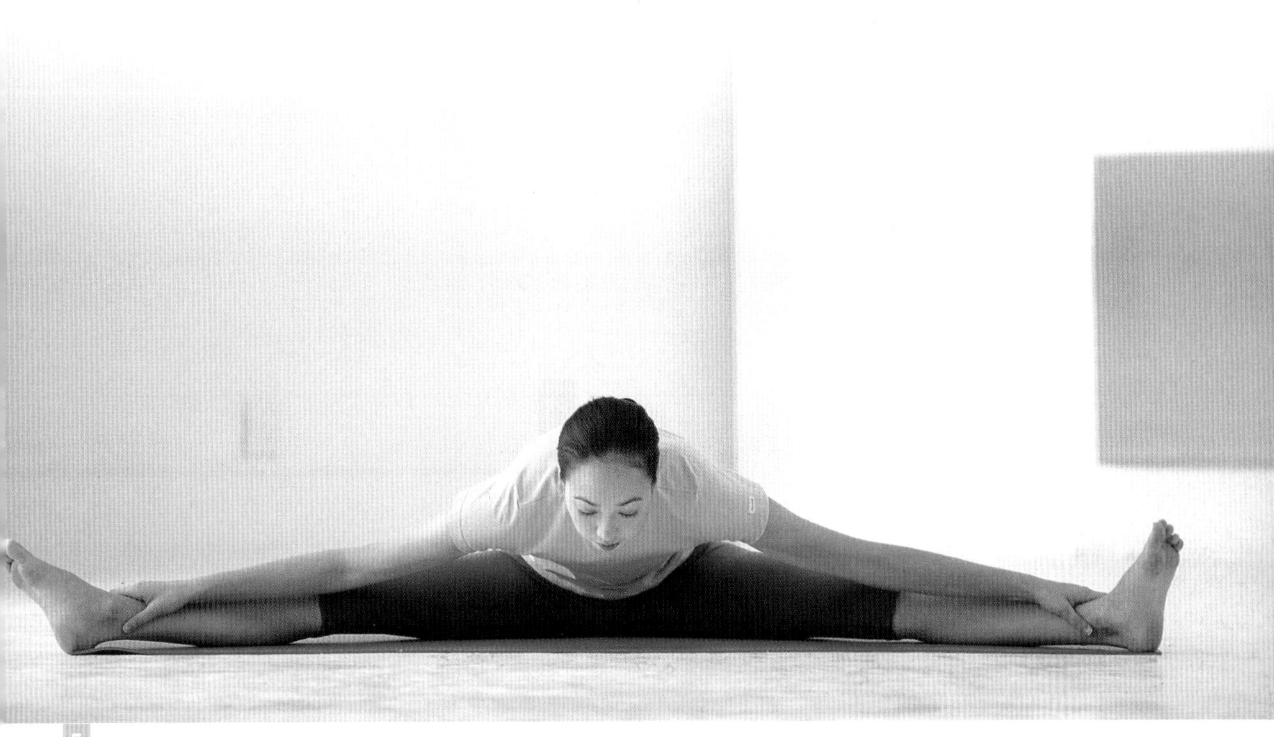

5 Inhale and lift up to the centre and exhale down. Then stretch your hands out towards each ankle and bring your chest close to the ground, lengthening the spine as you do so. Hold the downwards stretch and begin either deep breathing or Breath of Fire for 1 minute. Then inhale and hold the breath for a few seconds.

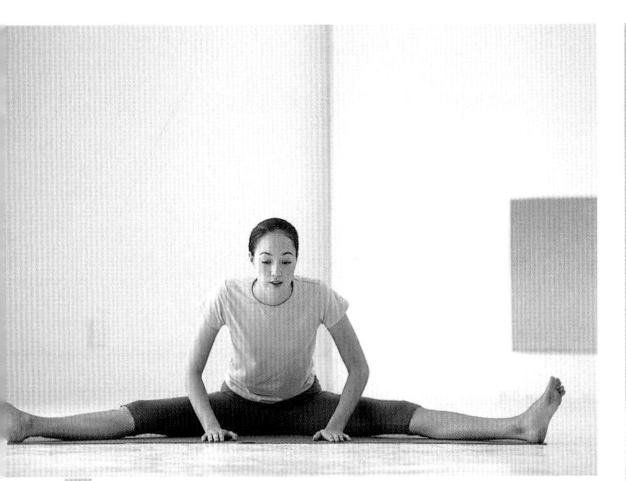

6 Exhale and slowly sit up. Push with your hands on the ground to bring yourself back to a sitting position to avoid straining the lower back.

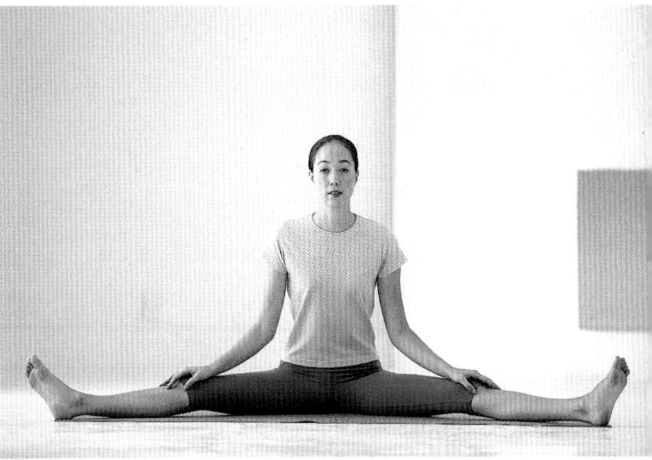

7 Inhale deeply as you return to the upright position. Then exhale and relax out of the position. Only stretch as much as feels comfortable in this exercise if you are not flexible.

KNEELING SUN SALUTATION

This series of postures is a modified version of the classic Sun Salutation. By regularly practising the Kneeling Sun Salutation, you will find it easier to practise the Moon Salutation *(p.79)*. The Kneeling Sun Salutation will flex your spine in every direction, stretch your limbs, deepen your breathing, and enable you to experience a place of peace.

As you become familiar with moving body and breath together in a Vinyasa, you can add in other poses at certain points. For example, add Upward Facing Dog (step 6) after Downward Dog (step 5) in this set.

When you move from one pose into another in a set – inhaling into one pose, exhaling into the next, and so on – the set is referred to as Vinyasa. This dynamic style of yoga practice allows your body to get used to the postures gently and gradually. As you move, the Vinyasa allows you to focus your breath on different parts of your body and heighten the intensity of the effect of each movement. Once you get a feel for it, it becomes a beautiful yoga dance of your body and your breathing.

Lean back slightly if it feels natural, but do not arch deeply or hyperextend your neck

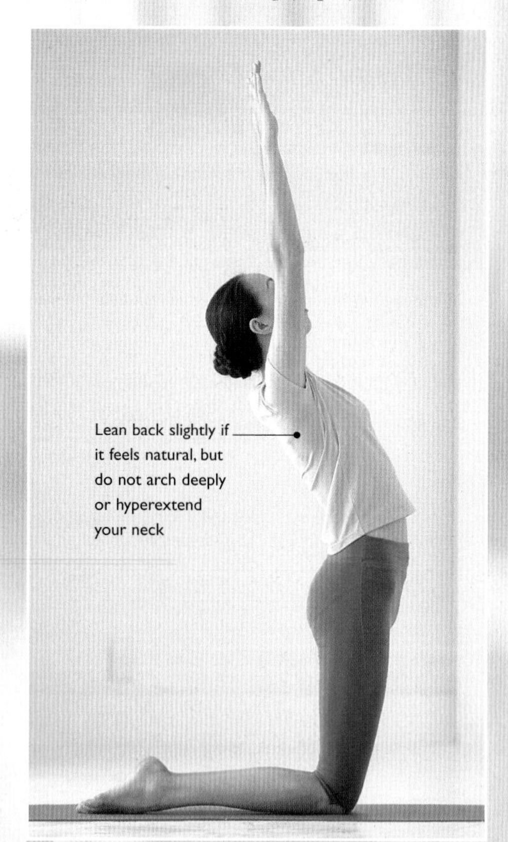

1 Sit back on the heels in Rock pose *(p.20)* and place your hands on your thighs. If this is uncomfortable, kneel up so that your body forms a straight line from the knees upwards.

2 As you inhale, kneel up slowly and lift your arms out in front of your body and upwards. As you complete your inhalation, kneel fully up with your chest lifted and arms extended overhead. Pause the breath for a few seconds. For those with lower back difficulties, sweep your arms out to the sides of your body and then upwards.

Pause briefly at the end
of each movement to
maintain your awareness
of your body movements

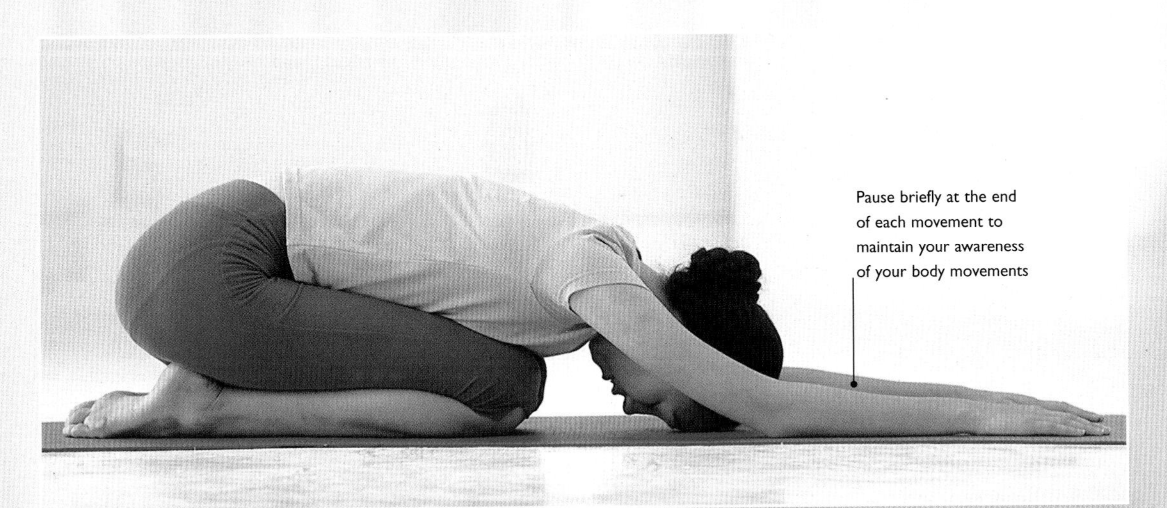

3 As you begin to exhale, slowly sit back on the heels once again while you bring your arms back down in front of your body. As you near the end of your exhalation, round the back and bring your forehead to the ground in an extended Child's pose, with your arms stretched out in front of you on the ground. Hold the exhale and remain still for a few seconds. To protect your lower back, sit back onto the heels before bringing the arms down just in front of your knees. Then as you bring your forehead to the ground, stretch your arms out in front of you and finish the exhale.

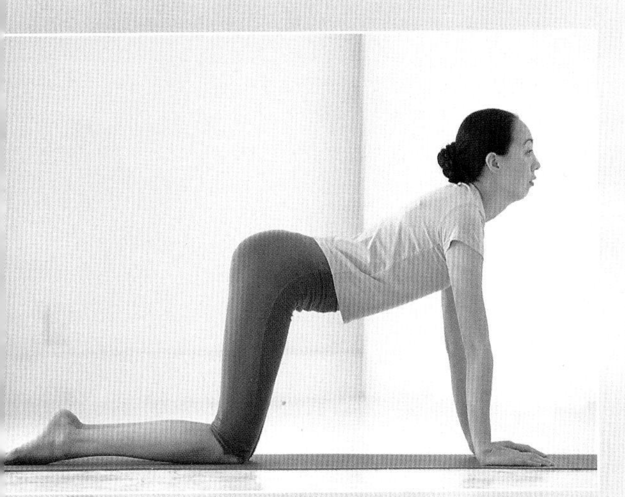

4 Inhale and lean into your arms as you lift your body forwards onto your knees and hands, with your buttocks up. Your spine curves towards the ground and your head is lifted with the shoulders relaxed. Lengthen your spine and press the tailbone back as you complete the inhalation. This is called Cow pose.

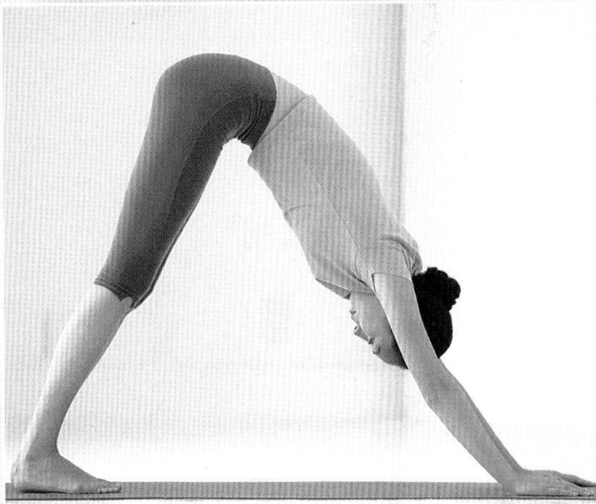

5 As you exhale, keep the hands in place while you come onto your feet and hands in Downward Dog. Your body forms a triangle with your buttocks at the highest point. Straighten the legs and press the heels to the ground. Stretch your spine away from the ground. Your hips will move towards the ceiling and back away from your hands. This will give your arms, spine, and legs a deep stretch.

6 Either go on to step 8 or move into Upward Facing Dog: position your feet a little further back as you begin inhaling. Lower your body down until it is just above the ground. Press into your arms and lift your chest and head in Upward Facing Dog pose as you finish the inhalation. Keep your movements fluid.

To protect a delicate lower back, bring your knees to the ground

Keep your arms strong, with palms flat and fingers together

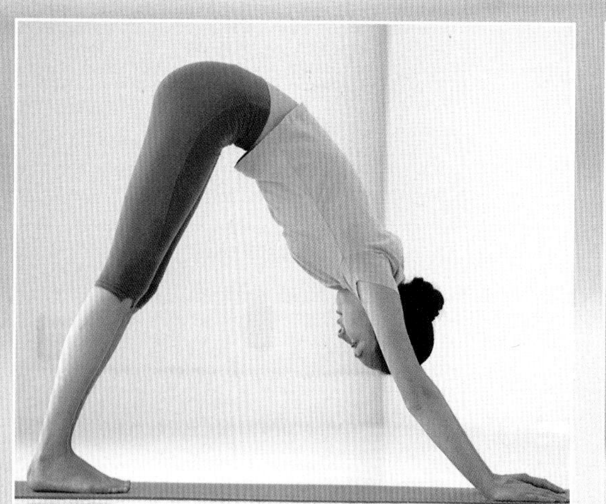

7 Exhale as you return to Downward Dog (step 5), lifting the pelvis upwards and pressing it back. You may need to adjust your feet again, bringing them forwards a few steps.

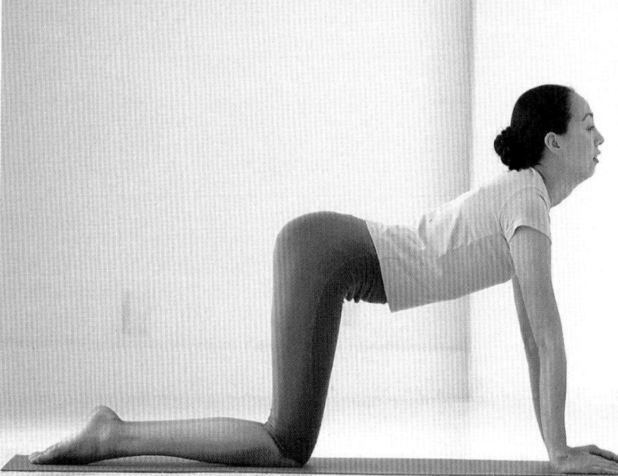

8 Begin to reverse the order of the Vinyasa: as you inhale, gently come onto your knees into Cow pose (step 4).

KIM'S STORY (USA)

I have had health problems for most of my life. At age four I had my first operation, for hip dysplasia, and was in a body cast for several months. At 35 years old, after 18 operations of various sorts, I developed fibromyalgia.

My massage therapist kept encouraging me to go to her yoga classes. I put her off for over a year, thinking how crazy it was to imagine a person like me, who could barely walk some mornings, being able to do yoga. I finally gave in and joined her senior citizens' class, which was the best choice for my extreme tightness. After attending for just a few weeks, I found myself hurting less and sleeping better. My coordination, posture, and tension release have improved greatly. When I feel my muscles start to tighten I practise yoga to release the tension rather than taking a pain-reliever.

The best part is that I truly feel better. I never dreamed I could be so in tune with my body. I try to incorporate yoga into all I do. For example, besides practising yoga in the morning and night, during the day when I wash dishes I practise standing poses. When I drive I practise yogic breathing, which actually helps my concentration, and when I fold laundry – Forward Bends!

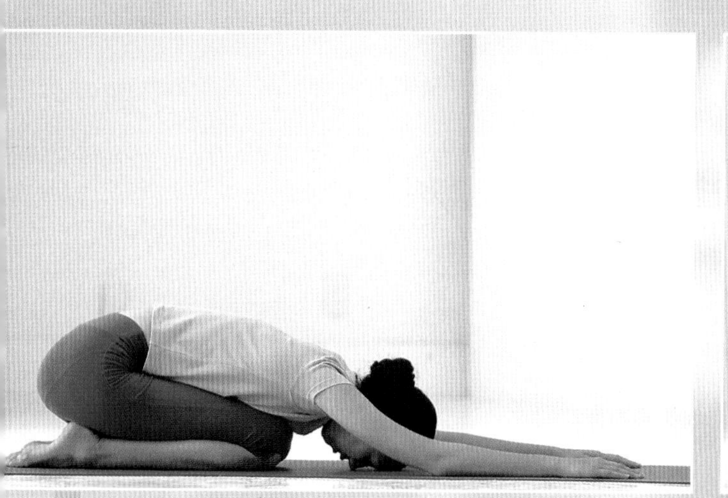

9 Then exhale back into the extended Child's pose, following the sequence described in step 3.

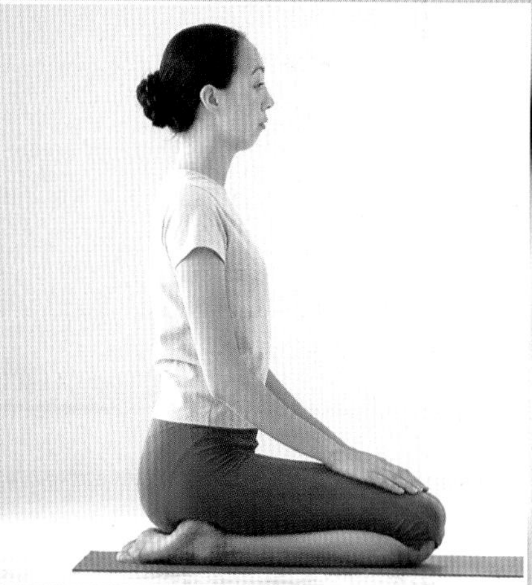

10 Inhale and exhale into Rock pose – back to step 1 – to end one round of Kneeling Sun Salutation. Inhale and repeat the sequence from step 2 for as many rounds as you like.

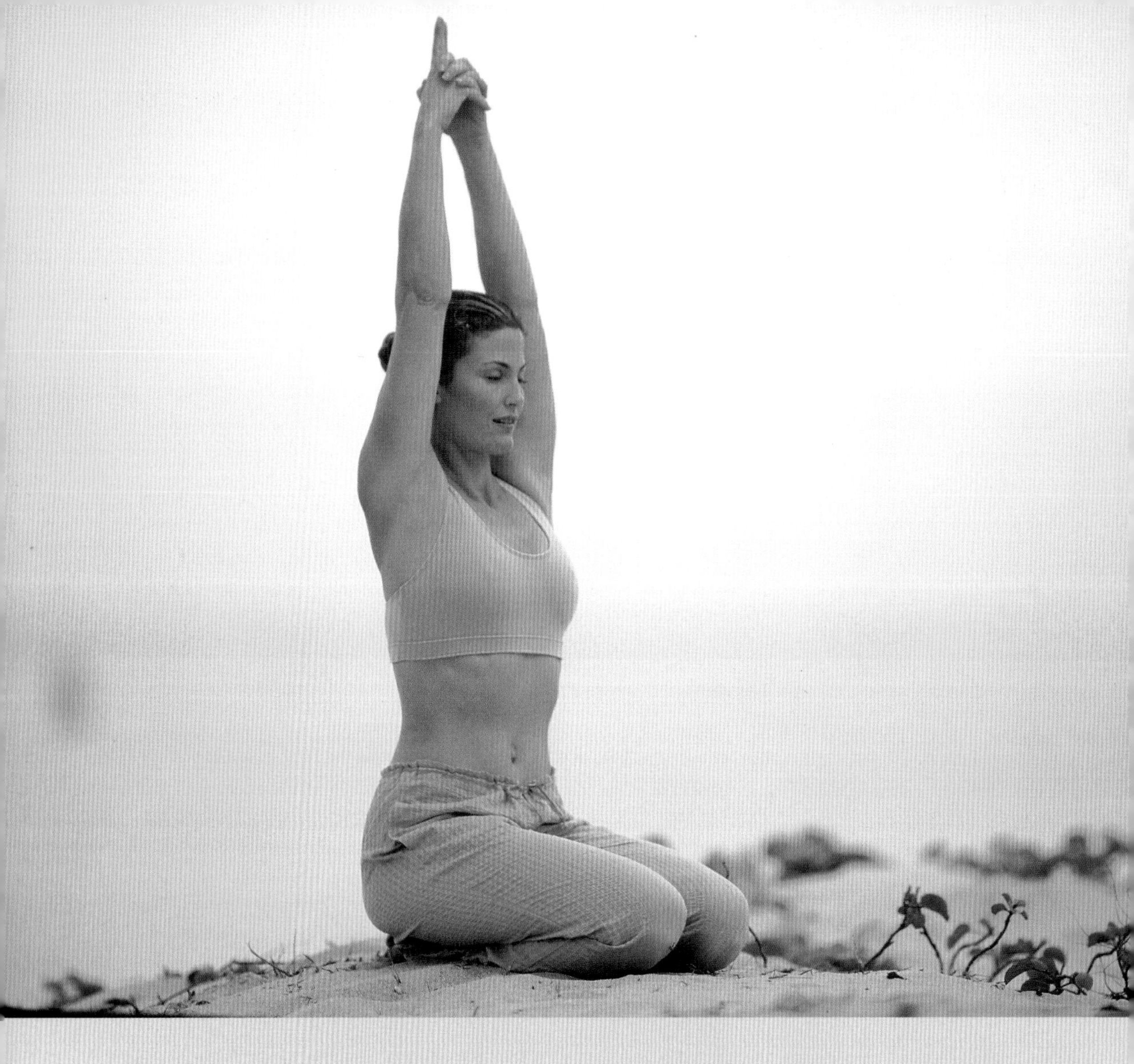

ESPECIALLY FOR WOMEN

All yoga is good for women – as for men – but some poses especially resonate with the physical and mental make-up of women. As a woman, it is imperative for your health and happiness for you to exercise every day. If you begin to find yourself feeling moody or easily frazzled, you need to move your body! This helps move your mind into new and brighter places. The poses explored here can all be practised with either deep breathing or Breath of Fire. Some women like to practise them as a daily routine, others prefer to add a few as warm-ups before a yoga set, or spontaneously practise a few postures in between busy moments in the day. Whatever your method, you will experience rejuvenation and relaxation from these poses.

CAT AND COW

This exercise brings great flexibility to the spine, including the cervical vertebrae, and circulates the spinal fluid. A great warm-up exercise, Cat and Cow Stretch will prepare you for the other postures in this chapter.

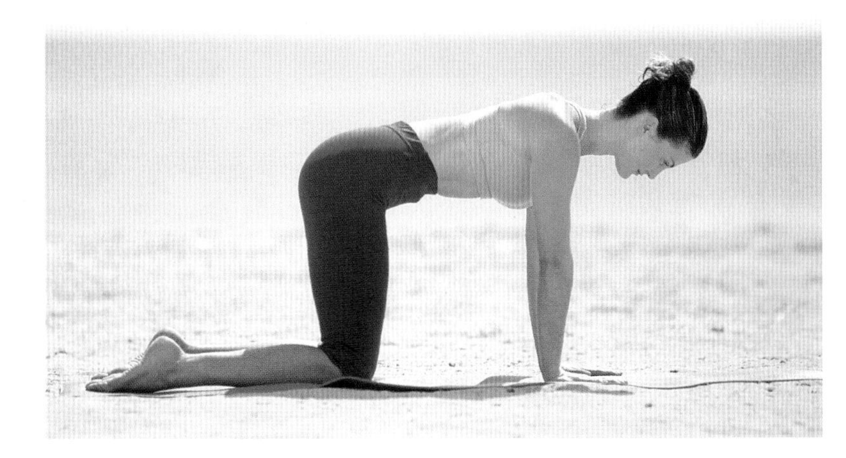

1 Position yourself on your hands and knees, with your knees under your hips and your hands under your shoulders. As far as possible, keep your elbows straight and your arms and legs stable throughout the exercise as your spine curves in each direction.

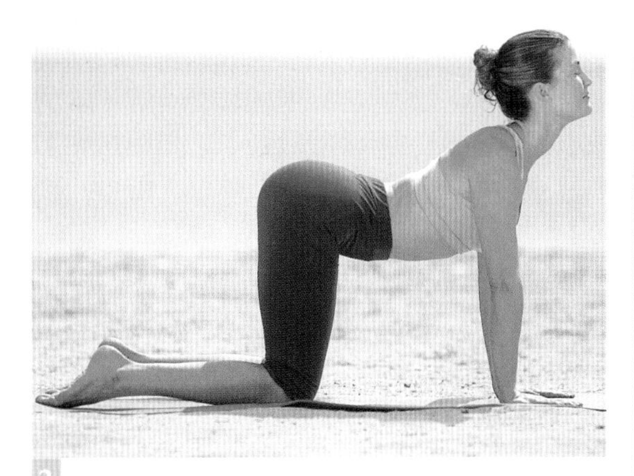

2 As you inhale, dip the spine towards the ground and bring your head back. This is Cow pose.

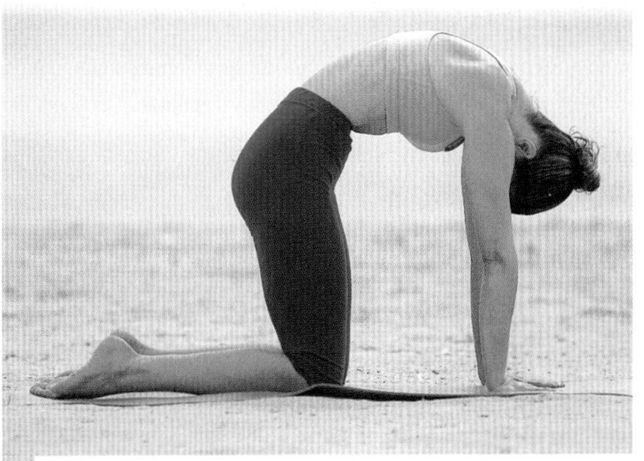

3 As you exhale, flex in the opposite direction so that your back is arched upwards in Cat pose and your head comes down so that your chin is close to your chest. Alternate between Cat and Cow poses, gradually increasing in speed and in the power of each breath as you continue for 2–3 minutes.

LIFE NERVE STRETCH

In yogic teachings, your sciatic nerve is also called your life nerve. Keeping your life nerve strong and stretched is important for the health and flexibility of your body.

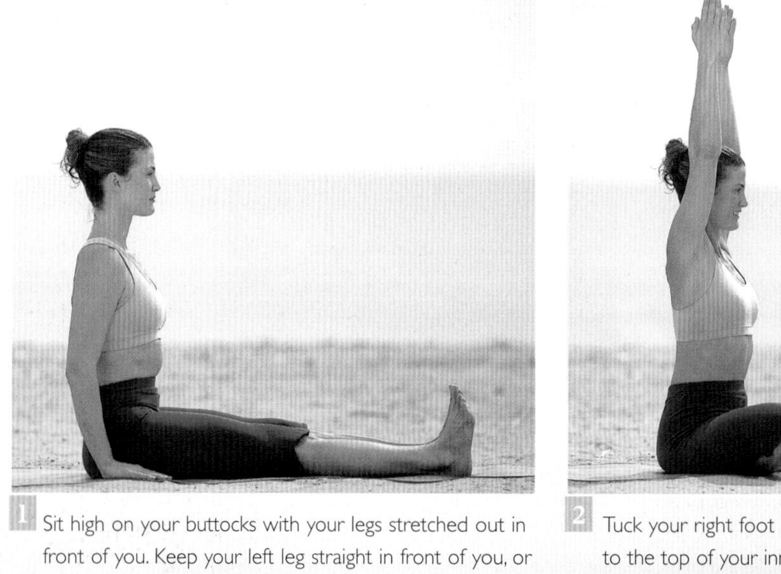

1 Sit high on your buttocks with your legs stretched out in front of you. Keep your left leg straight in front of you, or slightly to the side.

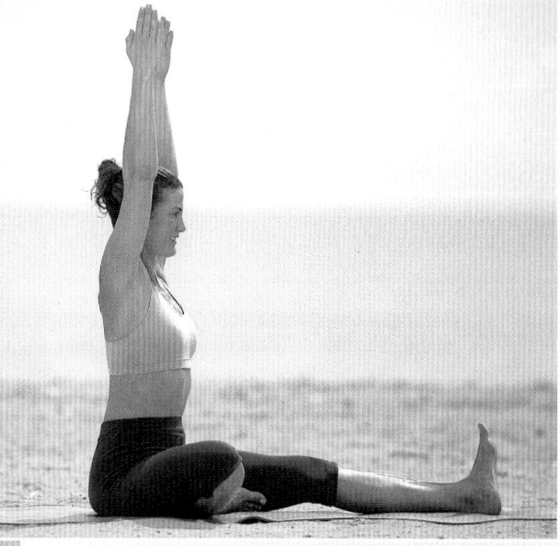

2 Tuck your right foot into the groin, with the heel as close to the top of your inner thigh as is comfortable. Inhale and stretch your arms up overhead, lengthening your spine.

3 Exhale and bend forwards, reaching your hands to your toes or any part of the leg that you can reach to give you a good stretch without straining. Hold the posture and breathe deeply for 1–2 minutes. Repeat on the other leg.

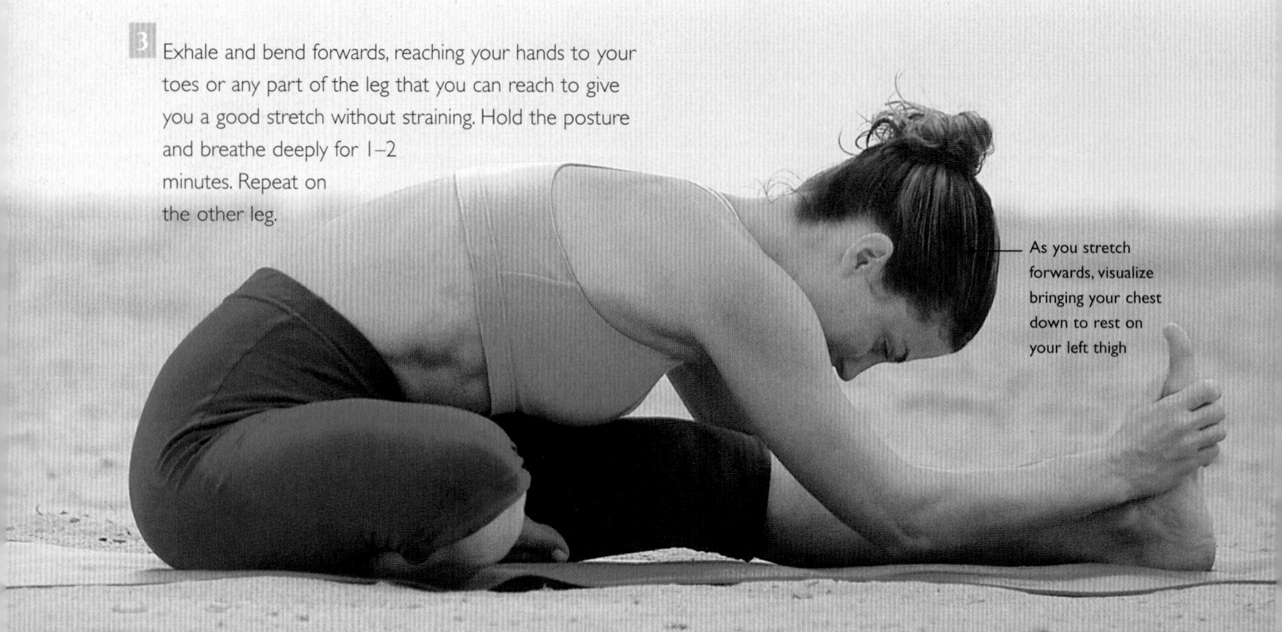

As you stretch forwards, visualize bringing your chest down to rest on your left thigh

LOCUST

This exercise strengthens the lower back, allows energy to flow to the spine, opens the nerve channels in the solar plexus, and tones the legs, buttocks, and stomach. It is excellent for releasing premenstrual tension.

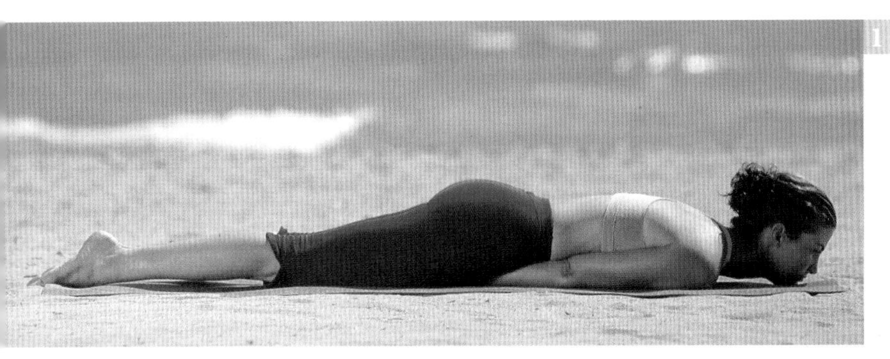

1 Lie on your stomach with your heels close together and your chin on the ground. Make fists of your hands and tuck them into the spot where they fit comfortably just inside the pelvic bones (where the legs and pelvis meet). Your hands will act as a fulcrum for raising your legs.

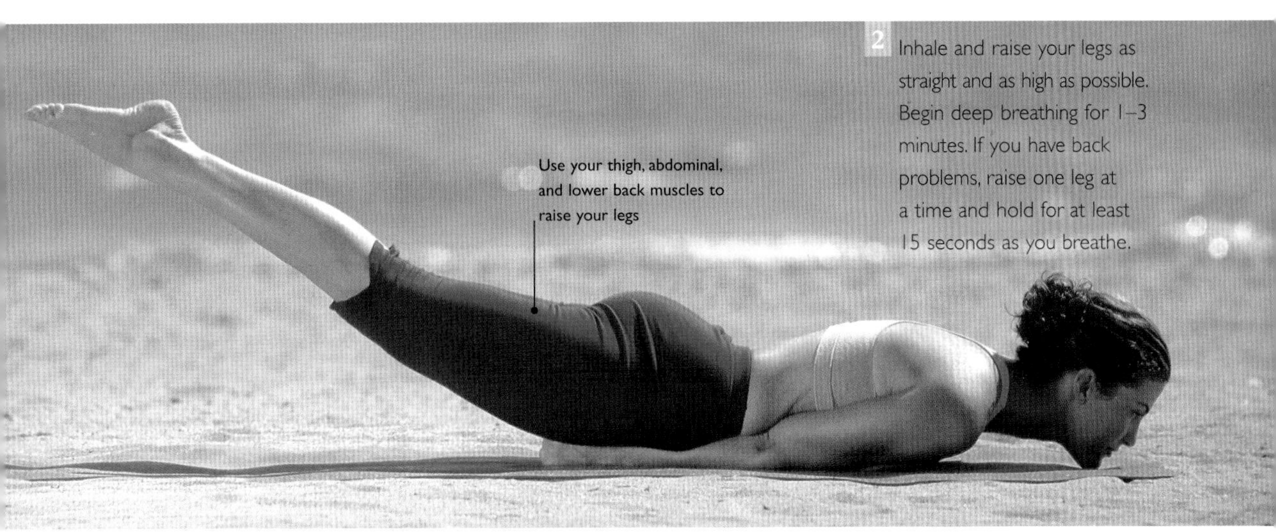

Use your thigh, abdominal, and lower back muscles to raise your legs

2 Inhale and raise your legs as straight and as high as possible. Begin deep breathing for 1–3 minutes. If you have back problems, raise one leg at a time and hold for at least 15 seconds as you breathe.

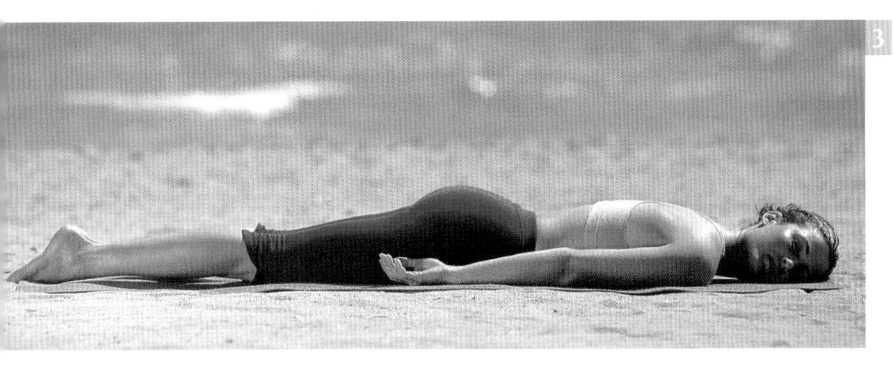

3 Then relax down, bringing your arms to rest at your sides, and turning your head to one side. Breathe deeply for a few moments.

BOW

This posture massages and invigorates the internal organs, strengthens the abdominal muscles, and expands your breathing capacity. It helps to prevent digestive and bowel disorders, and reduces fat around the waist area. Bow pose also stretches the thigh muscle which, according to yogic science, controls the calcium–magnesium balance in the body. This balance is necessary for both physical and mental wellbeing.

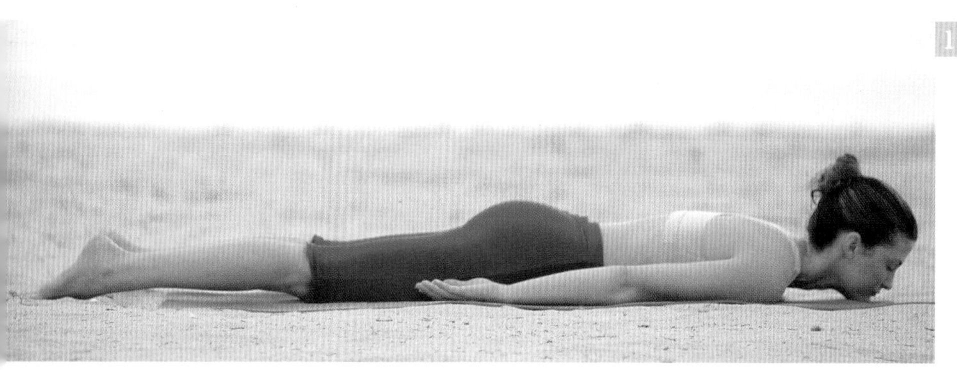

1 Lie on your abdomen with your chin on the ground and arms resting at your sides.

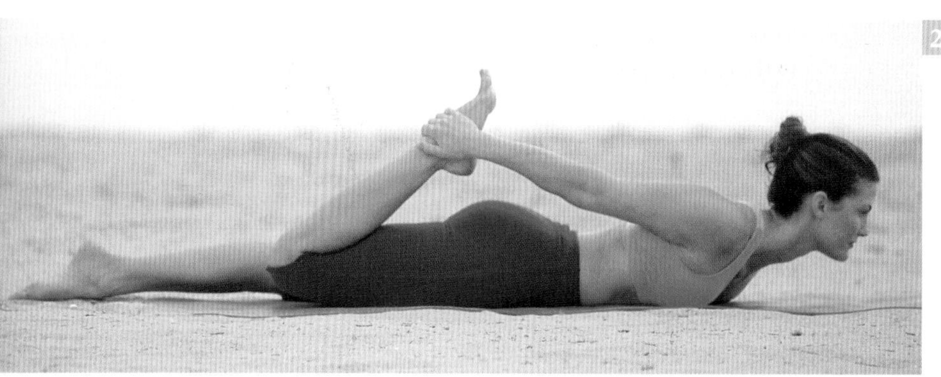

2 Bend your right leg at the knee. Reach back with your right hand and grasp the right ankle.

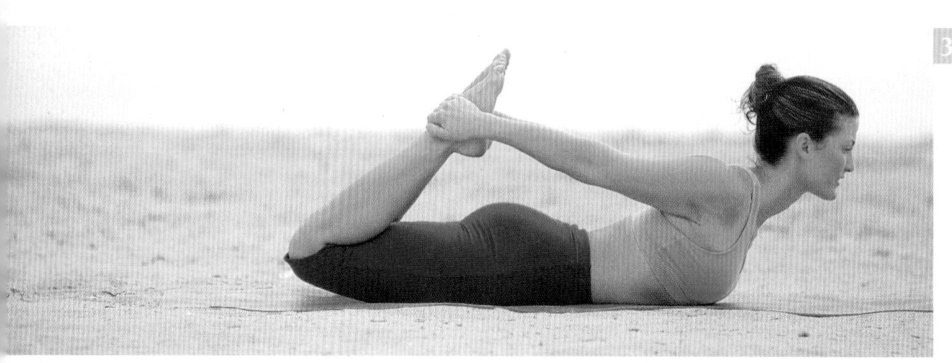

3 Bend your left leg at the knee and reach back with your left hand to grasp the left ankle.

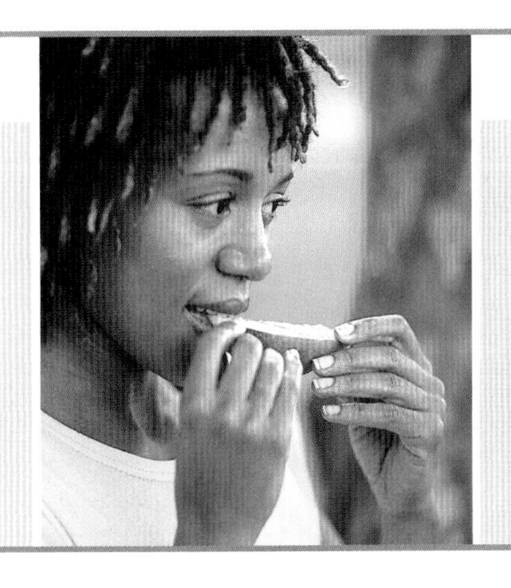

EAT MANGO FOR HEALTH

Mango is wonderful for women. It helps with menstrual problems and is a tonic for the digestive system. Mango lassi ("lussee"), a yogurt-based drink, is delicious for breakfast, or as a mid-afternoon pick-me-up. Combine in a blender 2 cups of plain yogurt, 2 medium, ripe mangoes, peeled, stoned, and sliced, 2–3 tablespoons of maple syrup or honey, 6 ice cubes or 150ml (5fl oz) water (a few drops of rose water are optional, available at Asian stores, to add a fragrant touch). Blend until smooth. Makes about 4 cups for sharing.

4 Inhale and lift your body upwards, raising your head, chest, and thighs off the ground. Create a tension between the straight arms and the legs to stretch higher. Breathe deeply, expanding the chest on the inhale, relaxing it on the exhale. Continue for 1–2 minutes.

EASY-DOES-IT VERSION

If you can't reach your ankles, use a prop such as a belt around the ankles to grasp onto. If you can reach them but can't stretch and hold, inhale as you stretch up and exhale as you relax down. With steady practice you will be able to do the full pose.

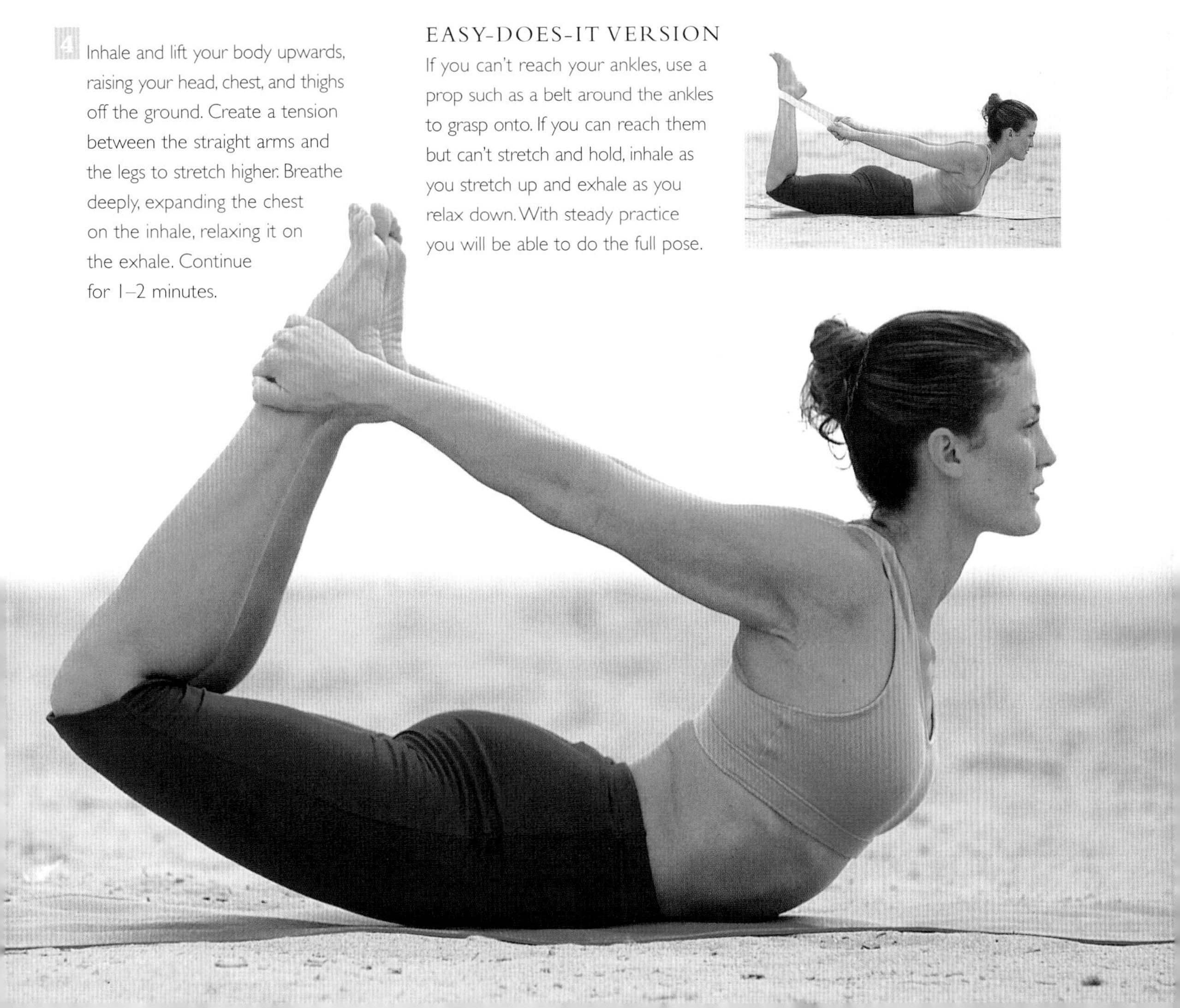

CAMEL

This pose builds strength in the muscle groups of the back, helping to prevent sciatica and slipped discs. Camel pose also helps to balance the navel chakra, which is your energy centre of personal health and willpower, and relieves the stomach from the effects of overeating. According to yogic teaching, whoever does Camel pose regularly has control over hunger and thirst, just as a camel would. Camel pose stretches the thigh muscles which, according to yogic science, controls the calcium–magnesium balance in the body. This balance is necessary for both physical and mental wellbeing.

GOLDEN MILK

This is wonderful for the spine and lubricates the joints.

Boil ¼–⅓tsp turmeric in 85ml (3fl oz) water for 8 minutes. Add 250ml (8fl oz) organic milk and 1tbsp raw almond oil. Remove from heat and add honey to taste.

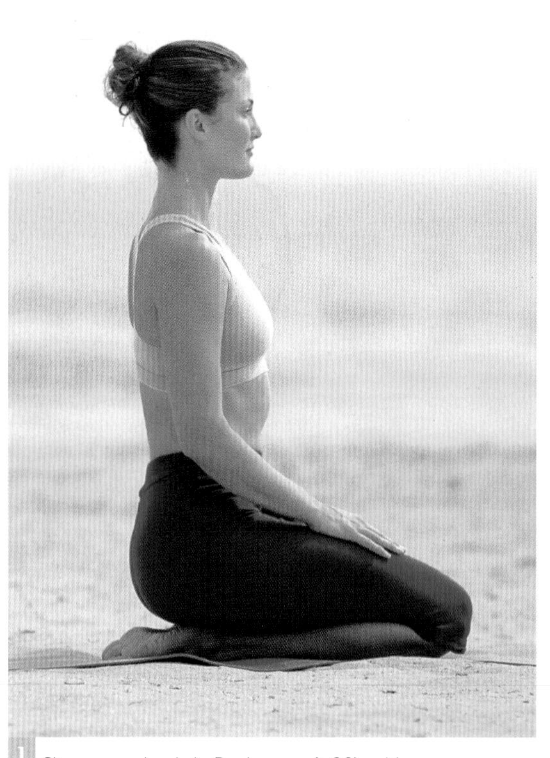

1 Sit on your heels in Rock pose *(p.20)*, with your spine straight and hands on your thighs.

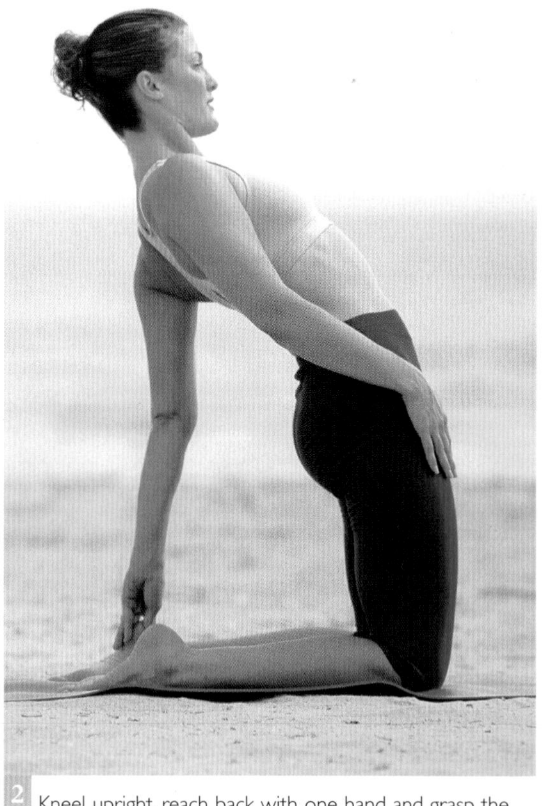

2 Kneel upright, reach back with one hand and grasp the heel on that side, then repeat on the other side.

Relax your face, neck, throat and shoulders
Lift and expand your chest more fully with each breath

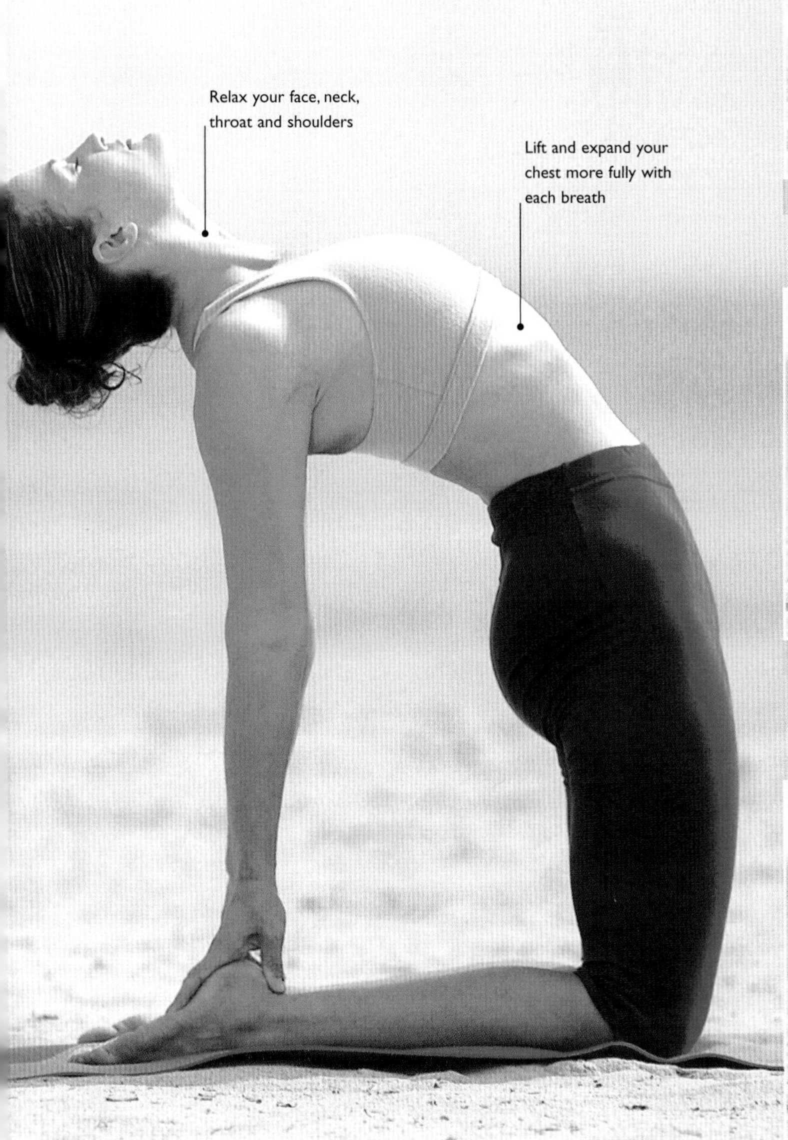

3 Press the hips and thighs forwards to steady the pose, and to create a deeper stretch. The chest is lifted up and the head is tipped back but not dropped fully. Relax your face, neck, throat, and shoulders. Breathe deeply or use Breath of Fire *(p.24)* for 1–2 minutes.

EASY-DOES–IT VERSION

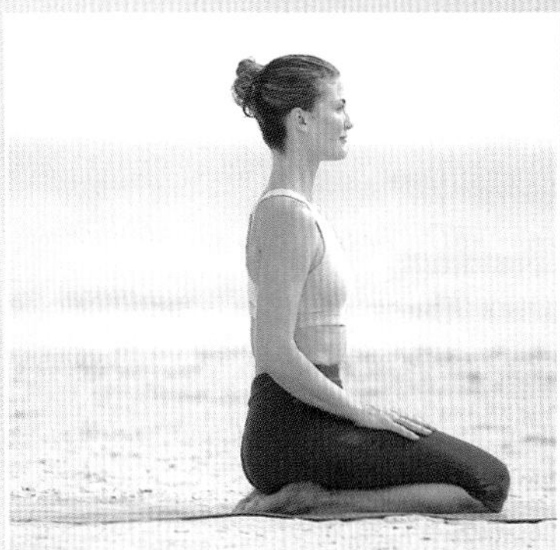

1 Sit on your heels in Rock pose with your spine straight.

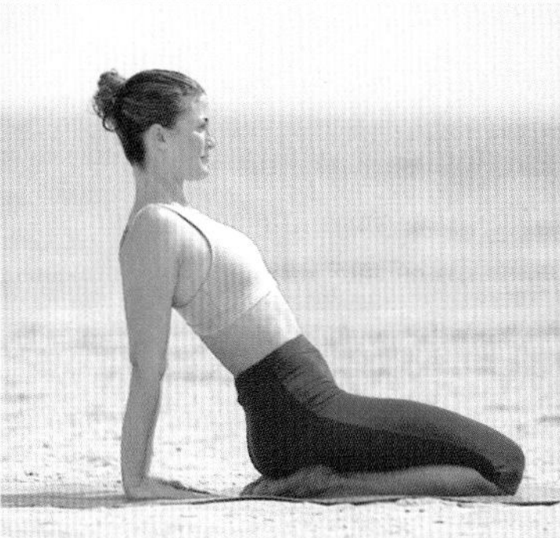

2 Lean back onto your hands, keeping the chest lifted. Point your fingers either towards or away from your body.

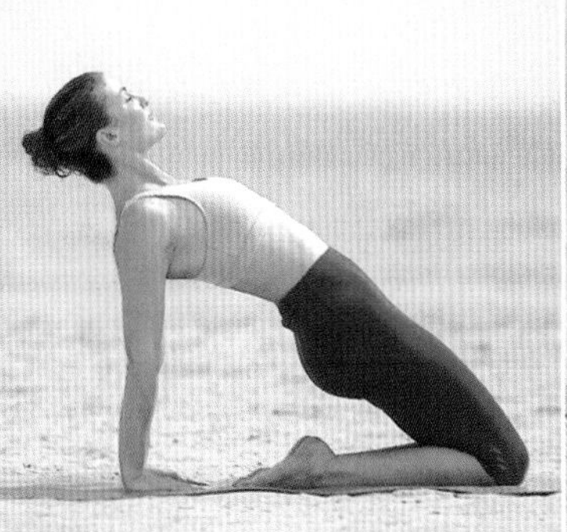

3 Lift your buttocks off the ground as high as possible as you press the hips and thighs forwards. Continue for 1–2 minutes.

CHILD'S POSE

Child's pose is a resting pose that allows the effects of previous yoga poses to be assimilated. Pressing your forehead to the ground activates the sixth (intuitive) centre between the eyebrows. Child's pose also acts as a counterpose to Bow pose *(pp.46–47)*, relaxing and curving the spine in the opposite direction. If needed, add a small pillow or rolled towel under the head or under the buttocks for comfort in this pose.

YOGI TEA

This health-promoting drink is delicious. The spices used are particularly beneficial to internal health.

To 1 litre (1¾ pints) of water, add:
15 whole cloves
20 green cardamom pods (crushed slightly)
15 black peppercorns
8 slices ginger root or
5 5cm (2in) sticks of cinnamon. Cover and boil gently for 30–40 minutes (add water as it evaporates). Add ½tsp black tea and 750ml (1¼ pints) organic milk (dairy or non-dairy) Bring to a boil. Turn off heat, add honey to taste.

After Camel pose *(pp.48–49)*, rest in Child's pose. Rest your buttocks on your heels and bring your forehead to the ground and your arms alongside your body, with the palms facing upwards in a relaxed manner. Breathe gently for 1–2 minutes or two, relaxing the entire spine and shoulders.

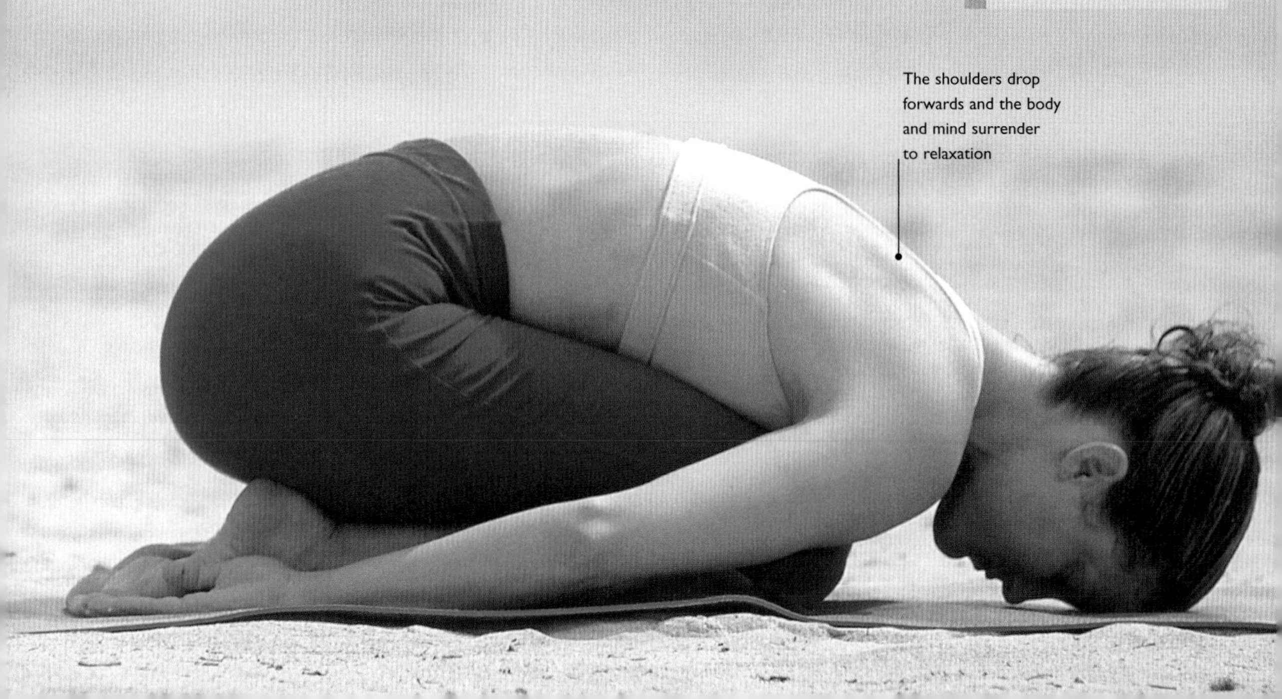

The shoulders drop forwards and the body and mind surrender to relaxation

STRETCH POSE

Stretch pose is known to adjust and balance your navel point, which increases stamina, willpower, and wellbeing. When your navel point is strong and balanced, you have a steady pulse centred at the navel – not left, right, above or below it. You can check your navel pulse by bringing your thumb and fingers of one hand together and pressing deep into the skin surrounding the navel. As an experiment, check your pulse before, then again immediately after, practising Stretch pose for 1–2 minutes, and notice what differences you discover. Generally, your pulse will be deeper, stronger, and more evenly centred at the navel point after practising Stretch pose.

According to yogic tradition, the navel is the focal point for all 72,000 nerves in the body. So Stretch pose tunes up the whole nervous system as well as the digestive and reproductive systems.

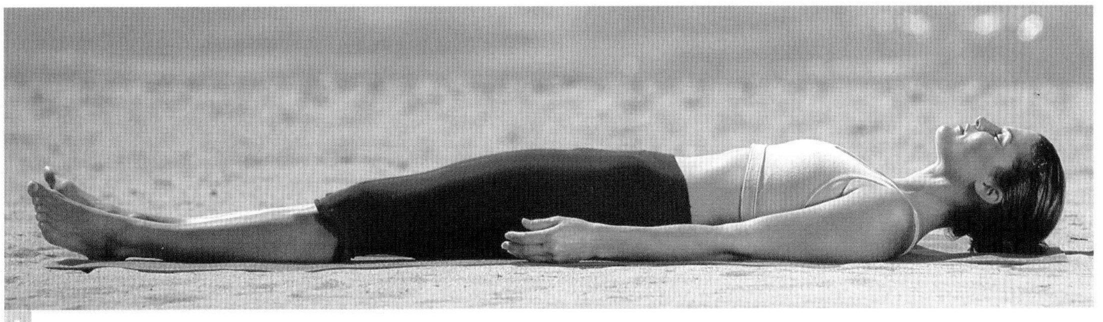

1 Tuck your pelvis forward to take any pressure off the lower spine before coming up into Stretch pose. This will help to ensure that when you lift your legs up it will be your abdominal muscles rather than your back muscles that are supporting your lift. Before lifting your head, consciously relax your neck muscles and prepare to use your upper back, chest, and abdominal muscles to lift your neck and head. This will avoid straining your neck in any way.

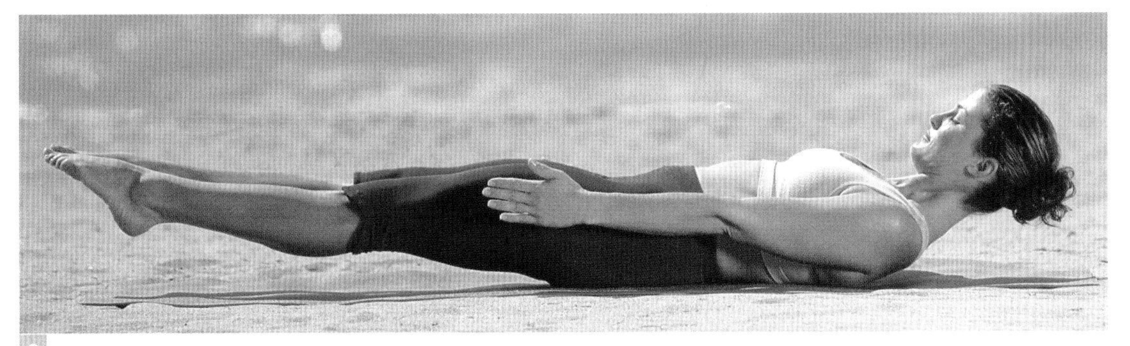

2 Keep your heels close together and raise them 15cm (6in) from the ground with straight legs. Raise your head 15cm (6in) and fix your eyes on your pointed toes. Stay mindful of keeping the neck and lower spine relaxed while holding the pose. Your arms are held at your sides, palms facing the thighs but not touching. Hold this position for 1–2 minutes while doing Breath of Fire *(p.24)*. Then relax down for a few seconds.

SHOULDERSTAND

Shoulderstand is said to benefit the entire body, especially the throat, thyroid, and circulation. Shoulderstand increases flexibility in the cervical region of the spine, and helps prevent varicose veins. The muscles of the back, shoulders, and arms are stretched and strengthened, too. It also provides an inverted gravitational pull, which suspends and relaxes all your internal organs. Make sure that you read through all the instructions before attempting this pose.

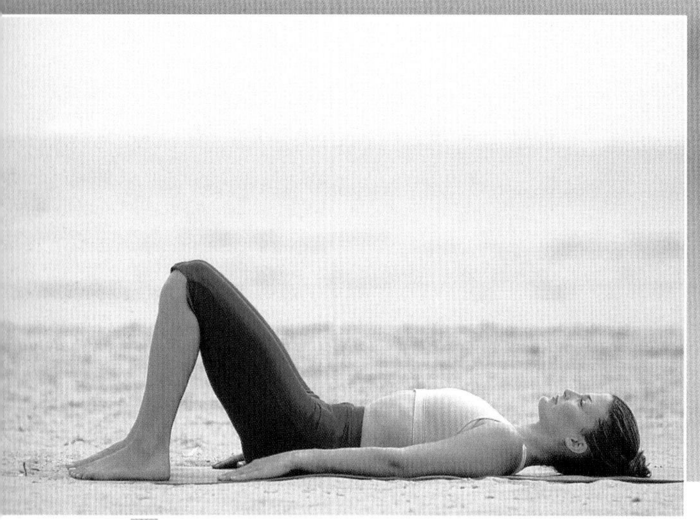

1 Lie on your back with your legs bent at the knee and your feet flat on the ground. Your arms are at your sides with your palms facing downwards.

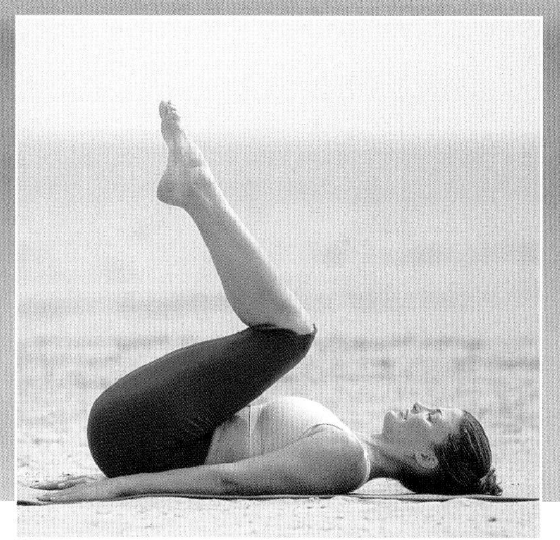

2 Keeping your arms and hands in the same position, raise your legs to a 90° angle.

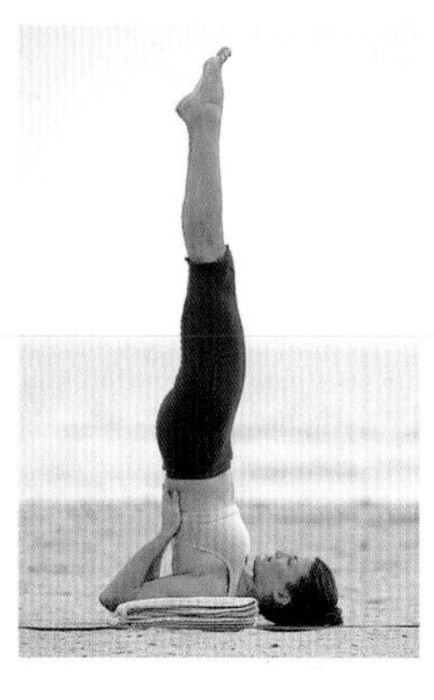

USING PROPS IN SHOULDERSTAND

To relieve pressure on the neck area in Shoulderstand, place one or two thick felt blankets under your shoulders and upper back, just at the edge where your shoulders meet your neck. The blanket should be large enough so that you can also rest your elbows on it and feel stable. Your neck will then have room to relax and straighten when you come up into Shoulderstand. Another alternative and a good preparation to Shoulderstand is found in Pelvic Tilt Position 2 *(p.64)*.

After Shoulderstand rest on your back for a minute or two, either with your legs out straight or, if there is pressure on the lower spine, lie with your knees bent and tip your pelvis slightly forwards, or put a firm pillow under your knees.

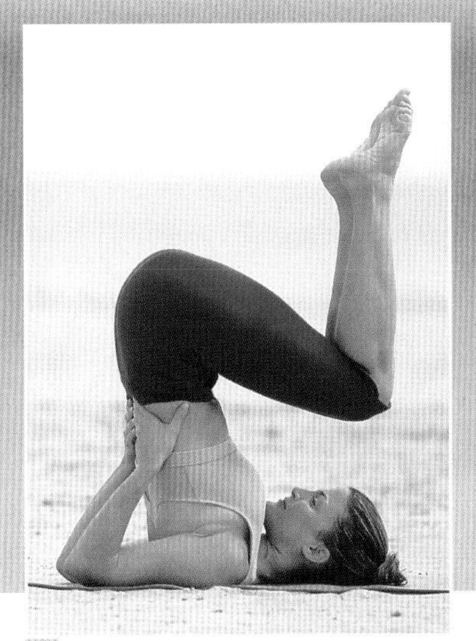

3 Begin to push your body up so that your legs are as straight as possible while supporting your back with your hands and your elbows, which remain firmly on the ground.

4 Relax and stretch up higher on your shoulders. Adjust your hand positions: the further your hands move towards your upper back, the straighter your spine will be. Your chin should rest on your neck. Breathe for 1–2 minutes.

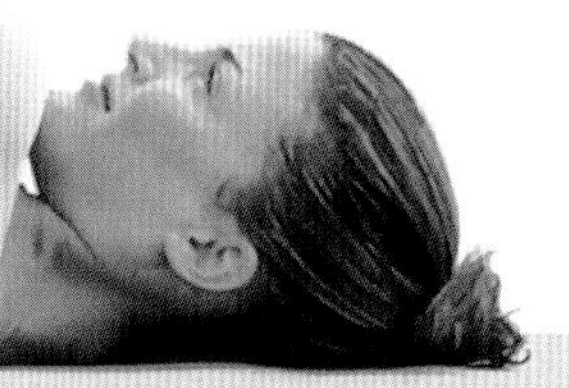

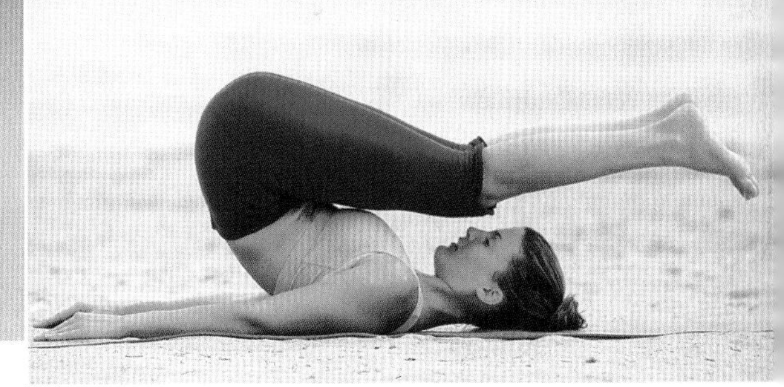

5 To come out of the pose, lower your legs over your head into a modified Plough pose, keeping your knees close to your head. As you roll out slowly place your arms on the floor beside you, or continue to support your spine with your hands on your back. Exhale deeply.

ARCHER

Archer pose develops the quality of courage in the face of a challenge. It balances and strengthens the nervous system and your electromagnetic energy field, or aura. Every one of your chakras is activated in this pose: the leg position works on the first, second, and third chakras, the stretch across the chest and the arm positions work to activate the heart centre, while the turned neck stimulates the throat chakra. The gazing and strong breathing work on the intuitive (sixth) centre and the crown centre.

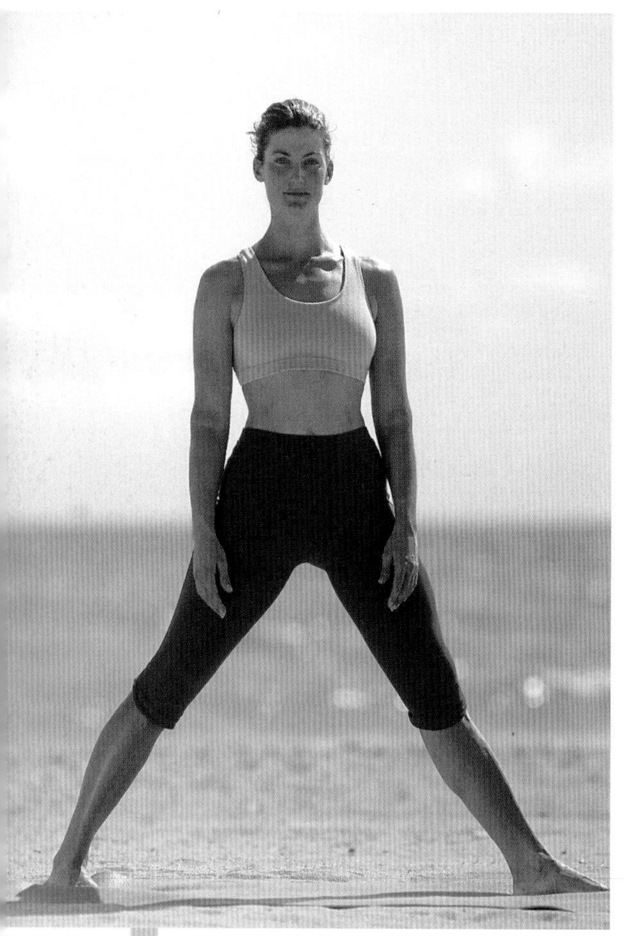

1 Stand with your legs straddled about 75cm (30in) apart, with your left leg forwards, foot turned to the side, and your right leg back at a 45° angle to the front foot. The right foot should face forwards.

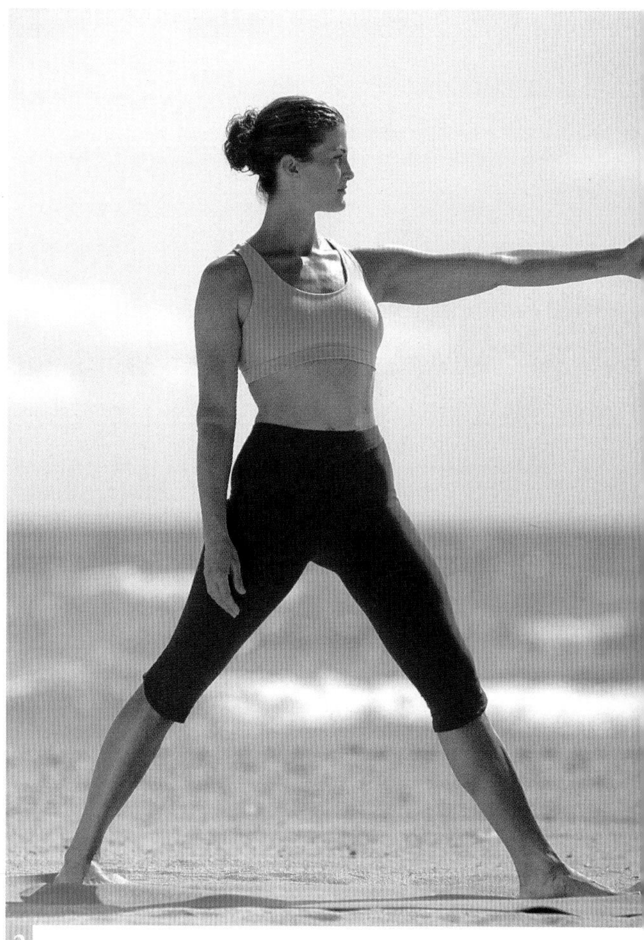

2 Raise your left arm straight out in front, parallel to the ground, and make a fist as if grasping a bow while pressing the thumb forwards. Turn your head to face forwards and fix your eyes above your fist on the horizon.

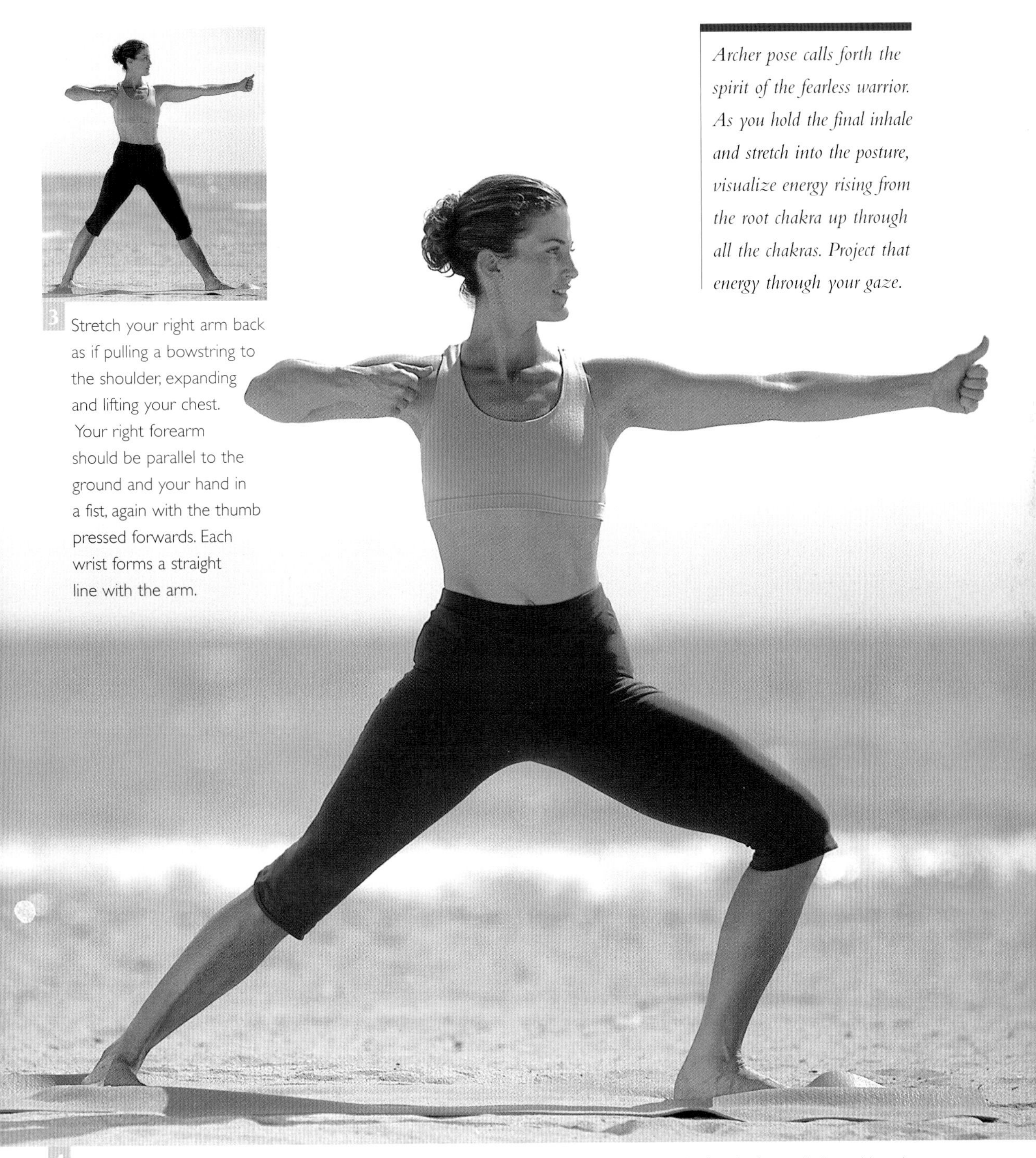

Archer pose calls forth the spirit of the fearless warrior. As you hold the final inhale and stretch into the posture, visualize energy rising from the root chakra up through all the chakras. Project that energy through your gaze.

3 Stretch your right arm back as if pulling a bowstring to the shoulder, expanding and lifting your chest. Your right forearm should be parallel to the ground and your hand in a fist, again with the thumb pressed forwards. Each wrist forms a straight line with the arm.

4 Bend your left knee and lean into it so that you cannot see your left foot. Keeping your body centred, do not lean forwards but put 70 per cent of your weight on the front leg. Begin deep, full, slow breaths or Breath of Fire.

After 1–2 minutes inhale deeply, then exhale and lean into the pose as fully as you are able to without straining. Then, relax and switch legs so that your right leg is forwards at the starting position.

SAT KRIYA

This kriya, or set, practised with the chant *Sat Nam* *(p. 16)*, strengthens and balances the entire sexual system and digestive system. Your general physical health is improved since all the internal organs receive a gentle rhythmic massage from this exercise. Beginners should practise Sat Kriya for one minute, slowly working up to three minutes. After a time of steady practice, the period of Sat Kriya can be extended, and it is good to practise everyday for at least three minutes, but remember to approach this powerful kriya with respect. Ideally you should relax for at least the same amount of time as you have practised Sat Kriya, and it is recommended that you relax for up to twice that amount of time.

The chant, Sat Nam, *means "truth-identity", or "Truth is my essence". Chant in a constant rhythm about once a second.* Sat *should be said powerfully but not necessarily loud.* Nam *is short, the syllable is not extended, and it may be barely audible.*

BALWINDER'S STORY (CANADA)

No one could ever have told me that the experience of being a parent is like no other. When I was pregnant with my first child I would see other parents struggling with their toddler in the supermarket. I wondered why they were so impatient with their child, and imagined that my husband and I would be different with our child.

I no longer hold that opinion. I have two young children now. A good day used to be when I was able to shower. Now it is if my three-year-old doesn't stress me out. Yoga has been my saving grace. I recently underwent teacher-training for Kundalini Yoga. One of the kriyas that we were assigned and did religiously was Sat Kriya. As much as I disliked this kriya in the beginning, I have become fond of it. It has allowed me to process strong feelings such as anger and sadness, and has truly made me into something I cannot express.

On most days I am reminded by my children that what I am doing not only helps me but them as well. Often they mimic me by bringing their tiny hands up into position and chanting Sat Nam. Because of my daily practice I enjoy my role as a parent and maintain my grace even though there may be chaos around me.

Do not practise this
on a full stomach or
during menstruation

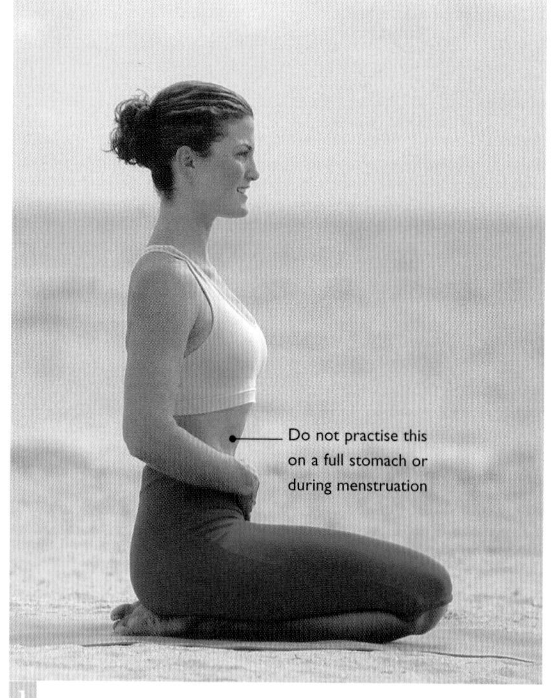

1 Sit in Rock pose. Place your hand on your abdomen and pull the navel up and in towards the spine while saying *Sat*. Your breath will go out as you chant. Then take a very quick and short inhale through your mouth as you relax your abdomen. Then chant *Nam* and begin again. Practise this step the first few times you try Sat Kriya to learn the internal movement. After that, begin step 2.

Mentally allow energy to flow up the body and out the top of the skull when you squeeze your muscles

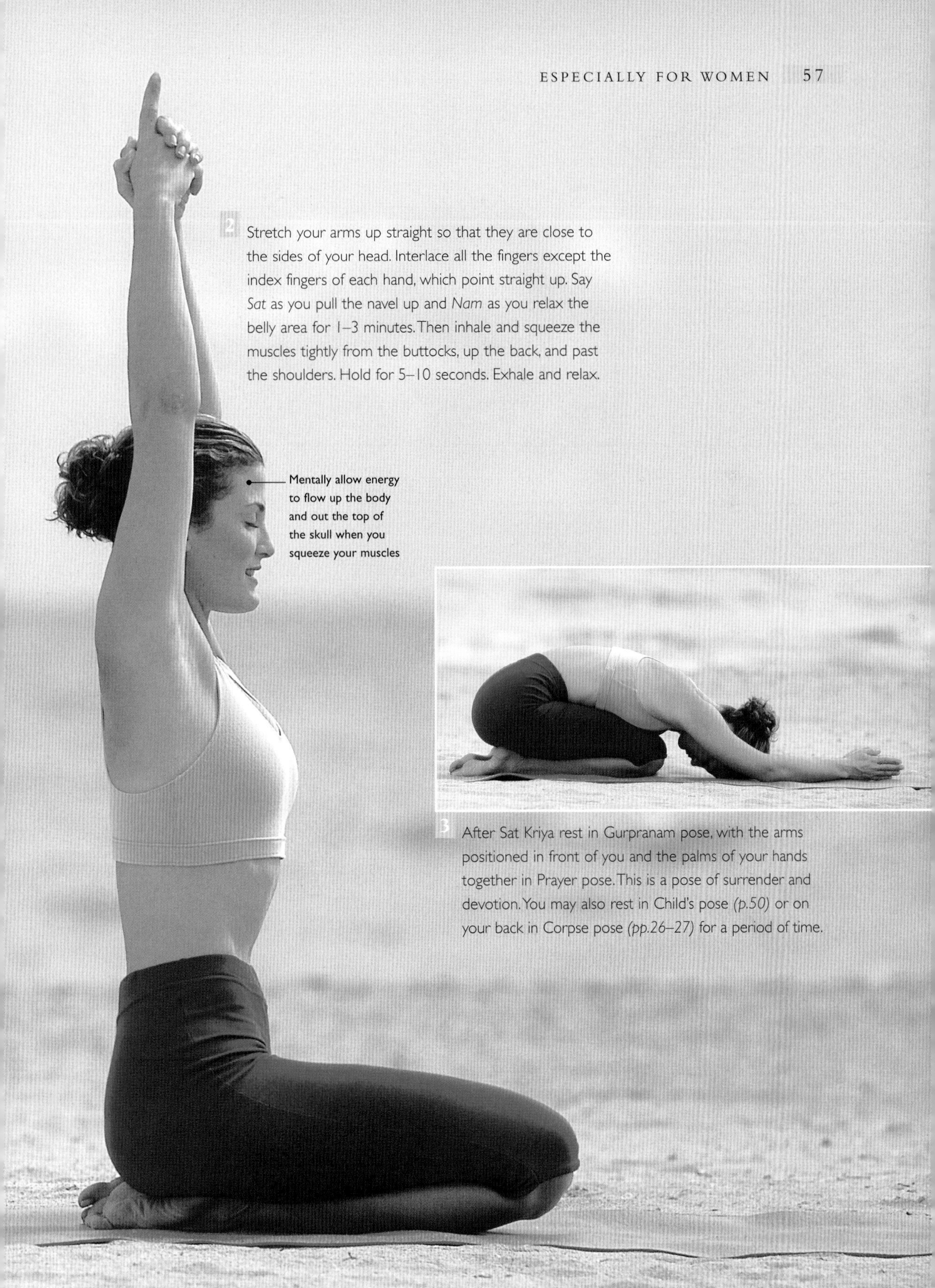

2 Stretch your arms up straight so that they are close to the sides of your head. Interlace all the fingers except the index fingers of each hand, which point straight up. Say *Sat* as you pull the navel up and *Nam* as you relax the belly area for 1–3 minutes. Then inhale and squeeze the muscles tightly from the buttocks, up the back, and past the shoulders. Hold for 5–10 seconds. Exhale and relax.

3 After Sat Kriya rest in Gurpranam pose, with the arms positioned in front of you and the palms of your hands together in Prayer pose. This is a pose of surrender and devotion. You may also rest in Child's pose *(p.50)* or on your back in Corpse pose *(pp.26–27)* for a period of time.

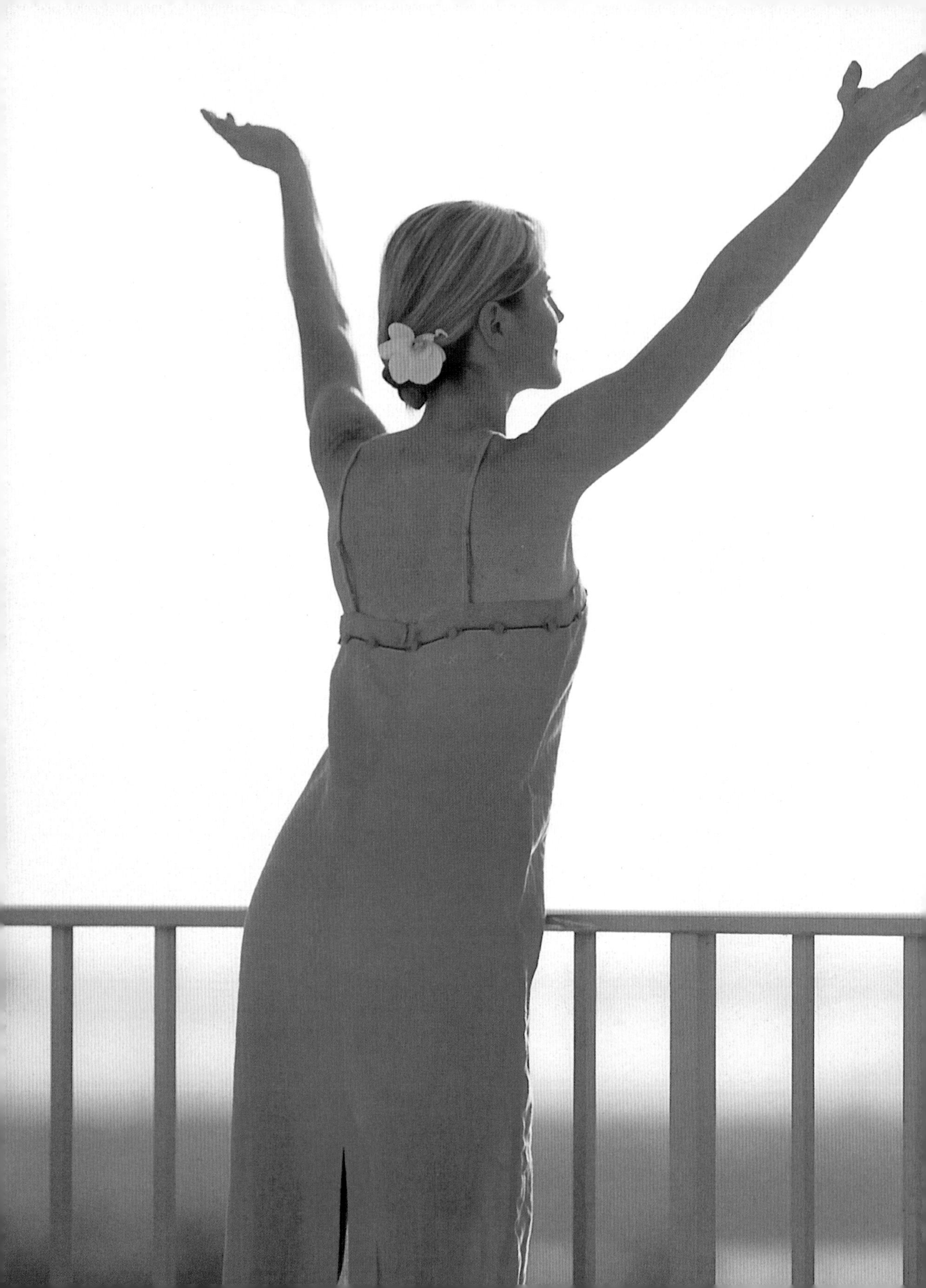

RELAXING & ENERGIZING

Experience the freedom and joy that is grounded in a steady yoga practice and a meditative mind. From this expansive overlook you are open to all the possibilities that life has to offer How does yoga accomplish this? Yoga fosters awareness. Through yoga you become aware of tension in your body and discord in your mind. You practise relaxing and releasing yoga. Or when you are tired and your mind is clouded, you choose yoga to bring physical energy and mental clarity. Eventually you'll be amazed to discover that yoga provides a deeply satisfying balance of true relaxation and, at the same time, an uplifting sense of energy.

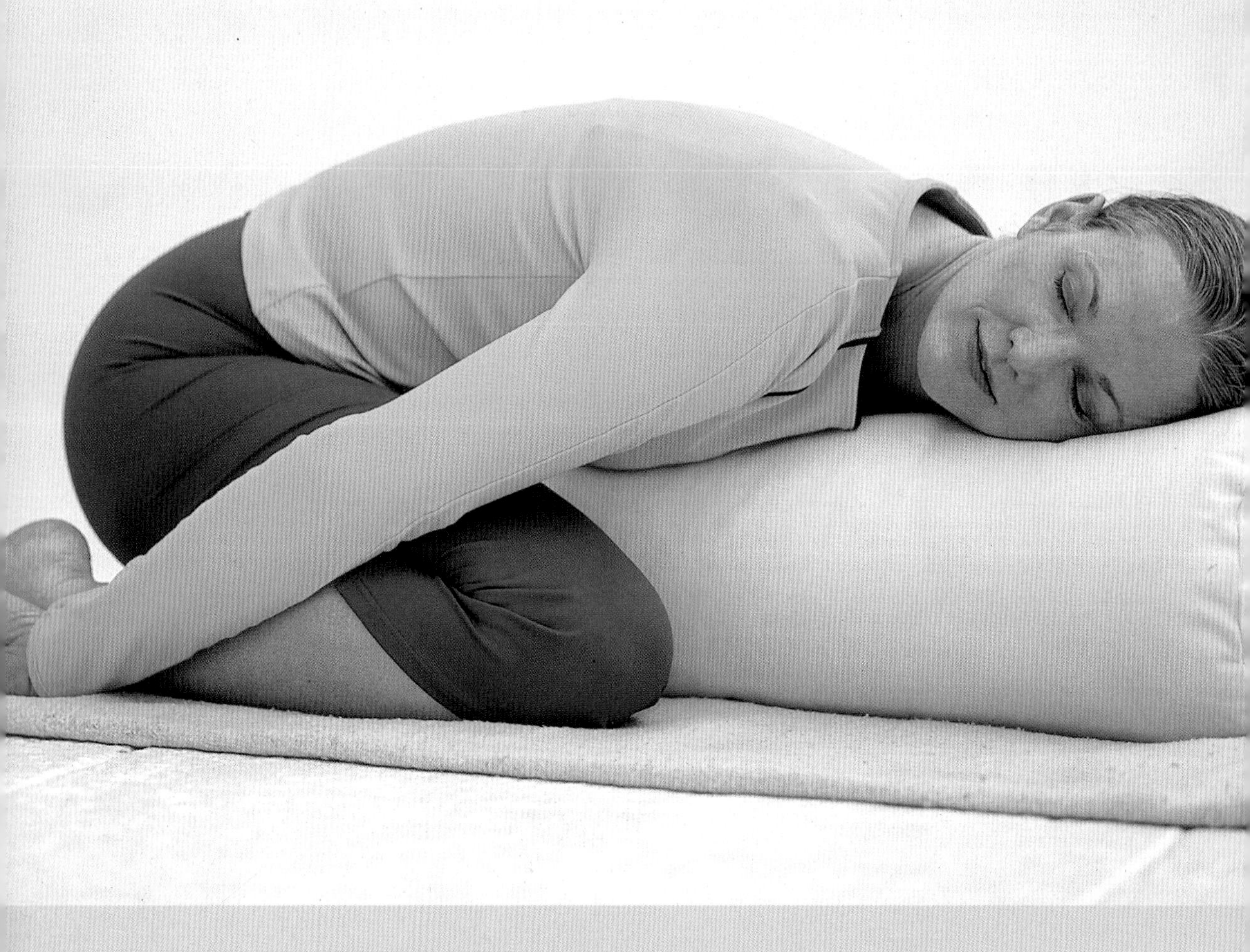

REJUVENATING YOGA

We have amazing powers of self-regeneration. Our challenge is to believe in our innate capacity to rebalance, and to do it with integrity and without guilt. When we are frazzled by the day's end, we know what will renew us – a few minutes of quiet time, a walk in the woods, a good book and a bath, or a small, candle-lit sanctuary for yoga.

This chapter, and to a great degree, this book, is designed to foster the self-regenerating capacity of woman through yoga. Here you will have the chance to unwind the tight muscles of your body and the restrictive pressures of your mind through restorative yoga, wall yoga, and a yogic technique called Alternate Nostril Breathing.

RESTORATIVE YOGA

Sometimes we need to stop doing and just be. That's when restorative yoga comes to the rescue. These soothing, quieting poses encourage your own natural healing processes to activate, whether it be relief from stress, back pain, high blood pressure, asthma, or any number of imbalances. The poses are wonderful tools for support and relaxation during menstruation, menopause, and pregnancy.

SUGGESTED PROPS

Bolster *A cotton-filled cushion with round ends. A thick blanket or sofa cushion may be substituted.*

Blanket *One or more firmly pressed felt-type woollen or cotton blankets.*

Eyebag *To relax the face and eyes. A folded face cloth may be substituted.*

Sandbag *To apply pressure to small areas of the body.*

BASIC RELAXATION

This helps lower blood pressure and heart rate, releases muscular tension, reduces fatigue, improves sleep, and enhances immune response. Use a bolster and rolled towel; an eyebag and blanket for warmth are optional.

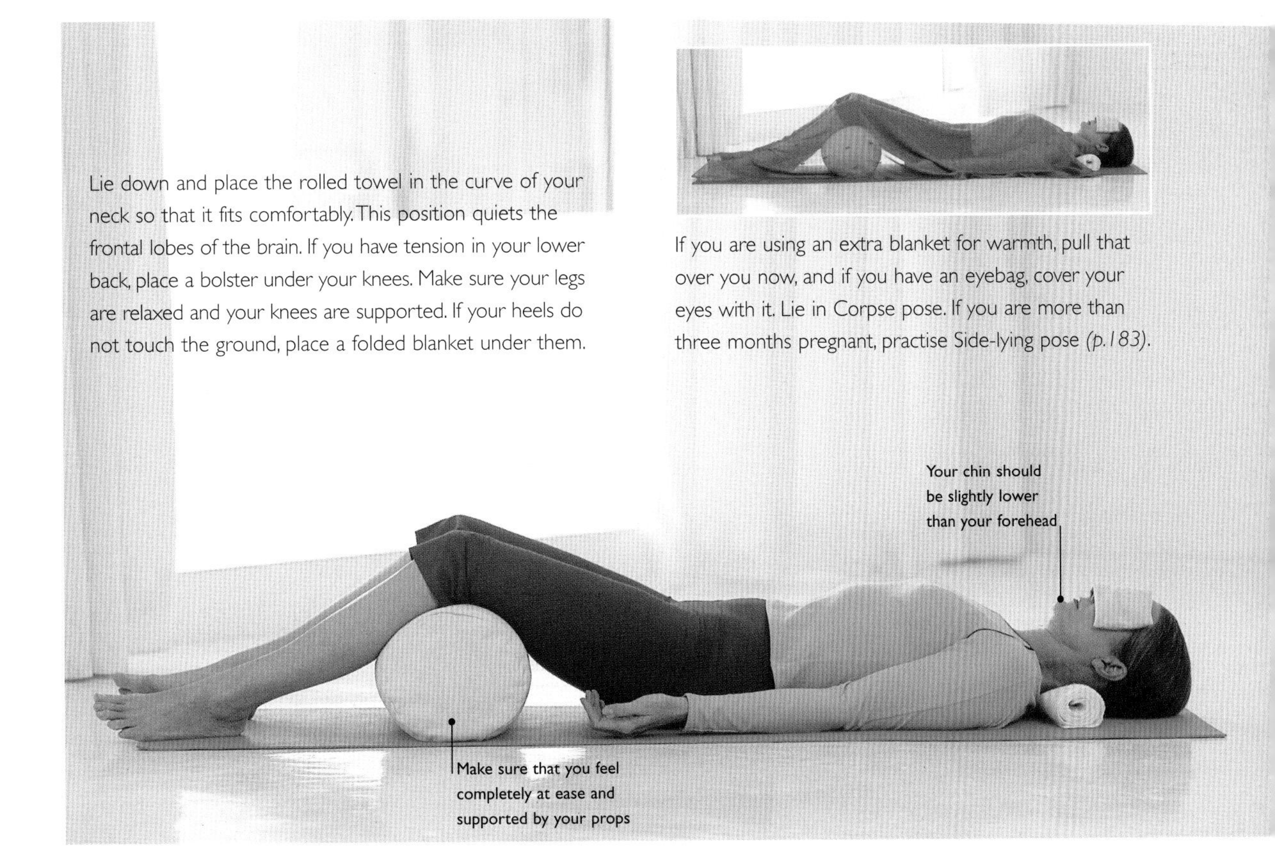

Lie down and place the rolled towel in the curve of your neck so that it fits comfortably. This position quiets the frontal lobes of the brain. If you have tension in your lower back, place a bolster under your knees. Make sure your legs are relaxed and your knees are supported. If your heels do not touch the ground, place a folded blanket under them.

If you are using an extra blanket for warmth, pull that over you now, and if you have an eyebag, cover your eyes with it. Lie in Corpse pose. If you are more than three months pregnant, practise Side-lying pose *(p.183)*.

SIMPLE SUPPORTED BACKBEND

This is a welcome remedy for the common habit of slouching forwards. The muscles of the middle and upper back stretch and relax, the rib cage is opened, and the organs of the upper body are rejuvenated. You will need one or two blankets, a towel, and a bolster.

Do not practise if you have lower back pain, disc disease, are more than three months pregnant, or menstruating.

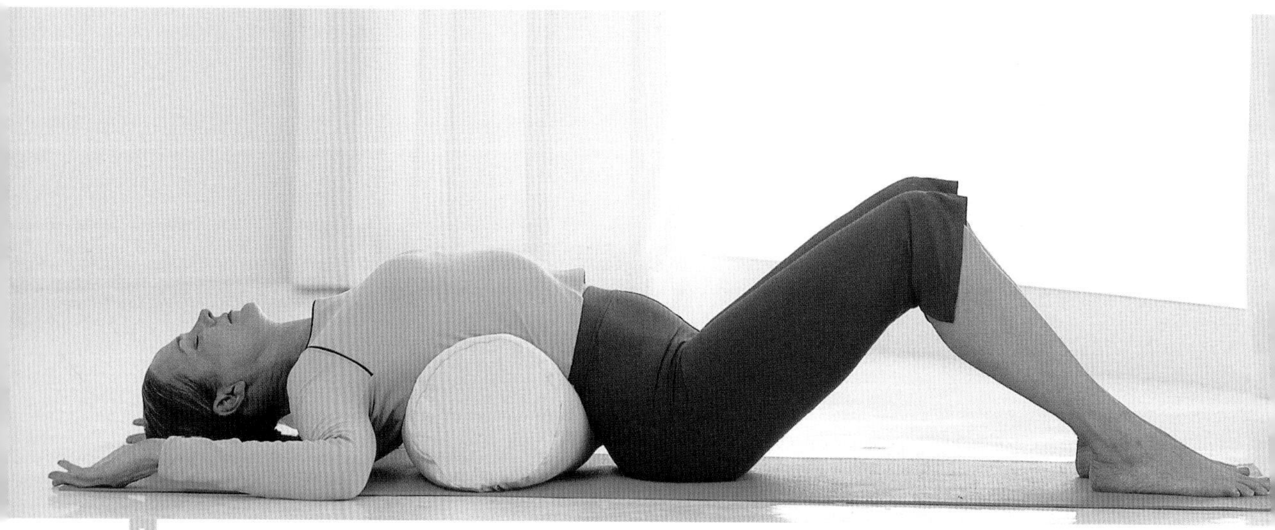

1 For neck support, roll a blanket or towel in a way that will maintain the natural curve of your neck. Position a bolster where your middle back will rest and a rolled blanket under your shoulders at a comfortable height. Bend your knees or place a rolled blanket under them to protect your back and relax the abdomen. Rest your arms on the ground above your head or to the sides, whichever is comfortable. Relax for up to one minute, gradually increasing the time.

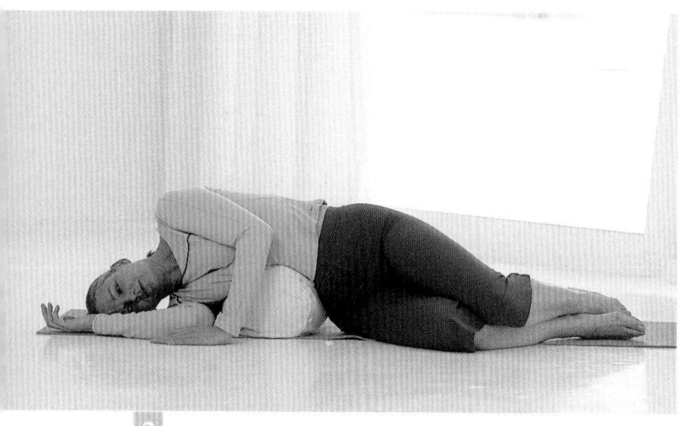

2 Roll onto one side and remove the props from under your neck and shoulders.

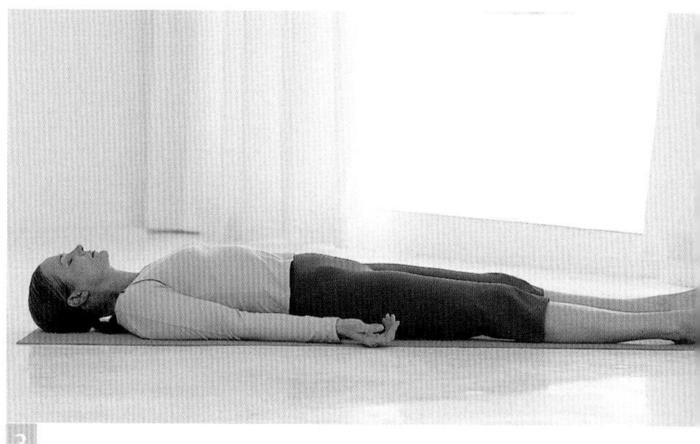

3 Remove the bolster and rest your lower back flat on the ground on for a few breaths.

SUPPORTED CHILD'S POSE

This gently stretches the lower back, eases tension in the abdomen, relieves shoulder tension, and quiets the mind. It is a good counterpose for backbends. Do not practise this if you have a chronic back condition or are more than three months pregnant.

You will need a bolster or a few blankets for stacking. Optional is a blanket to cover yourself with.

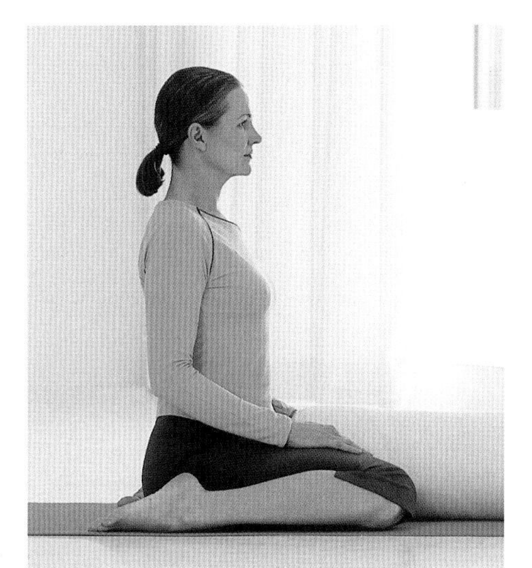

1 Kneel on a blanket with your knees apart and your bolster between your thighs. To avoid stressing the ligaments of your outer ankles, point your toes backwards, not towards each other. To take pressure off the knee joints, place a rolled towel towards the bend in the knees.

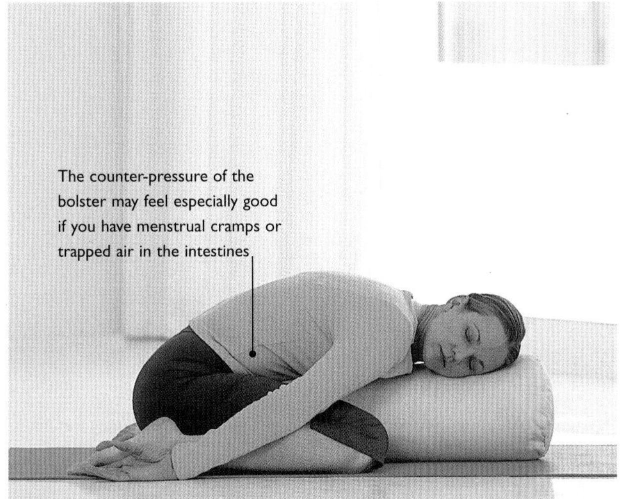

The counter-pressure of the bolster may feel especially good if you have menstrual cramps or trapped air in the intestines

2 Rest your chest gently on the bolster. If you need more height, add a blanket or pillow to the bolster. Let your tailbone drop towards your heels to lengthen your lower back as you relax. Turn your head to each side for a minute or so. Your arms may either reach back towards your feet or forwards around the edges of the bolster. Close your eyes. Practise for 2–3 minutes.

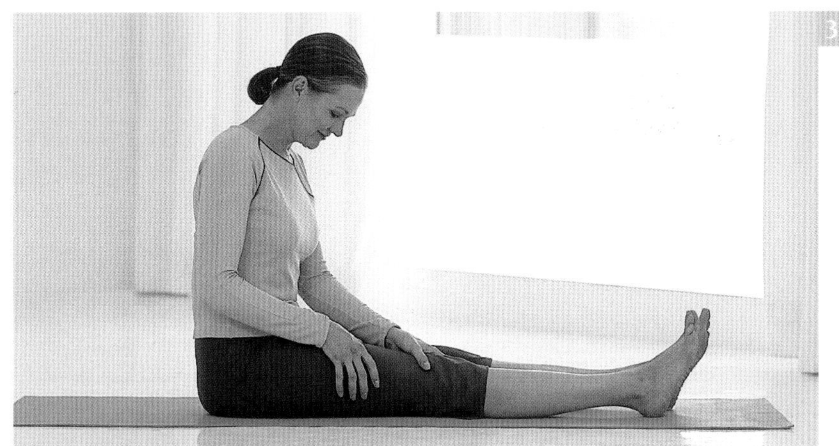

3 When you come out of the pose, stretch your legs forwards and massage or shake your legs, especially around your knees, before you stand up.

WALL YOGA

For each of these exercises, prepare your space by placing a yoga mat and/or a felt blanket or sheepskin on the ground up close to the edge of the wall. The mat should be long enough to fit your body and head. Do not practise these poses if you are more than three months pregnant.

PELVIC TILTS

As you straighten up and curl down you will feel a "rubber band" stretch in the body. The ground provides support for the spine as well as a gentle massage to individual vertebra as you curl and uncurl the spine.

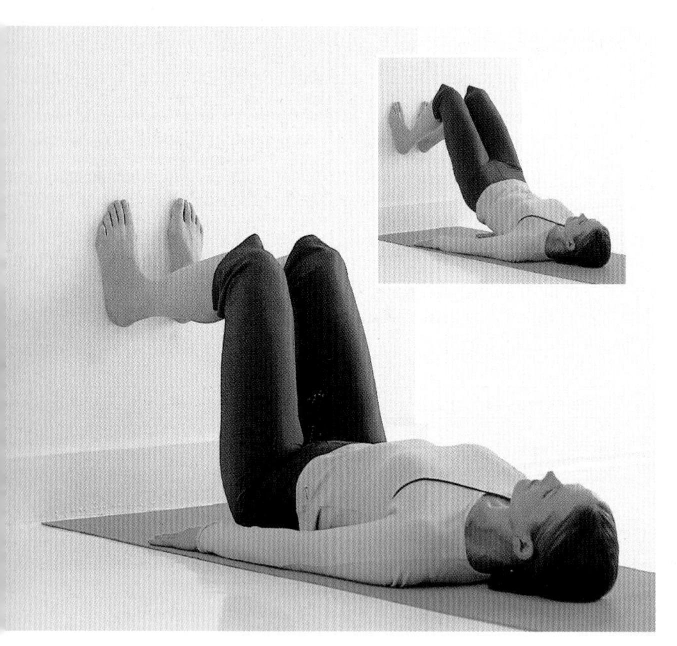

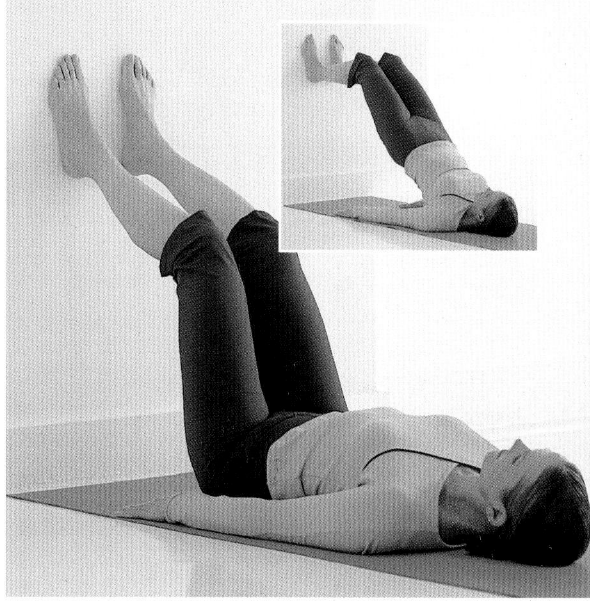

POSITION ONE

Lie on the mat with your buttocks about 30cm (12in) from the wall. Bend your knees and place your feet on the wall around 45m (18in) from the base of the wall. Place your arms on the ground at your sides, palms facing downwards. Inhale and lift the torso slightly off the ground, leading with your pelvis, and press your knees to the wall *(inset)*. Your spine will automatically straighten and lengthen. Exhale and reverse the motion.

POSITION TWO

Lie on the mat so that your buttocks are 30cm (12in) from the wall. Place your feet 1.1m (3½ft) up on the wall, about 20cm (8in) apart and parallel with each other. Inhale and lift the pelvis and torso high so that you are in a modified Shoulderstand *(inset)*. Press your hands against the ground. Hold the position for 5 deep breaths. Slowly roll down on the exhale: curve the upper spine towards the ground, then the lower spine.

NECK HELPER

This exercise trains your back, chest, and abdominal muscles to support the lifting of your head. In this way you avoid strain and your neck muscles are strengthened in the process.

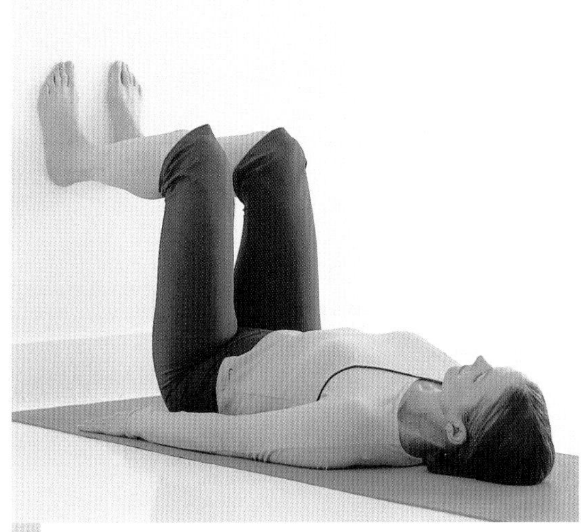

1 Lie on the mat so that your buttocks are about 30cm (12in) from the wall. Bend your knees and place your feet on the wall around 45cm (18in) from the base of the wall. Place your arms on the ground at your sides with the palms facing downwards.

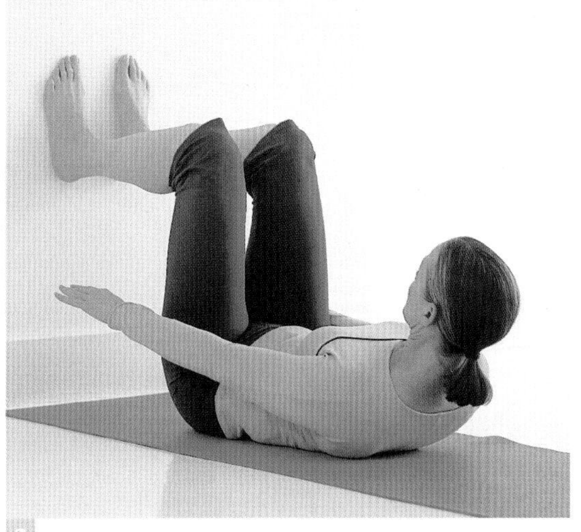

2 As you exhale begin to lift the chest, allowing the head to follow. Relax your neck and feel that your head is lifted by your upper body muscles. This allows the neck to lift without strain. Then inhale and lower your upper chest and neck, with the chest and back muscles supporting the neck.

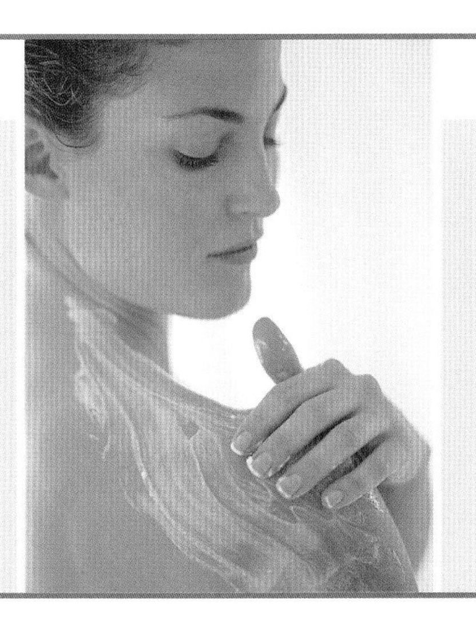

YOGURT BATH

For relaxing your body and nourishing your skin, take a yogurt bath. This is especially important following menstruation. It is a time for pampering yourself. Light a candle and have some soft, relaxing music playing. Warm some plain yogurt (preferably home-made) and steam up the bathroom first so that the bath is warm. Sit in the empty bath and massage yogurt all over your body, including your hair and scalp if you wish. Take your time, breathe slowly, and consciously relax. Continue for between 15 minutes and an hour, then rinse off the yogurt in a warm shower. Then lie down and relax for up to one hour.

TAILOR

This resting pose finds the spine, hips, and buttocks naturally aligned and well-supported by the ground and wall. It allows the hips and pelvis to relax and open fully. The thighs are stretched and opened as you gently press the knees towards the wall.

Lie on the ground with the buttocks against the skirting board. Cross your legs and tuck one foot towards the inside of your thigh. The other foot rests to the outside of your tucked leg. Continue for 1–3 minutes, then switch the inside and outside leg position to balance the hips.

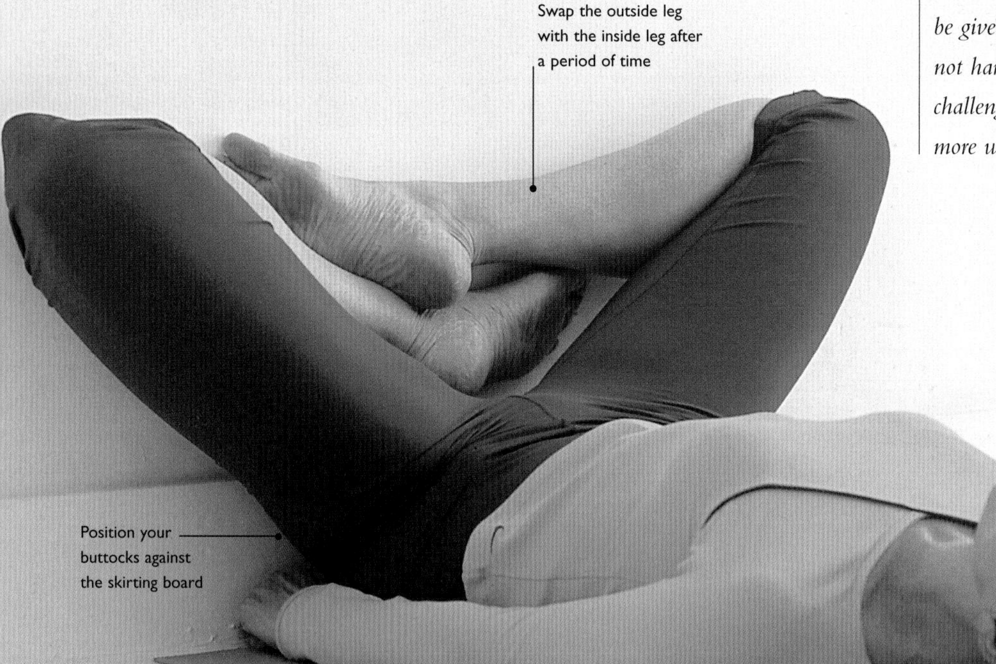

GUILT-FREE SELF-RENEWAL

In times of intense pressure my saving grace has proven to be guilt-free solitude. A walk among the trees calls me or a meditation will resonate with me, or I cry and laugh away my cares to a friend who knows them as well as I. Returning from solitude, my transformation is apparent to my family, friends, and co-workers. Self-trust grows into life trust. I know that I would not be given anything I could not handle, and that every challenge I meet makes me more wholly who I am.

STRENGTHENING INNER THIGHS

This exercise strengthens the inner thigh muscles, which are often weak and therefore easily injured. It also strengthens the nervous system. Do this exercise slowly, with conscious awareness of activating the power of the thigh muscles.

1 With your buttocks against the skirting board, straighten the legs against the wall. Consciously activate the inner thigh muscles by imagining you are hugging the muscle to the bone. You may feel a slight stiffening in the thigh muscles as you do this.

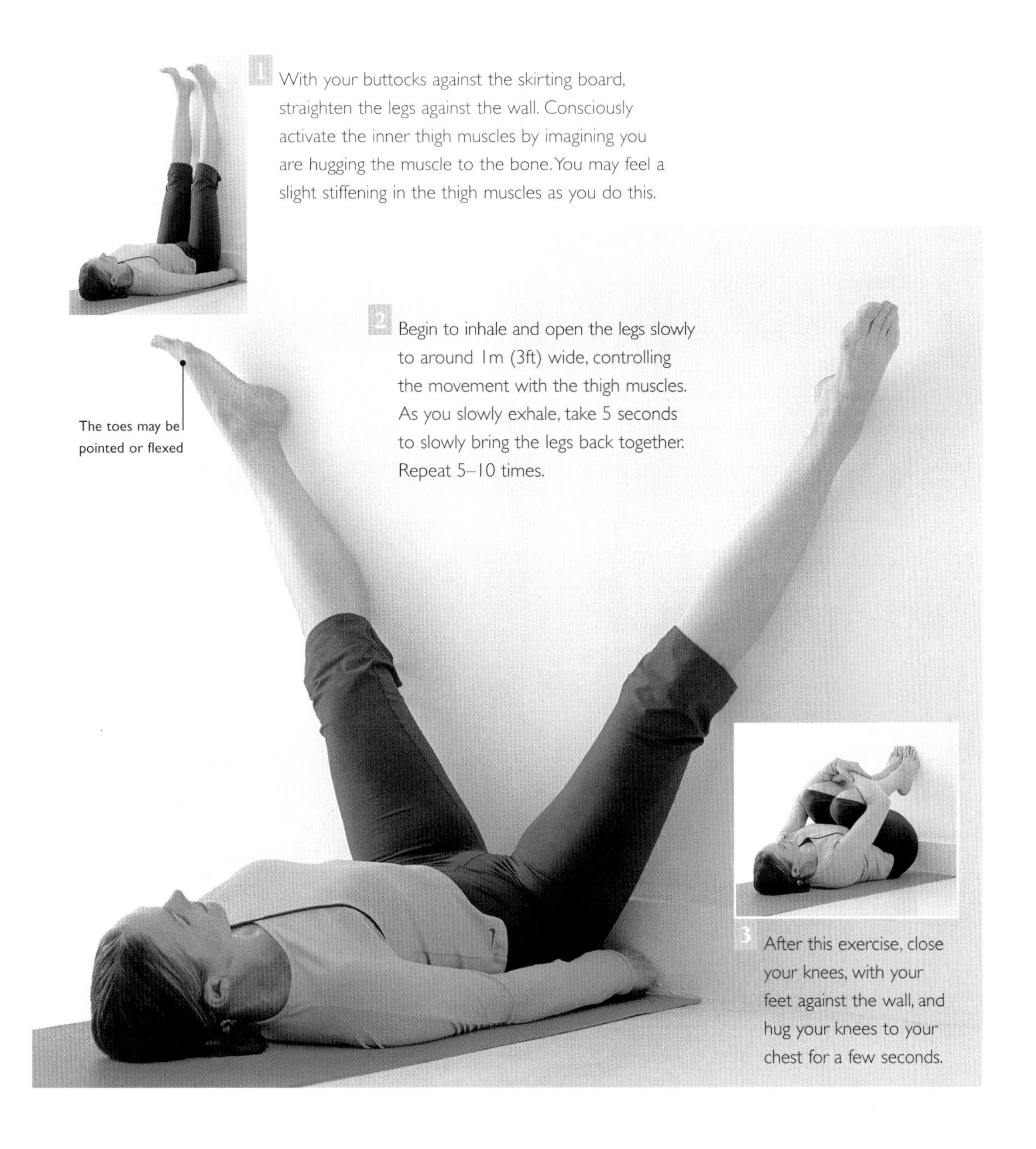

2 Begin to inhale and open the legs slowly to around 1m (3ft) wide, controlling the movement with the thigh muscles. As you slowly exhale, take 5 seconds to slowly bring the legs back together. Repeat 5–10 times.

3 After this exercise, close your knees, with your feet against the wall, and hug your knees to your chest for a few seconds.

ENDING WALL YOGA

Knowing how to move away from the wall when you are finished is important. The muscles and joints that you have exercised and stretched may be in a delicate state, so it is best to move slowly and follow the three steps below.

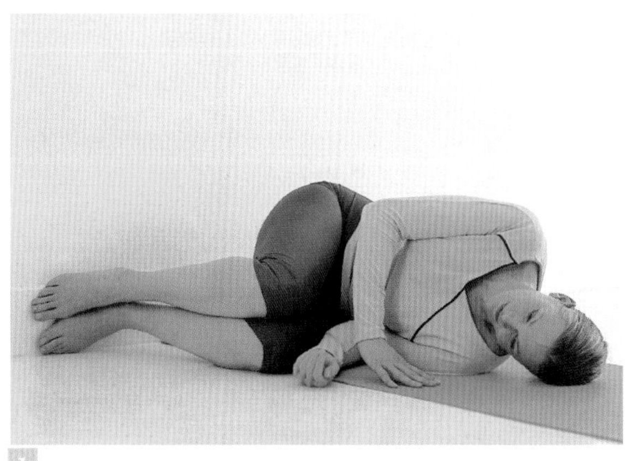

1 Bring your knees to one side and roll your body down onto that side. Steady yourself with one hand.

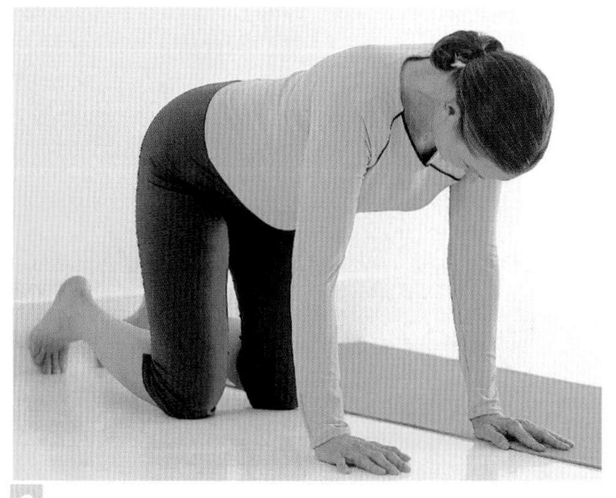

2 Making a smooth transition from step 1, come up onto your hands and knees.

3 You may like to counter-stretch for a minute in Child's pose, with your forehead on the ground and your arms relaxed on the floor by your sides.

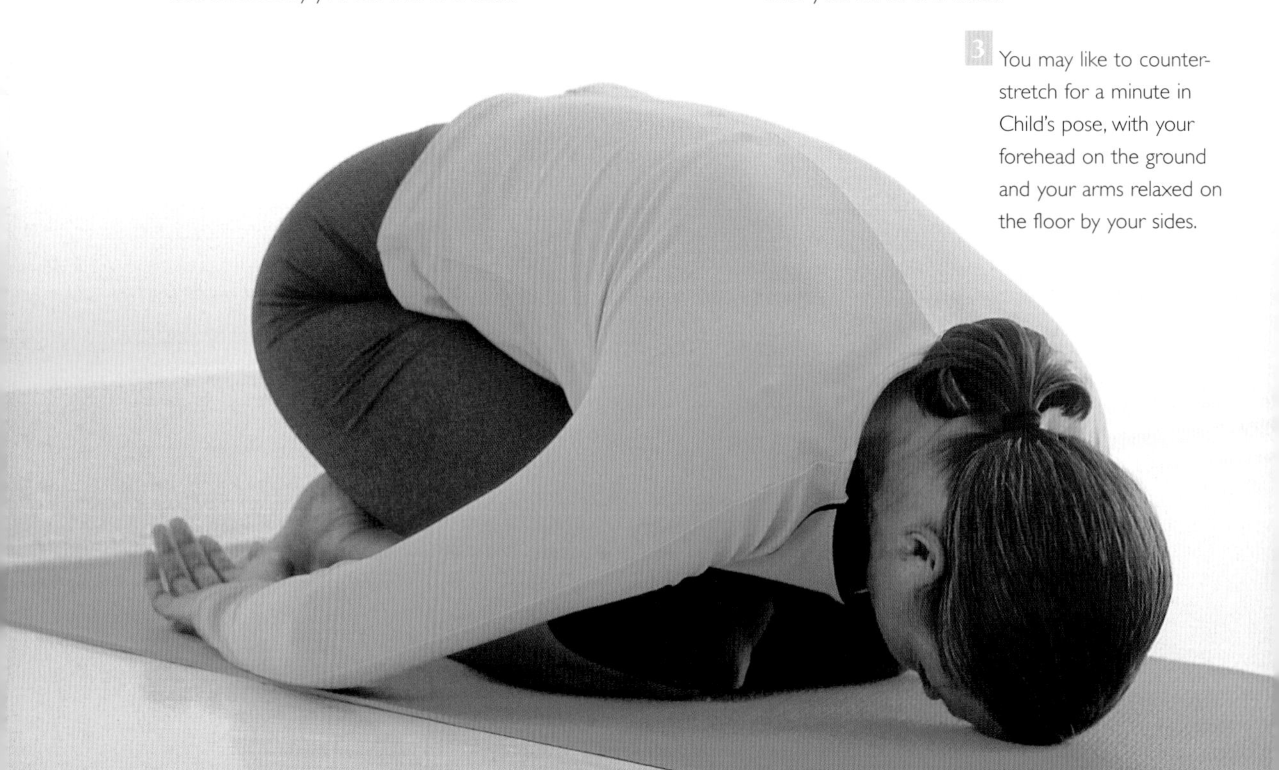

HOW TO DO ALTERNATE NOSTRIL BREATHING

According to yogic teachings, nostrils are gateways to vast energy within the body. The left nostril cools the air as it is drawn in, which relaxes you. The right nostril warms the air as it draws it in, energizing you. Breathe through one nostril at a time to calm or energize yourself.

In yogic science the left side of the body is the moon side: cooling, receptive, feminine energy. The right side is the sun side: warming, projective, masculine energy.

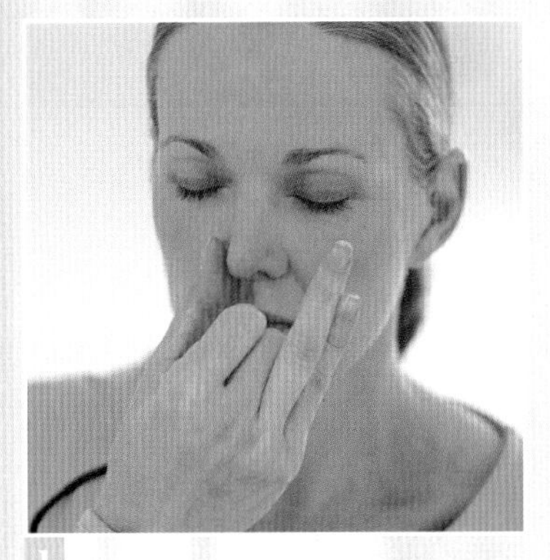

1 Sit with a straight spine. Using the right hand, extend the thumb, ring finger, and little finger. Fold the index finger and middle finger towards your palm. Block the right nostril with your thumb. Inhale through the left nostril.

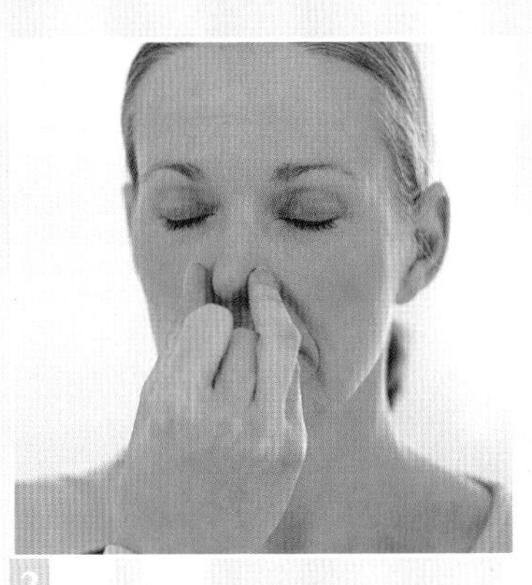

2 After you have inhaled, and your thumb is still gently pressing against your right nostril, bring your ring finger onto your left nostril so that both nostrils are now closed. Hold them closed for a few seconds.

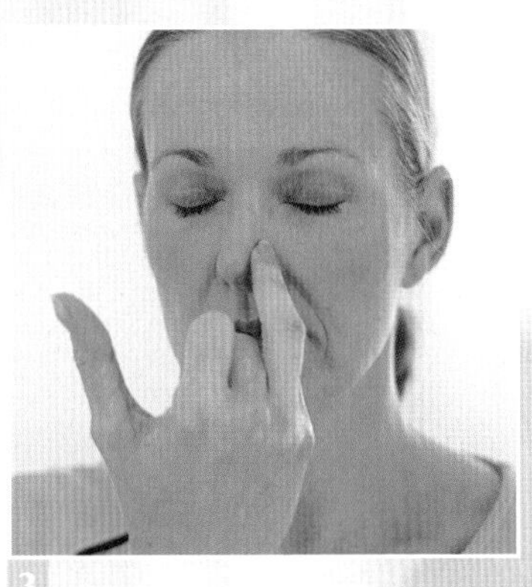

3 To exhale, lift your thumb and exhale through your right nostril. Empty your lungs, and begin again, inhaling through your right nostril and exhaling through your left nostril. Repeat for 5 minutes.

PAULETTE'S STORY (USA)

Fifteen years ago, I was diagnosed with psoriatic arthritis. Before that I had been physically active, running six to eight kilometres a day. I had three major operations, and was in and out of a wheelchair for two years. With great apprehension, I signed up for a Gentle Yoga class, and after one session I was hooked! I had found something good for my body that was adaptable to my aching joints.

Sometimes I would come to class in extraordinary pain, but would force myself to work through it. I used props and adapted my poses to take pressure off the damaged joints. Some poses I will never be able to do, and a teacher told me once not to dwell on those but concentrate on poses I can do and do them well. Some months I feel strong and practise regularly, but other months I can't because of operations or flare-ups of the disease. On bad days, just getting out of bed and getting dressed will be my goal for the day. I can accept that. I think of it as "two steps forward, one step back", but still, I've moved one step.

Because of my condition, I never thought of teaching until my teacher gave me the opportunity to teach a Gentle Yoga class. I considered it an honour to show others that no matter what limitations you have, yoga can help!

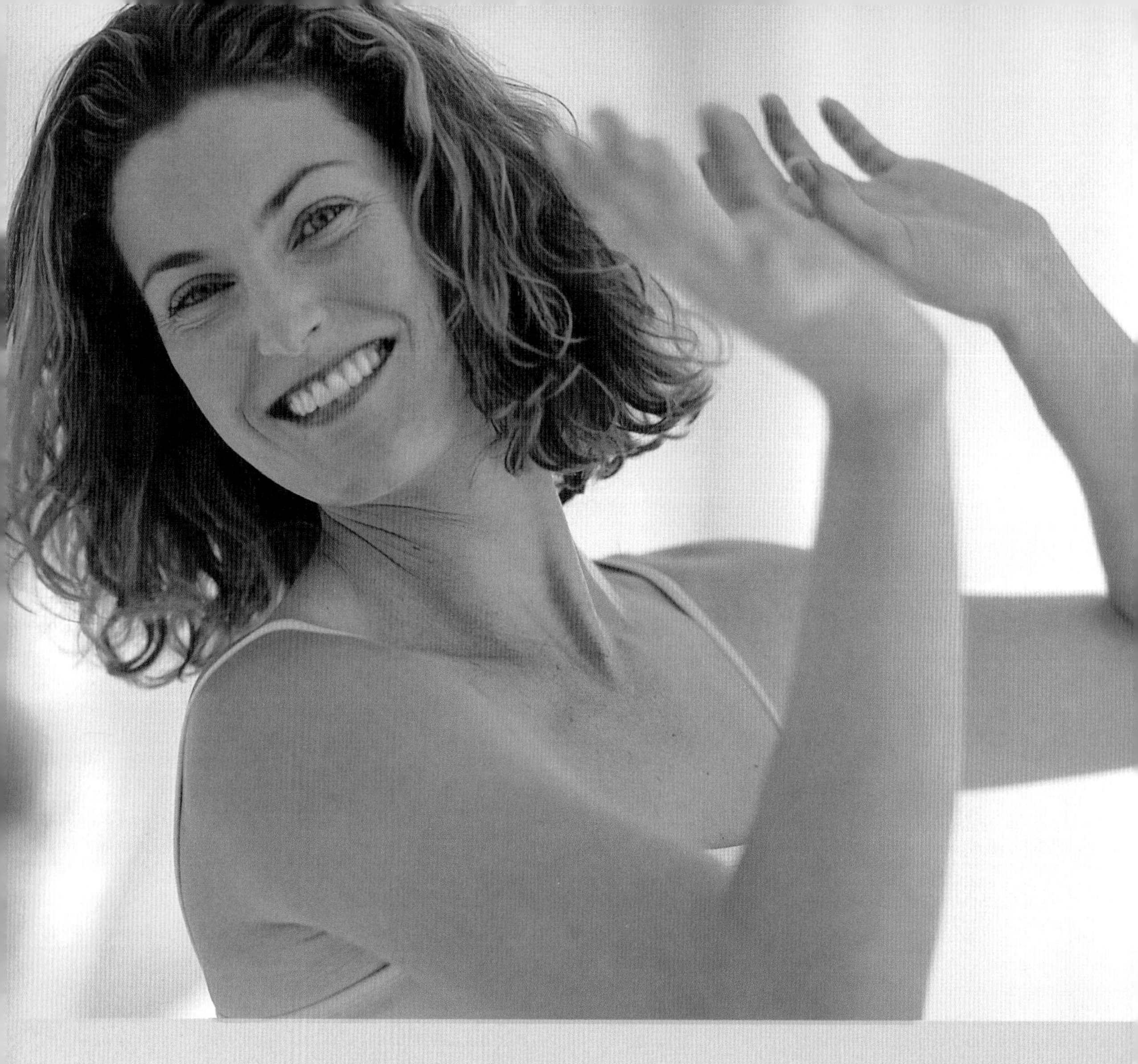

TO RELAX & REJOICE

It's easy to feel like rejoicing when you are relaxed. So getting relaxed is the first step – always. Take relaxation breaks throughout the day, even if they last for only a couple of minutes. Excuse yourself from your work and move outdoors or into a private room for a few minutes of quiet where you can hear yourself breathe and feel your body unwind as tension falls away. Strong exercise and breathing automatically lead to relaxation by releasing tension stored in the body. Whether you prefer working out, jogging, or free-form dance, moving your body moves out stress, and that is exactly what we will explore in the creative yoga practice contained in this part of the book.

MOVEMENT RELAXATION

Rhythmic, unforced, graceful, and free movement relaxes the entire body and mind, releasing everyday emotional traumas that leave their signature of tension in the body. If these areas are not relaxed, built-up stress can lead to physical and mental health imbalances. This simple set of yoga exercises, enhanced by meditative music, is a lovely process of self-expression and self-healing.

1 MOVEMENT

In the first part of this exercise you draw your awareness into your inner body. Then, as you dance from a place of inner awareness, your body and mind work as one. Use music *(p.224)* for steps 1 and 2, or just step 2.

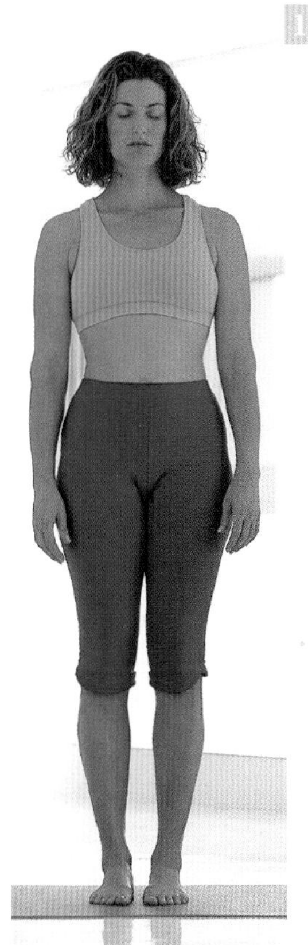

1 Stand up straight with your arms completely relaxed. Close your eyes. Become aware of each part of your body from the inside, starting with the feet and slowly working up to your head. Allow the tension to release in each part. Consciously let it go.

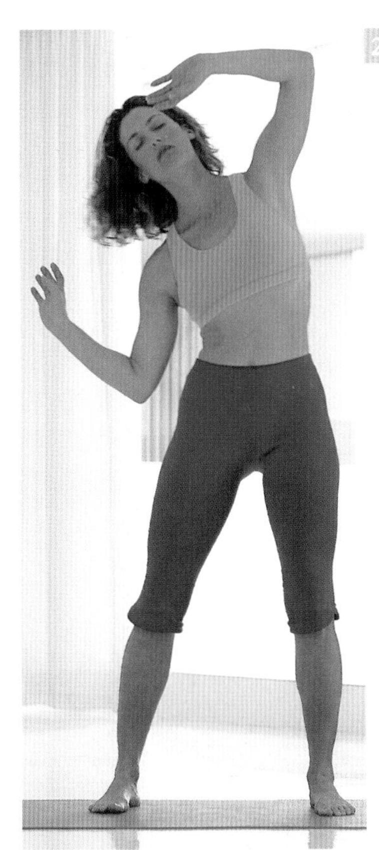

2 Keeping your eyes closed, begin to dance, swaying and moving each body part. Move in whichever way you want to. Express yourself through the movement of your body, continuing for 3–11 minutes or as long as you like.

2 TOUCH

Feeling the entire body confirms the reality of the relaxation, is self-healing, and smooths the aura (the energy field surrounding you, according to yogic tradition).

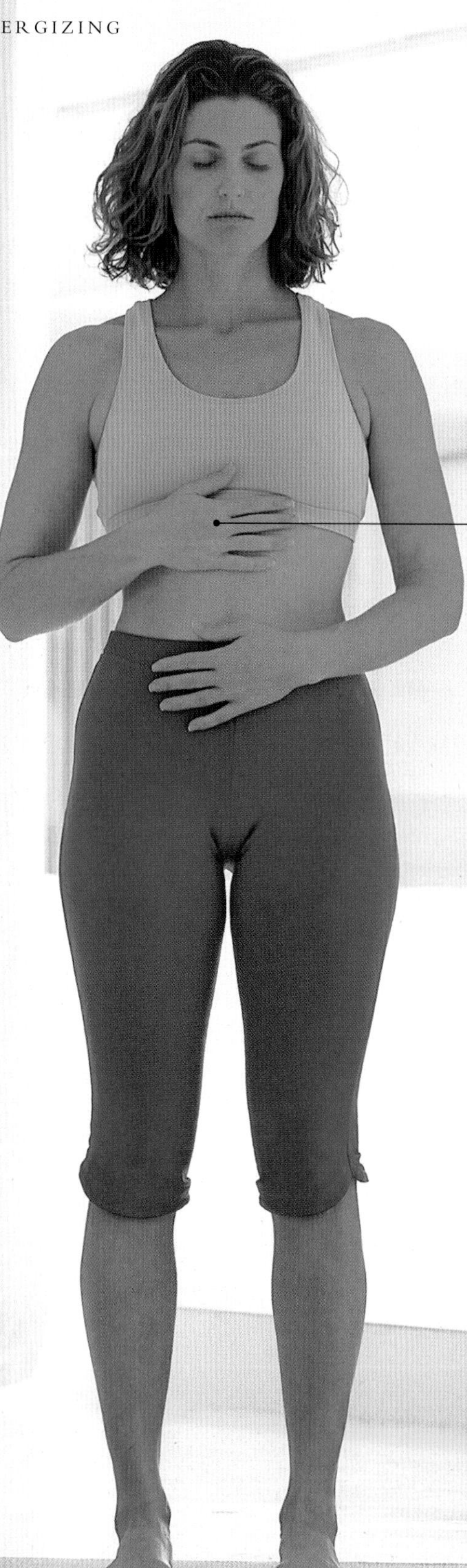

Feel sensitively with the palms of your hands, and bless yourself with your touch

Stand straight with eyes closed. With your hands, begin to lightly feel each part of your body without reservation, not forgetting the soles of the feet and the backs of the hands. Continue for 2–5 minutes.

BALANCE

My Viniyoga teacher has taught me much about balance: "Be like a deer in a forest. She stops, listens, feels. The deer is very still, at ease, yet alert. Everything is coming into her field of sensations and awareness. Watch the interplay between expanded awareness while being at ease, and you will understand the two essential elements of yoga: sukhum *(ease) and* sthiram *(alertness)."*

3 FORWARD & BACKWARD HANG

The last exercise in this set strengthens the heart and circulatory system. If this system is weak, tissues in the extremities and in the joints may build up toxins that can lead to illness.

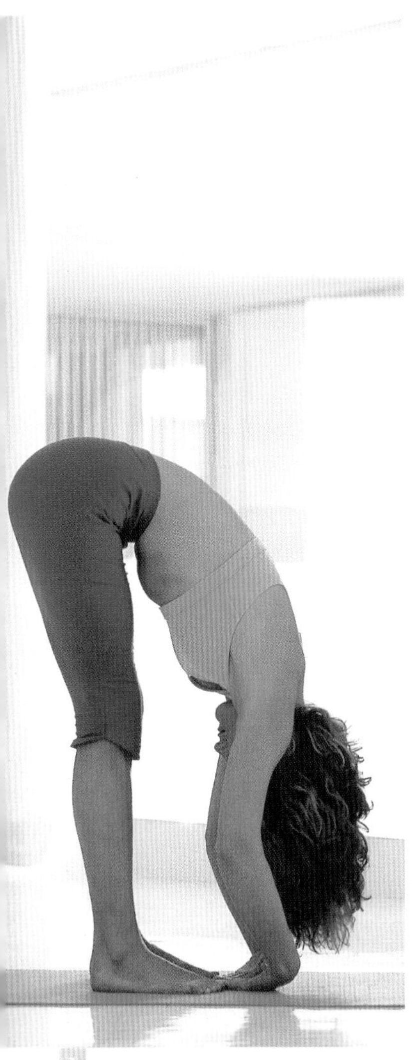

1 Lean forwards with arms completely relaxed and hanging down. Keep the knees relaxed and unlocked. Allow every muscle in your body to relax. Let your breath be relaxed and natural. Continue for 2–11 minutes.

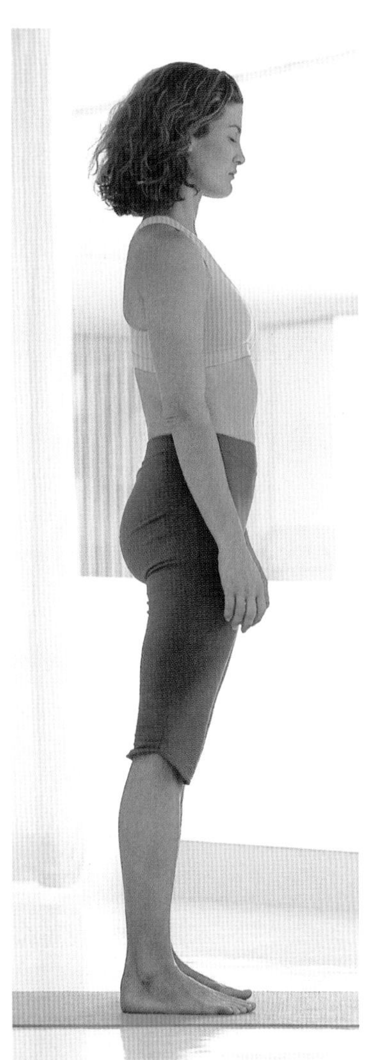

2 Inhale and exhale deeply several times, then slowly straighten up. Take 30 seconds to 1 minute to return to an upright position.

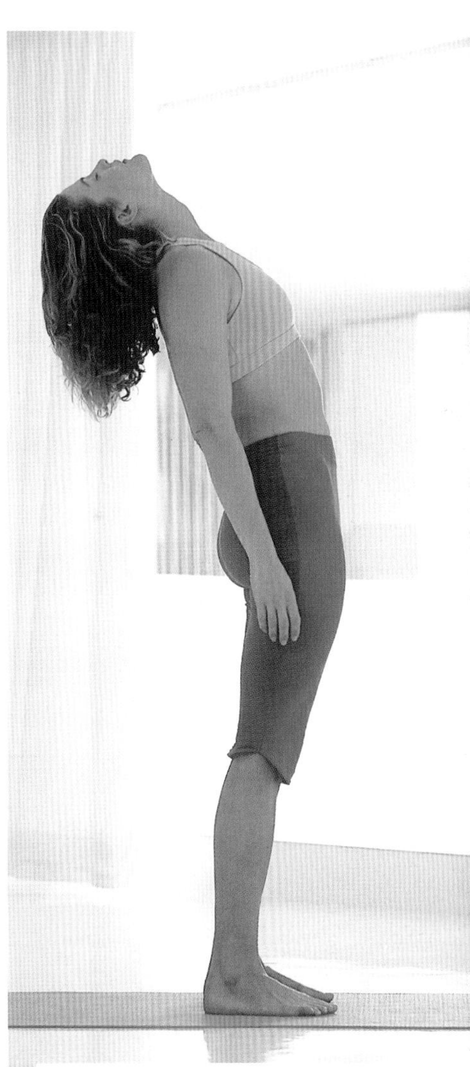

3 In a continuous motion, slowly lean backwards with arms hanging loosely. For neck problems, tip the head back only as far as is comfortable. Continue for 1 minute. Then slowly straighten and completely relax.

YOGA TO HELP YOU SLEEP

Sleeplessness has become a major problem in the West. In general, a practice of yoga will do wonders for relaxing the body and mind in preparation for sleep. Do the following exercises before bed, or anytime that sleep has been interrupted. Feel free to practise these together or individually. You may like to add in some relaxing poses from Rejuvenating Yoga (pp.60–69).

TABLE

This posture opens the pathway for spinal fluid to circulate to the brain as it strengthens the nervous system. It promotes deep relaxation through the tensing of muscles and the subsequent release of tension in the arms, neck, legs, and abdomen.

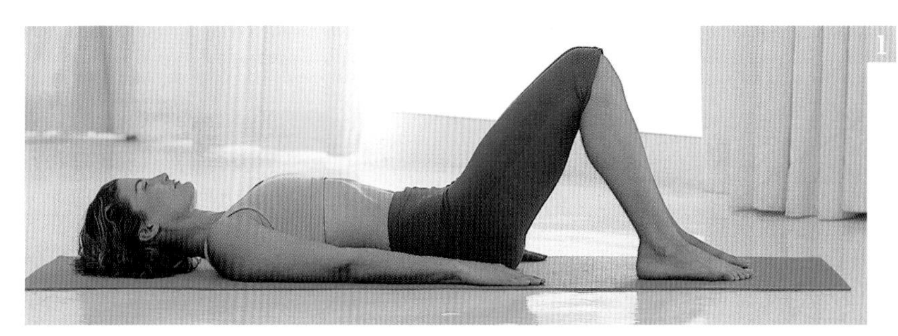

1 Lie down on your back. Bend your knees and put your feet flat on the ground and your arms at your sides.

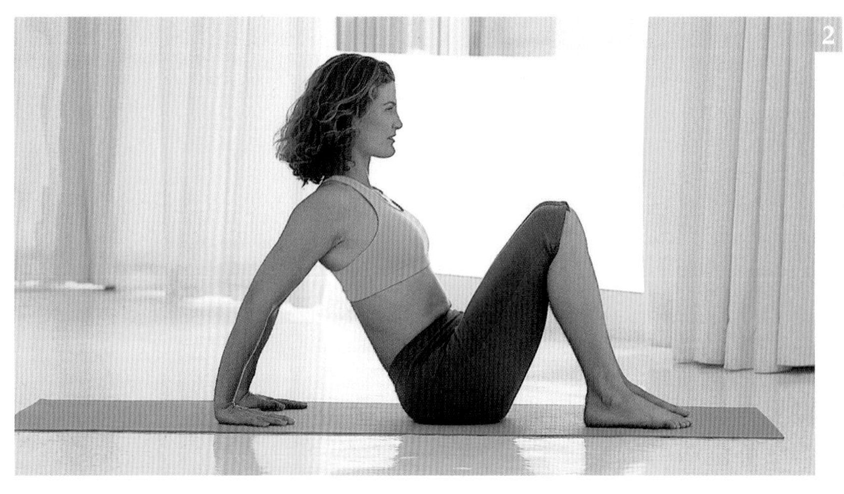

2 Keep your knees bent and sit up. Lean back slightly while keeping your chest lifted. Place your hands on the ground behind you with the fingers pointing inwards if possible.

DOERTHE'S STORY (GERMANY/SWITZERLAND)

There are days in my life when my schedule doesn't look like it will allow me more than one minute of yoga. But I know these are the days that are especially made for yoga! My practice becomes my little island surrounded by my busy life. I have learnt to take an hour for myself everyday without remorse. I find this daily practice helps me to create a positive day, and to learn to "be" instead of "do". After two years of intense yoga practice, I still have a lot of days where I think about the shopping list between inhaling and exhaling. Often in Downward Dog I give more attention to the dust underneath the sofa than to the alignment of my body. Every day is different – yesterday my practice was focused, today it is just a good stretch. My practice helps me to become an observer of myself without judgement. I still burn the potatoes on the stove and get impatient with my children. But yoga gives me tools to respond positively – to laugh at myself or breathe my anger away. My daily yoga practice gives me something to take into my life everyday.

3 Push yourself up into Table pose. Your body forms a straight line from your head to your knees. Your neck is in line with the rest of your body, and is not dropped fully back. Begin Breath of Fire or deep breathing for 1–3 minutes.

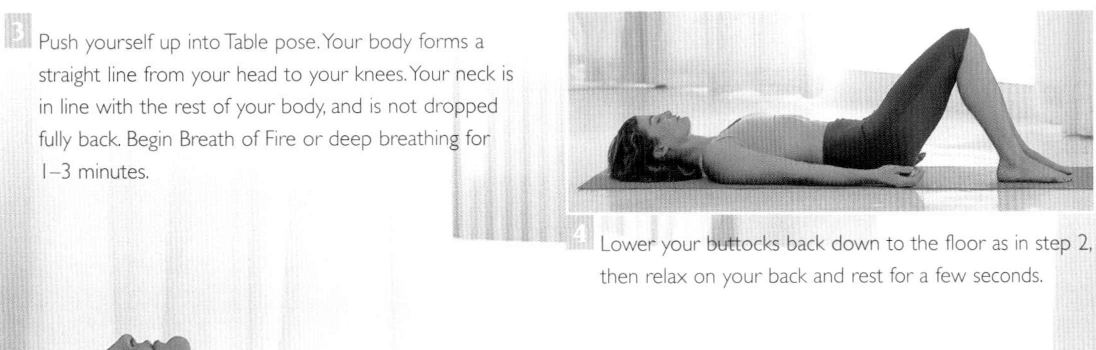

4 Lower your buttocks back down to the floor as in step 2, then relax on your back and rest for a few seconds.

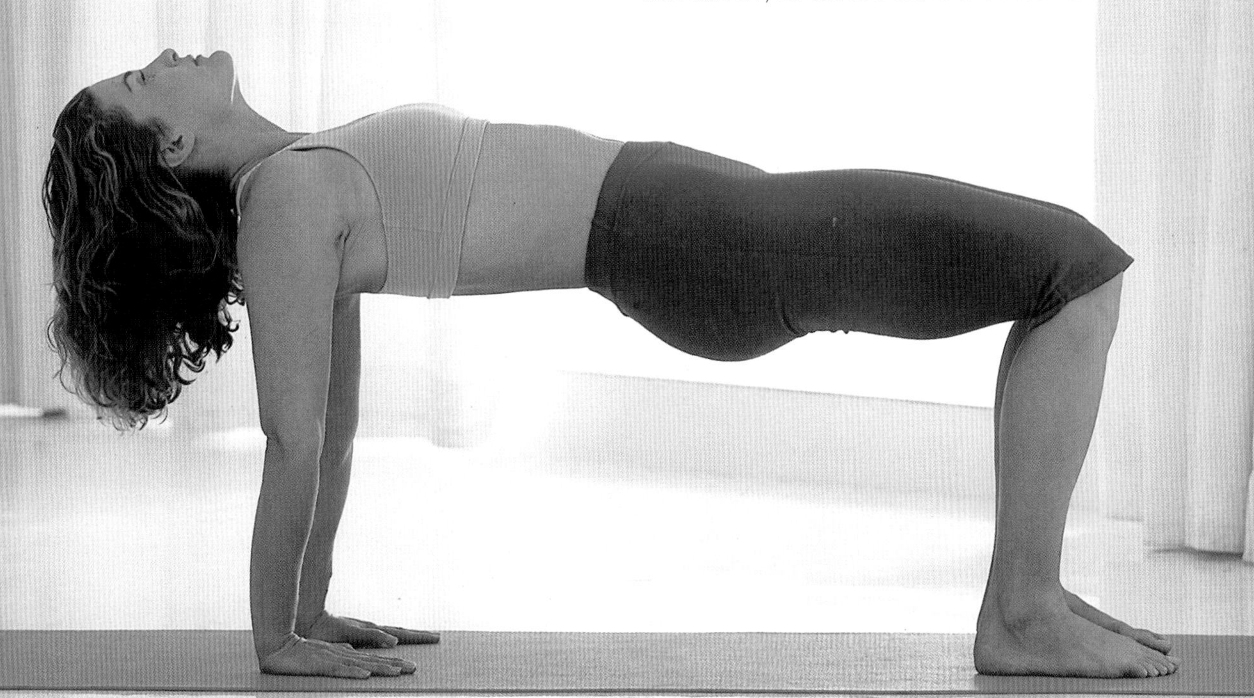

TENSION RELEASER

In this exercise a strong tension is created, then released all at once. It strengthens the nervous system, releases built-up tension, and is excellent to do before going to bed. The more tension you can put into the action, the deeper your relaxation will be afterwards.

Open your fingers wide, then close them tightly, as though you are grasping something

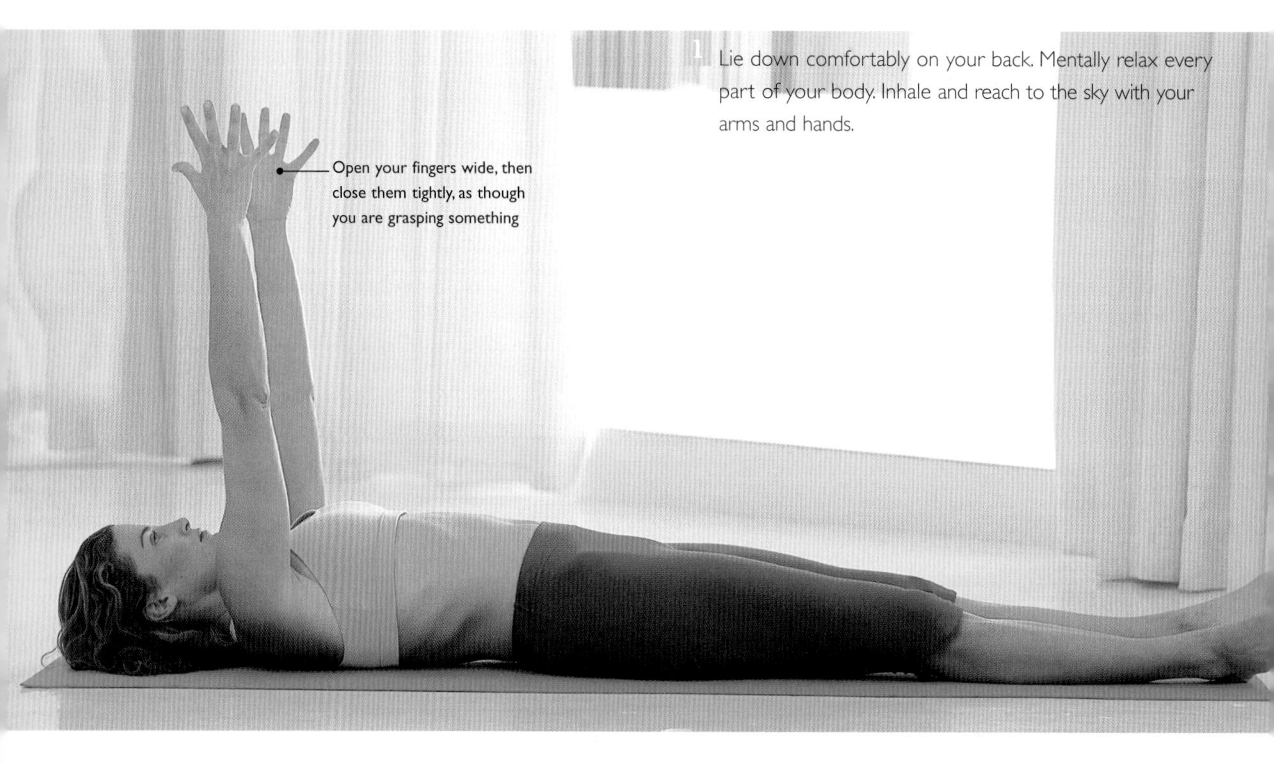

1 Lie down comfortably on your back. Mentally relax every part of your body. Inhale and reach to the sky with your arms and hands.

Keep the rest of your body relaxed

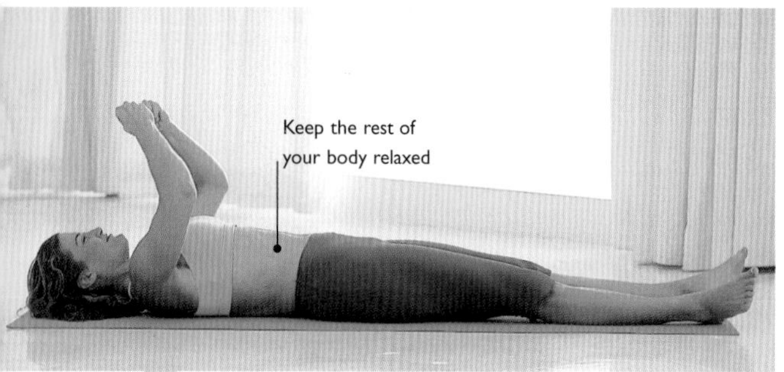

2 While creating as much tension as possible in your arms, hands, face, and upper chest, slowly pull your hands towards your chest. Let your arms shake. Hold your breath within you for the entire time you pull towards your chest.

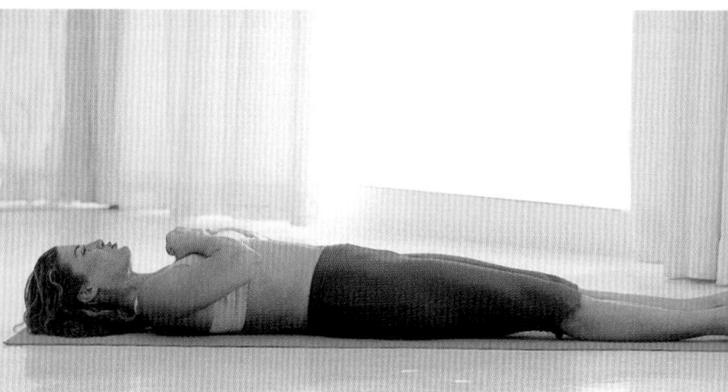

3 When your hands reach your chest, exhale all the breath out in an explosive breath through the mouth. Take one deep inhale and exhale as you relax totally. Then repeat the exercise a few more times.

COOLING BREATH

The Cooling Breath is helpful in soothing the mind and releasing emotions such as anger, frustration, and anxiety. It also relaxes the muscles, brings the mind to a state of tranquillity, and is great to practise before going to sleep since it generates a feeling of contentment.

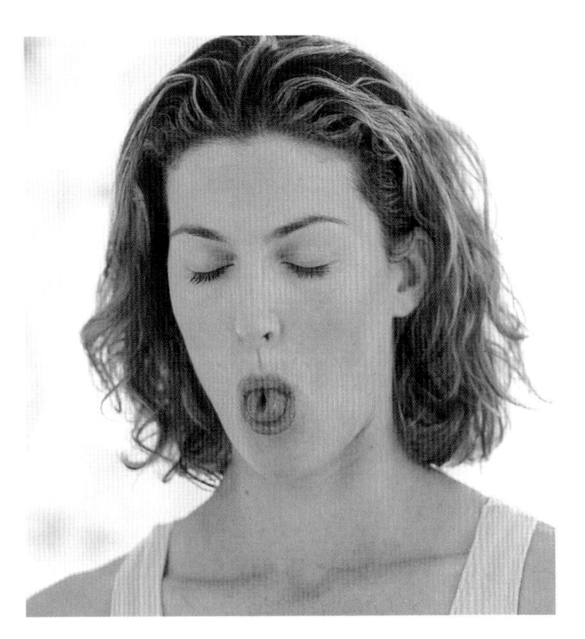

Sit in Easy pose *(p.19)*, with a straight spine. Straighten the arms and rest the hands in Gyan Mudra *(p.21)*. Open your mouth and extend the tongue out. Curl the sides of the tongue upwards and inhale through the mouth. The breath will produce a sound like rushing wind. Close the mouth and exhale through the nose. Continue for 3–11 minutes. If you cannot curl your tongue, shape your mouth like a circle and extend your tongue out while inhaling.

JAW RELEASE

This action relaxes and adjusts your jaw, and helps improve jaw tension, which often occurs from stress-related habits such as clenching and grinding the teeth. It also releases tension around the ears and neck.

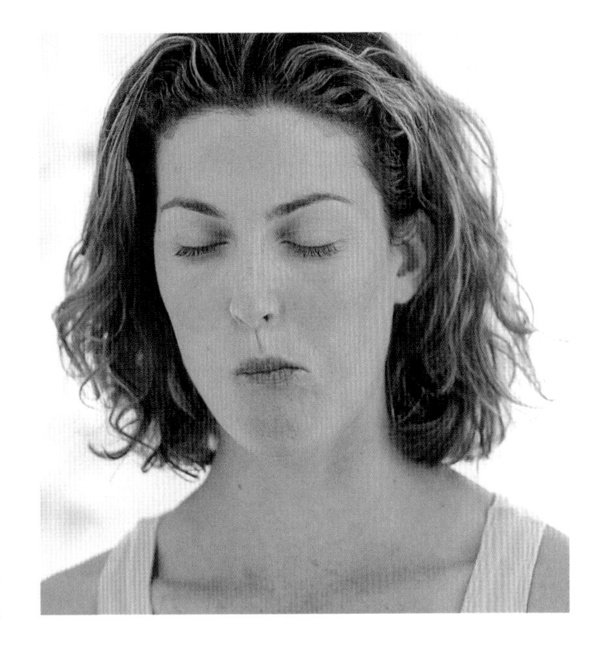

Lie down or sit in Easy pose *(p.19)*. Begin to roll your tongue in a wide circle around the outside of your teeth while keeping your mouth closed. Move slowly, stretching your tongue as far as you can to reach every corner. Circle 5–8 times in one direction, then 5–8 times in the opposite direction.

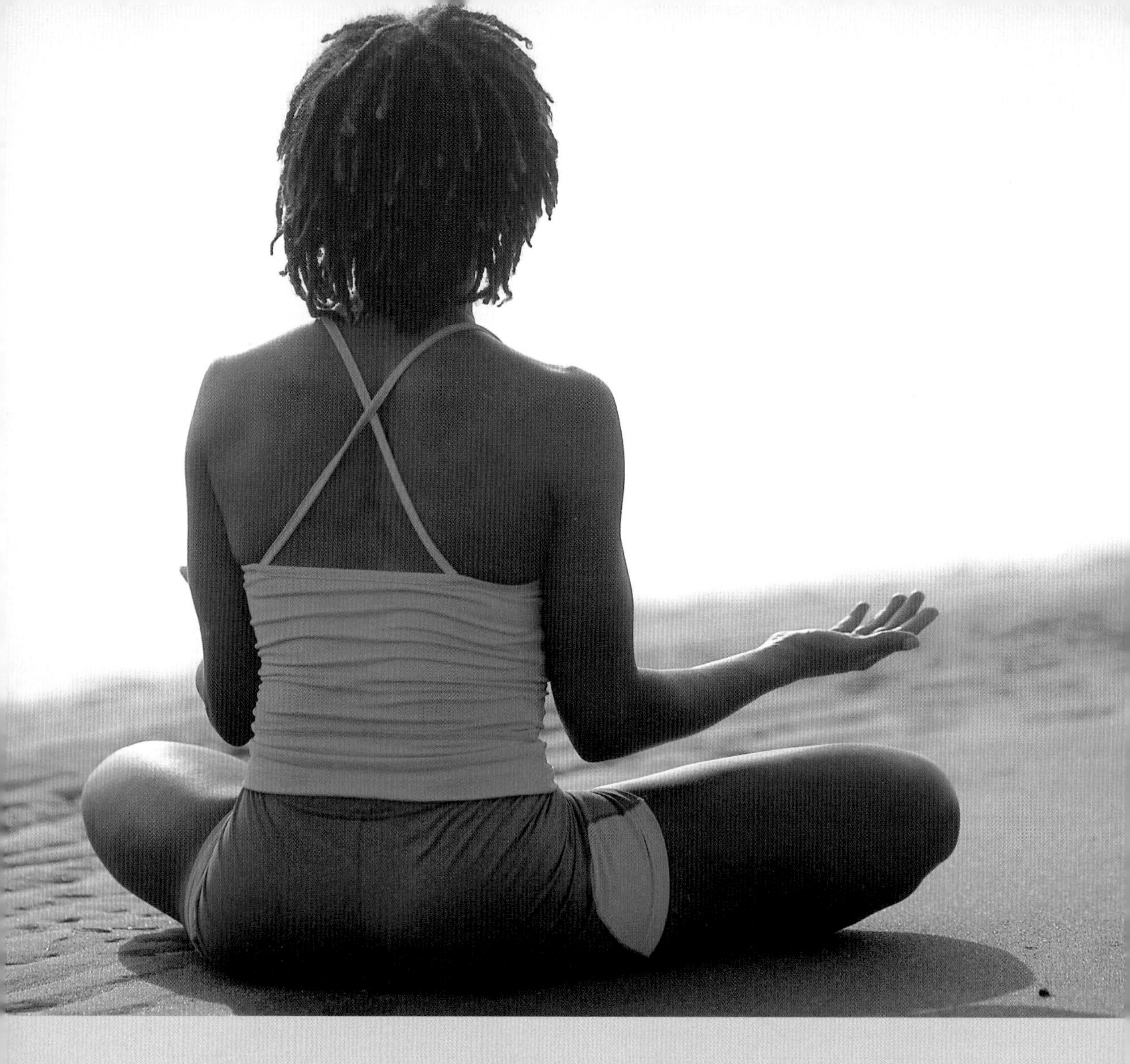

HEALING POWER

Healing is as natural as breathing for a woman. Throughout the ages we women have healed through every aspect of ourselves; through the compassionate touch of our hands, our poignant songs and art, the deep wisdom of our counsel, the conscious preparation of herbs and food, the life-giving milk that flows from our breasts... women's healing ways are infinitely creative and diverse. And through our deepest meditation we become the empty cup – a space that spirit fills to overflow. A woman in this state of consciousness heals with her presence. Her capacity to give is great, and she will often look to heal others before herself. Yoga and meditation serve to restore her so that she can go on healing the world.

MOON SALUTATION

The connection between women and the moon has always been strong. We women resonate with the energy of the moon through our monthly menstrual cycles, and reflect the moon's pattern in the waxing and waning of our thoughts and feelings. For this reason, many women find the practice of Moon Salutation holds special meaning for them. Practise 4–12 rounds of this strenuous sequence.

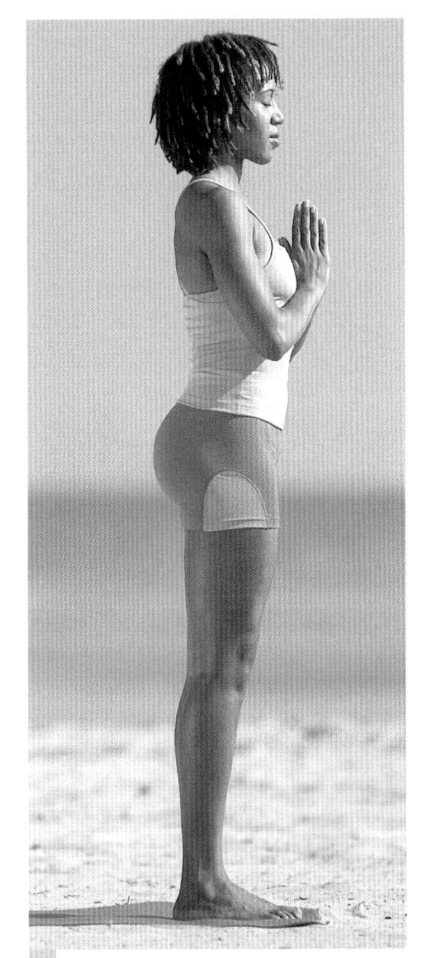

1 Stand upright with the feet close together. Bend the elbows and bring the palms of the hands together at the centre of your chest. This centres the mind and calms the body.

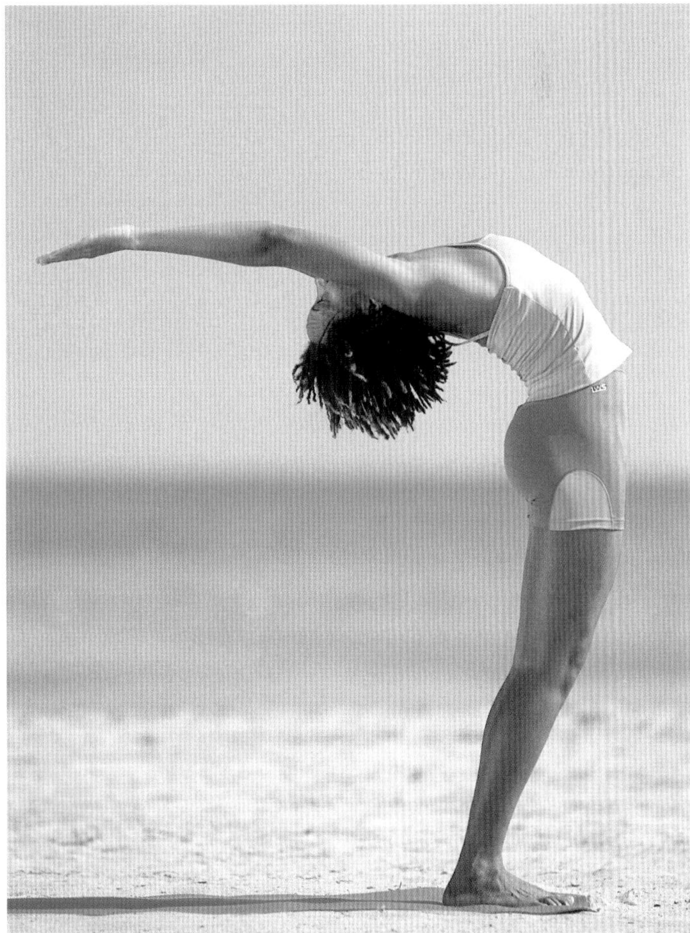

2 Inhale slowly and deeply as you raise and stretch both arms above your head. At the same time, arch your upper body backwards in one smooth, unbroken line, as far as possible without restraint. Bend only to your capacity, without strain. This stretches and tones the abdominal area, improves digestion, and opens the lungs ready for step 3.

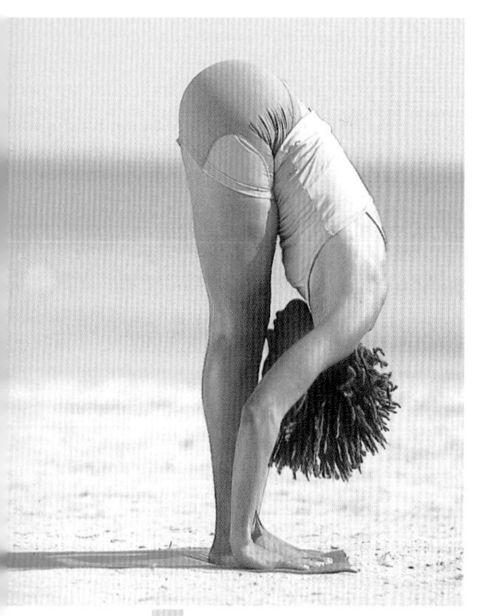

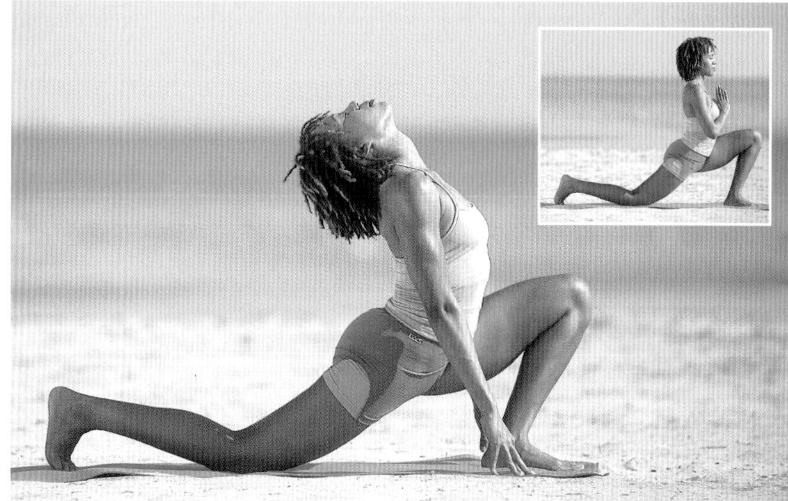

3 As you exhale slowly, bend forwards until your fingers touch the ground to either side of the feet. Bring the head to the knees as far as possible without straining.

4 Inhale, stretch your right leg back as far as possible, and drop your right knee to the ground as you bend your left knee. The weight of the body is supported on both hands, the left foot, and the toes of the right foot. Lift your chest, arch your back and head upwards, and bring your inner gaze to the brow point. This stretches and strengthens the muscles and nerves of the legs. Maintaining your balance, exhale and bring your palms together in front of your chest *(inset)*.

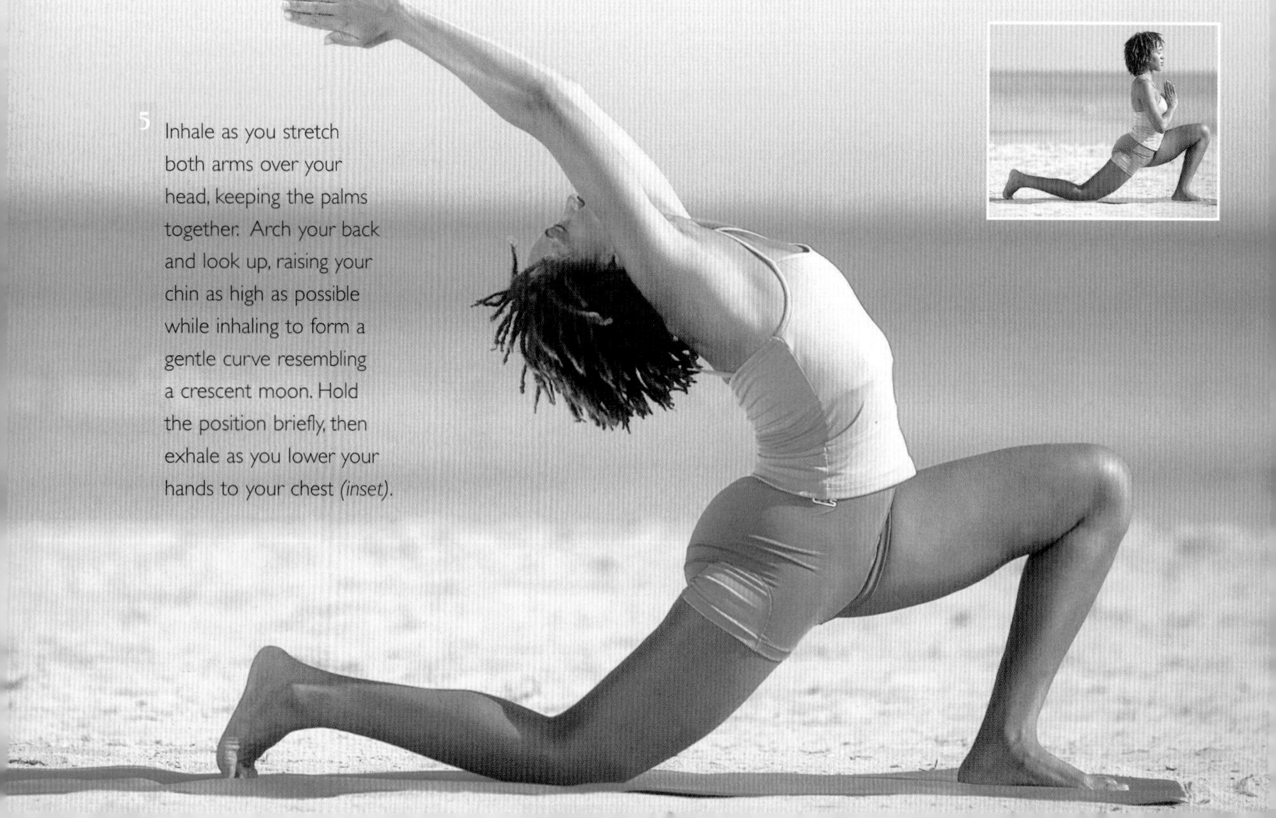

5 Inhale as you stretch both arms over your head, keeping the palms together. Arch your back and look up, raising your chin as high as possible while inhaling to form a gentle curve resembling a crescent moon. Hold the position briefly, then exhale as you lower your hands to your chest *(inset)*.

SHERIE'S STORY (USA)

When I decided to relocate my life and work, I left behind a very active healing practice, many friends, family, and my spiritual community. I set about starting up a new practice, but money was running out and I was feeling too under-confident to go out and meet the people who could use my services. Although I trusted that making this big a commitment was exactly what was being asked of me, I still experienced a great deal of fear.

I had studied several forms of Hatha Yoga, and knew yoga as a friend that could help me through all aspects of life. So I reconnected with yoga, this time with Kundalini Yoga, and it helped me find support not only in body, mind, and spirit, but also by providing a world community of holistic and spiritually minded people. The physical strength and flexibility gained from the postures energized me. The peace I experienced from within helped bolster my flagging inner security.

I especially love the incredible inner vibrating of the chanting, the soothing beauty of the sound of human voices blending together in yoga classes and in the early morning meditation practice. The chanting, an integral part of Kundalini Yoga, helped connect me more firmly with one of my inner truths: that I am part of the river of healing. I have known for years that all creatures have an amazing ability to heal themselves, even of things supposedly reversible. I have seen over and over again that miracles happen every day, and I feel grateful to be able to participate in some of them. I honour the practice of yoga and meditation for their roles in providing support and structure in my life and through my community.

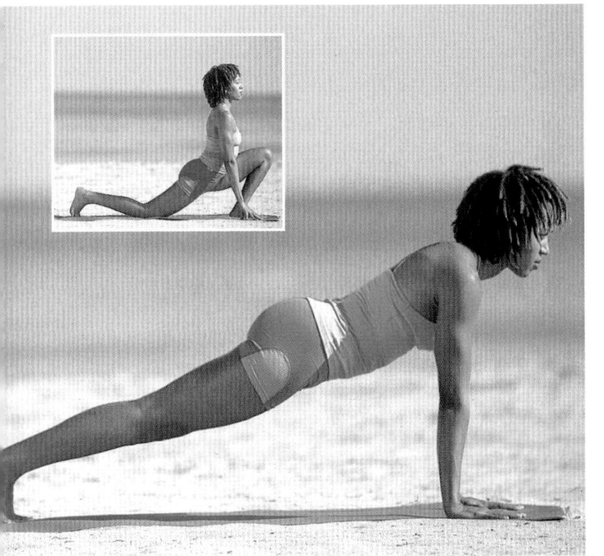

6 Inhale and return your hands to each side of your left foot *(inset)*. Retaining the breath, bring your left leg back and place your left foot next to the right, with the toes pointing forwards. Your arms are straight. Keep your head and hips in line with your spine. Your body should now be in a straight line, as in a push-up position.

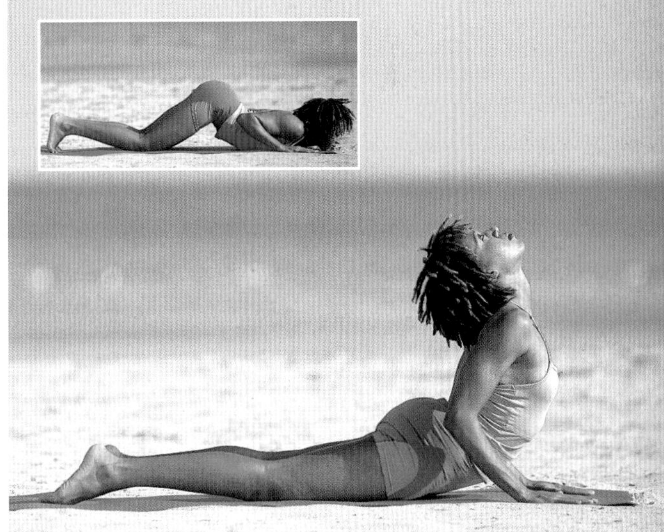

7 Exhale, lowering your knees, chest, and chin to the ground *(inset)*. If this is not possible, first lower the knees, then the chest, and finally the chin. Inhale as you slide your body forwards until the hips are on the ground. Arch your chest up and bring your head back into Cobra. Keep your elbows slightly bent as you curl back.

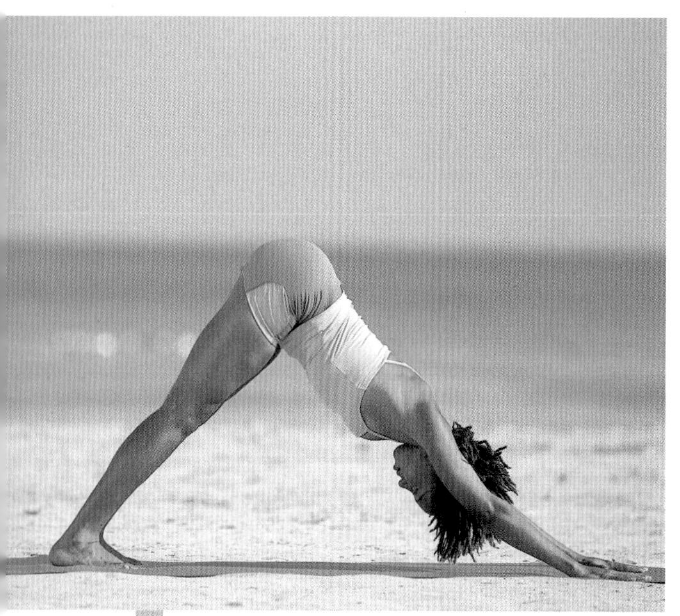

8 Keeping your hands and feet where they are, exhale and come onto the soles of your feet, lifting your hips into Downward Dog by pushing them up and back, away from your hands. Push your heels towards the ground and keep your knees straight. Stretch your spine and move your head inwards, towards your feet.

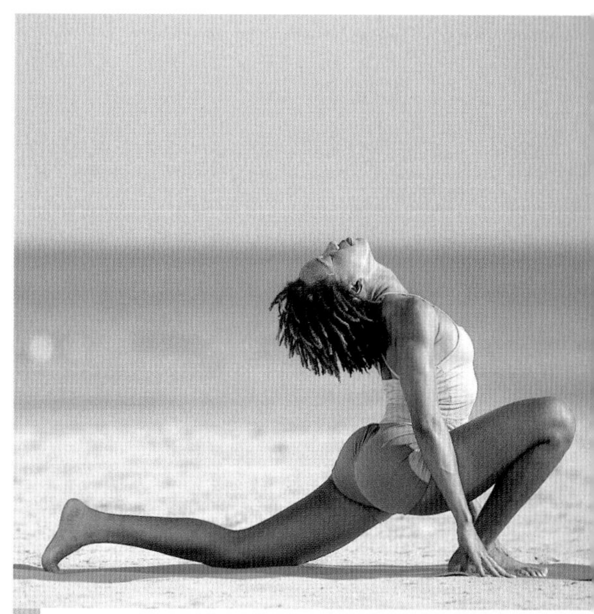

9 Inhale and change legs, bringing your right foot forwards between your hands. Drop your left knee towards the ground and stretch your head up. If when you bring your foot forwards it does not align with your hands, slide your hands towards your body so that they frame the foot.

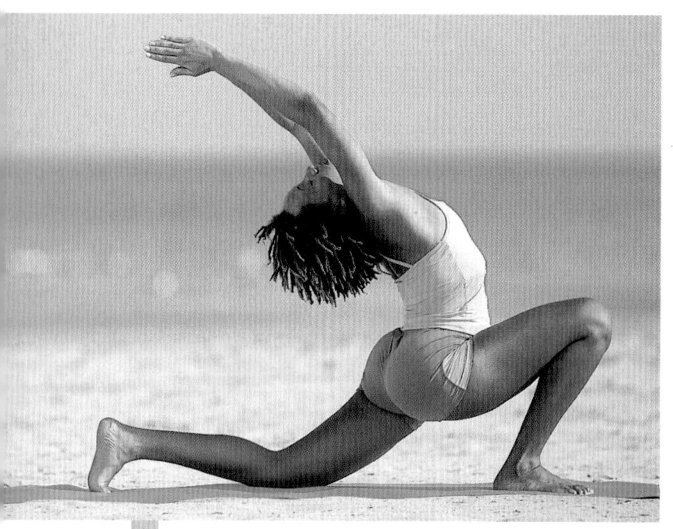

10 Maintaining your balance, exhale and bring the palms together in front of your chest. Then stretch both arms over your head, keeping your palms together. Arch your back and look up, raising your chin as high as possible while inhaling.

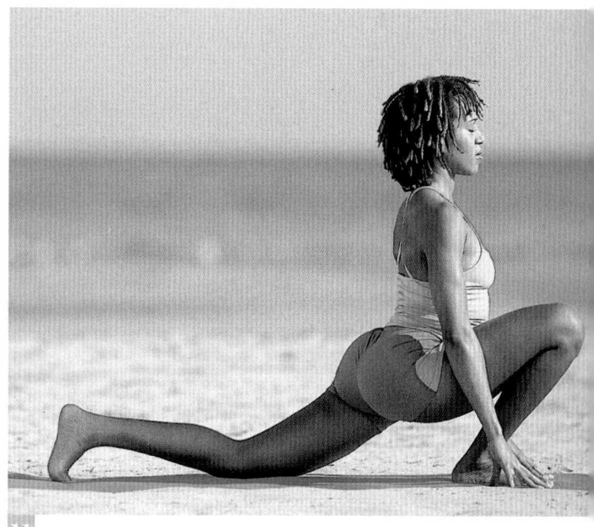

11 Exhale as you lower your hands to your chest, then inhale once again and return your hands to each side of your right foot.

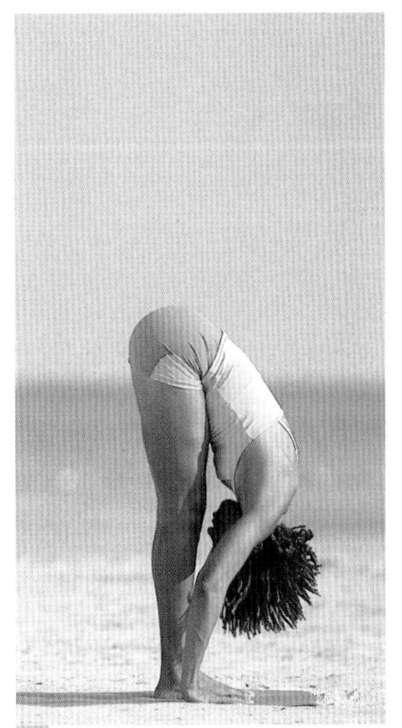

12 Exhale slowly as you bring your left foot forwards, straighten your legs, and stand up. Then bring your head down towards your knees.

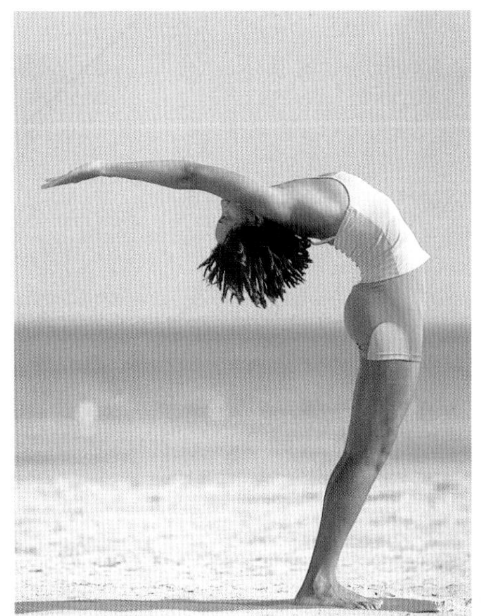

13 Inhale as you slowly bring your arms up over your head and stretch back. Tip the head back only as far as is comfortable.

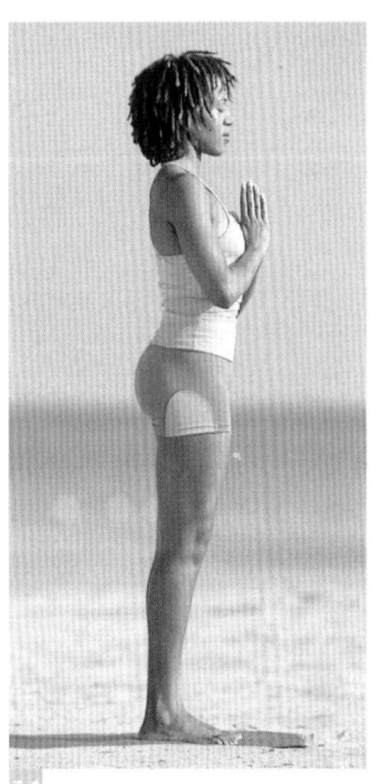

14 Exhale as you stand upright with your palms together at the centre of your chest in starting position. Repeat the sequence or end the set.

HEALING MEDITATION

The healing mantra Ra Ma Da Sa, Sa Say So Hung *(the "a" in the first part of the mantra sounds like mama) translates as "Sun, Moon, Earth, Infinity – I am Thou".*

To practise, sit in Easy pose with a straight spine. Place a firm pillow under your buttocks if necessary. Bend the elbows and draw them into the sides of the rib cage. The palms of the hands face upwards and are as flat as possible, creating a pressure at the wrists, and tipped at a 45° angle outwards to the sides. Close your eyes and focus between the eyebrows. Repeat the mantra once on each breath. Feel the navel pull slightly on the first Sa *and on* Hung. *This is a strongly-voiced, powerful chant that uses all the breath for each repetition (for a musical version, see* Music Resources, p.224*).*

Continue the meditation for between five and 30 minutes. Then inhale, hold the breath, and focus your healing energy towards the person(s) that you are concentrating on for healing. Then relax quietly for a minute.

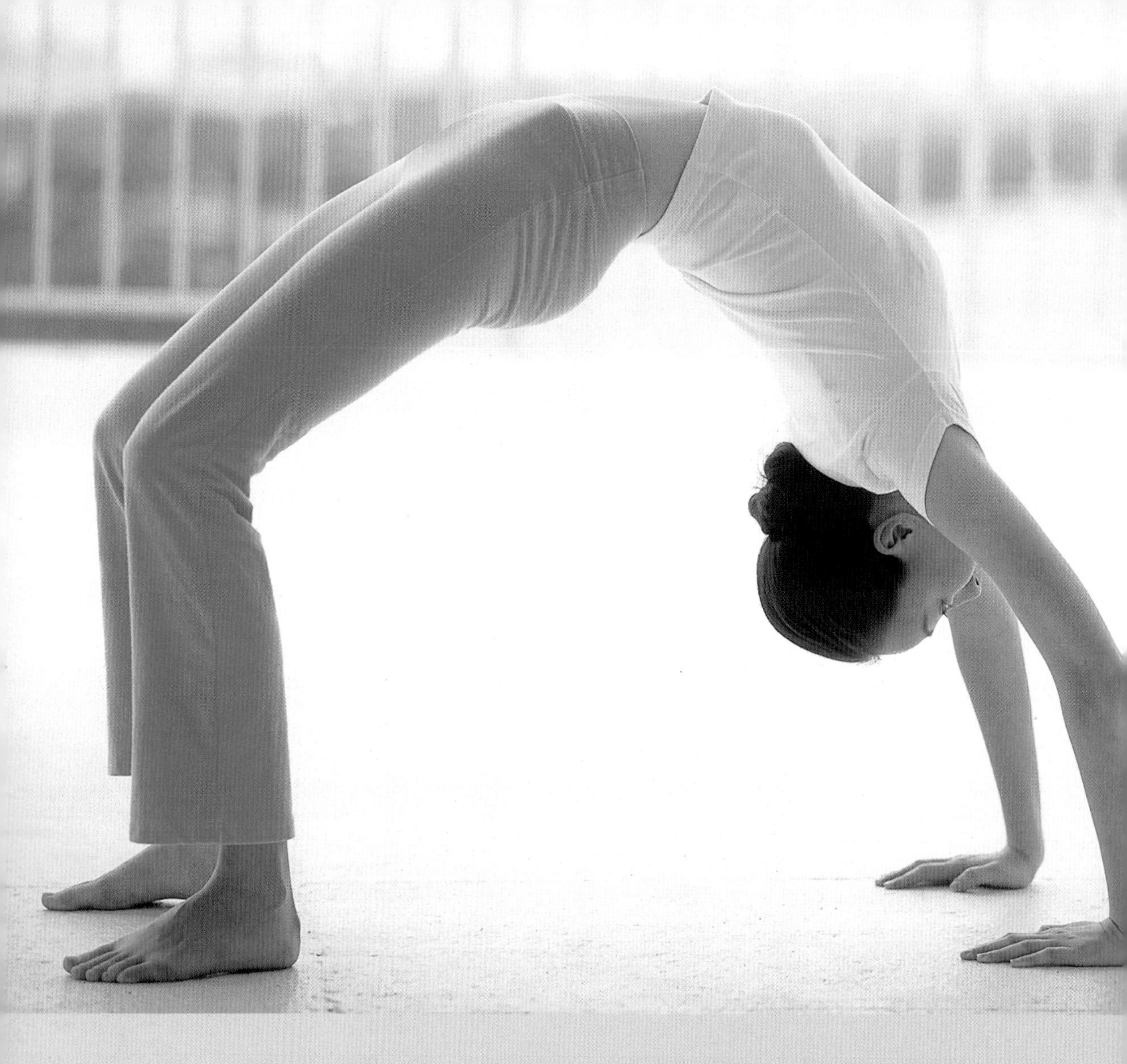

ENERGY FOR LIFE

When you have energy, you feel good and life looks good. Positivity is effortless. When you feel drained, it's a different story. Short tempers and emotional outbursts abound. Or you switch over to automatic pilot in a zombie-like attempt just to get through the day. Instead of reaching for a chocolate bar or coffee, take a couple of minutes to breathe and practise a few of the exercises explained here. They can be practised individually or together to energize body and brain. If you have no more than a couple of minutes to spare, try the quick-fix meditation on page 89, making sure that you leave time to rest deeply afterwards. And in case you need a reminder, you deserve to feel good!

BRIGHTEN UP

This fast-acting energizer can be done any time you need a pick-up. It increases the flow of energy and oxygen to your brain and brightens up your outlook. In yogic science, each area of the hand corresponds to a certain area of the body or brain. Your thumbs relate to your ego or unique personality. Stretching your thumbs upwards activates a positive ego.

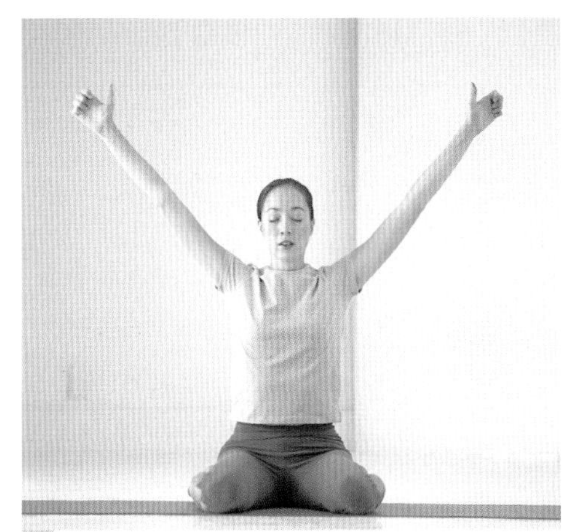

1 Sit between your heels, or alternatively on your heels. Lift your chest as you raise your arms to a 60° angle. Begin Breath of Fire. After 1–3 minutes, inhale deeply and hold the breath.

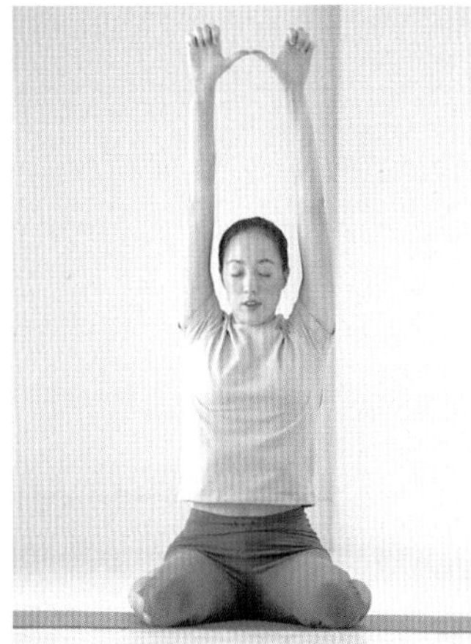

2 Slowly draw your thumbs together overhead on the held breath until the tips of your thumbs meet.

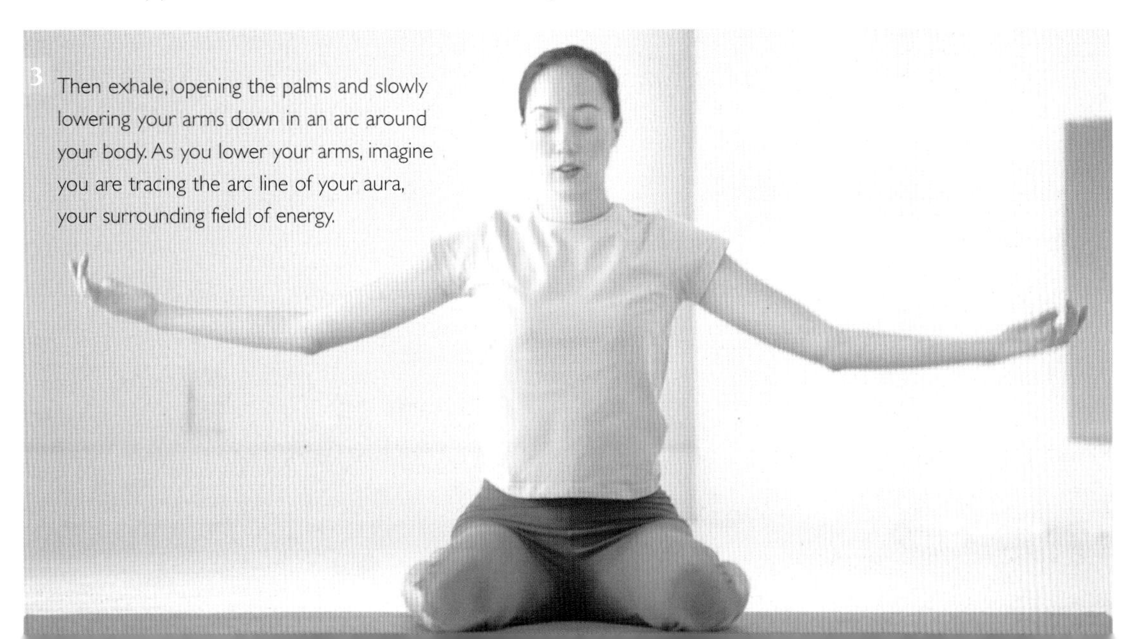

3 Then exhale, opening the palms and slowly lowering your arms down in an arc around your body. As you lower your arms, imagine you are tracing the arc line of your aura, your surrounding field of energy.

ROASTED MILLET

Millet helps to stabilize blood sugar levels. Eaten regularly, it can help you to stay even-tempered and calm.

250g (8oz) millet
750ml (24fl oz) water

In a skillet or saucepan, dry roast the millet on a medium–high heat. Stir for two minutes. Add water and cook covered, without stirring, on a medium heat for 20 minutes, then turn down the heat to low for the last five minutes, or until all the water is absorbed. Add a little almond or olive oil, butter – or even chopped garlic, basil, and parsley – and serve.

SPRING BACK

Physically, this exercise works on revitalizing all body systems, and can be a great aerobic workout. Mentally, it gives you the ability to spring back into life. It gives you an edge because it helps you to think fast. A woman must be physically active in order to have this edge.

2 As you exhale, punch forwards with the left arm while simultaneously springing off the ground and bringing the left leg forwards and the right leg back into a front stance position. During the jump, your right fist pulls back to the left side of your chest.

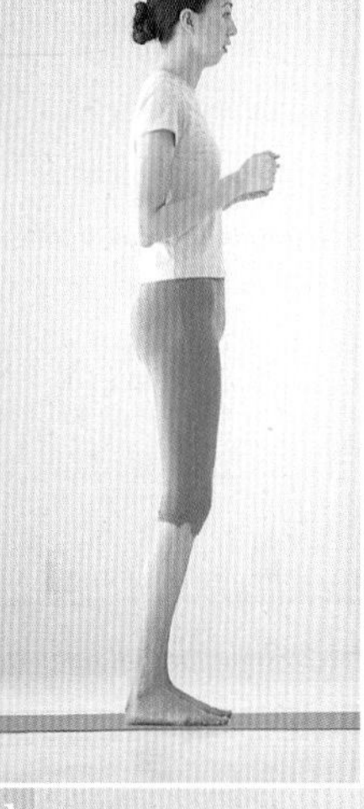

1 Stand with your feet shoulder-width apart and knees slightly bent. Your hands are in fists, with the palms facing each other in front of the chest.

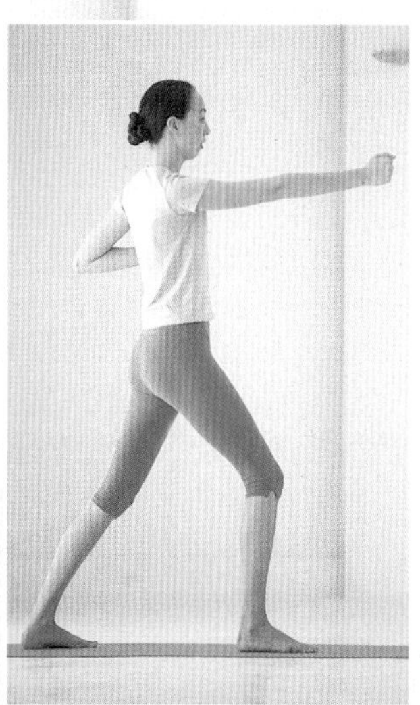

3 Spring back to the original position (step 1) on your next inhalation. Continue this action on the same side for 1–2 minutes. Then change sides. The jumping movement should be light and fast.

BUNDLE ROLL

The tightening of the body in Bundle Roll strengthens the nervous system as well as making your muscles stronger. It is good for relieving hyperactivity and anxiety in adults and children. Be sure to have soft padding underneath you as you practise Bundle Roll.

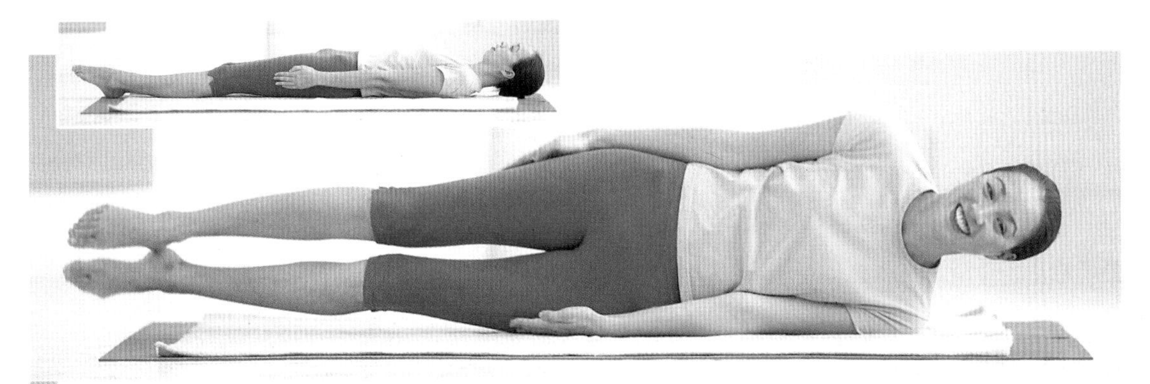

1 Lie down on your back with your arms straight at your sides *(inset)*. Stiffen your body, point your toes, and begin to rock from side to side until you flip over to one side. Keep your body straight.

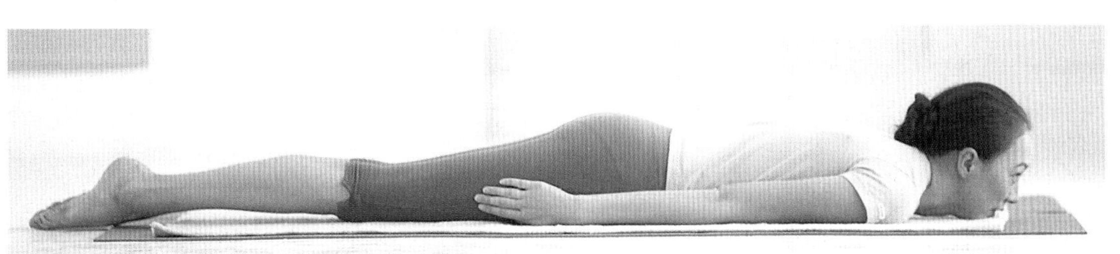

2 Flip onto your front, then roll from front to back and back to front, flipping over and over without bending. Maintain a tension in your entire body throughout. Continue for 2–3 minutes, then relax on your back or front for a minute.

GURUPRAKASH KAUR'S STORY (USA/INDIA)

I grew up with yoga. I remember getting up every morning to do yoga and meditation with my parents. I could bend right back in Cobra and bend my knees so that my feet were flat on my face. My parents would try their best to keep up with me, but of course I had the advantage of youth. Twenty years later I still have the advantage. Growing up with yoga, meditation, and conscious living has brought me to the ultimate place. At 22, I can actually say that I know who I am. I am happy and I am healthy. After practising yoga all my life, I have realized that the highest form of yoga is to teach. My hope is that I can take whatever knowledge and experience I have about this awesome science and touch the hearts and minds of everyone that I meet.

BRIDGE

This pose massages and invigorates the digestive organs, and is excellent for general strengthening of the ovaries and uterus. Bridge is a good preparation for Wheel *(p.90)*, or can be practised as an alternative to it.

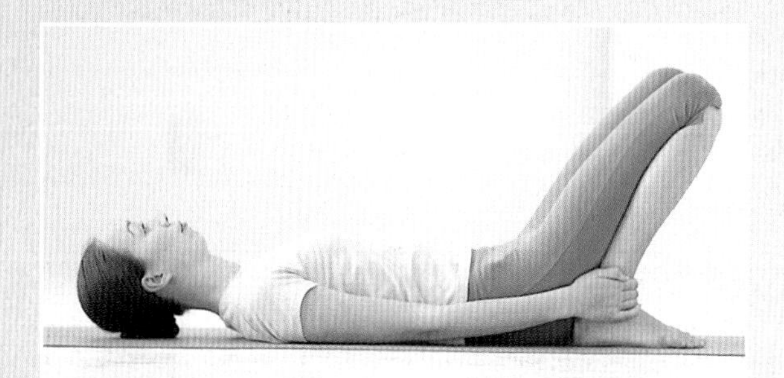

1 Lie on your back with your knees bent. Place the feet flat on the ground close to the buttocks. Reach down and grasp each ankle with the respective hands, or place your hands on the ground beside you with the palms down.

2 Keeping the feet, head, and upper shoulders on the ground, roll up. Start with your pelvis and follow with your upper spine. Lift as high as is comfortable as you inhale, then roll down as you exhale. As you roll down, lead with your upper spine, and follow with the lower. Continue for 1–2 minutes. Then stretch up and begin Breath of Fire *(p.24)* for 1 more minute.

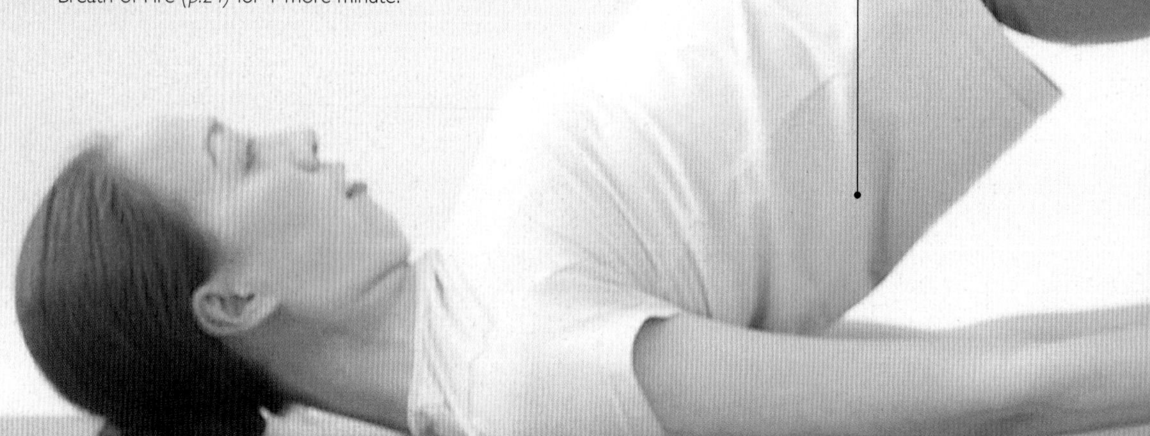

Rolling up and down enhances the elasticity of the spine and massages all the back muscles

COUNTERPOSE FOR BRIDGE AND WHEEL

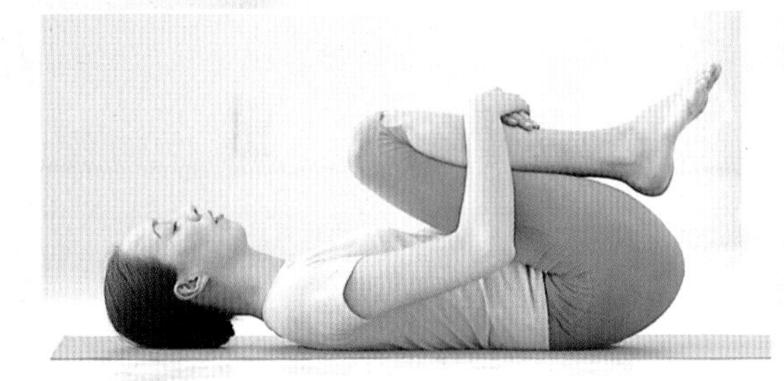

Tuck your knees into your chest with your hands on your shins, and breath deeply for 20 seconds–1 minute.

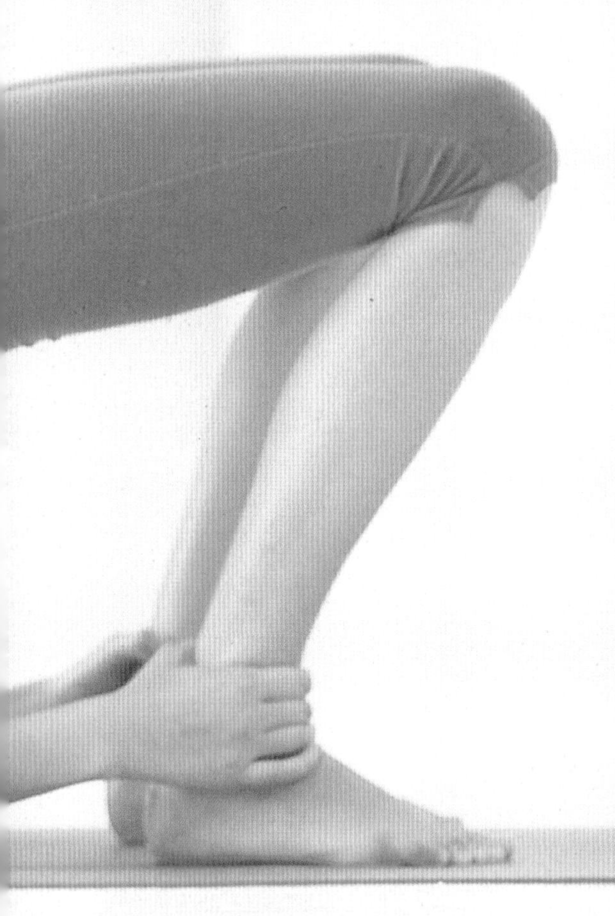

MEDITATION FOR ABSOLUTELY POWERFUL ENERGY

Only two minutes are needed to relieve "brain drain", or mental fatigue, with this meditation. It is important to allow resting time afterwards.

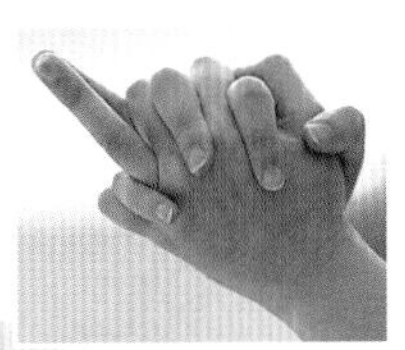

1 *Sit in Easy pose with a straight spine. Place your palms together. Keep your ring fingers together and extended as you interlace and fold down the other fingers.*

2 *Hold your hands a short distance from your solar plexus/diaphragm area. Your extended fingers point up at a 60° angle.*

3 *Close your eyes. Inhale deeply through the nose but keep your mouth open. Chant the mantra* Ong *(p.22), extending the sound through your nasal passages as* "Ooonnnnng"*. Sense the sound coming from the upper back area of your soft palate at the juncture of the throat and nasal passages. As you chant, your navel will pull back slightly towards your spine, and your attention will naturally flow upwards to the sixth chakra (your brow point). Repeat five times, or continue for longer if you wish. Then rest or go to sleep.*

WHEEL

Besides the Wheel's obvious benefits of increasing the flexibility of the spine and strengthening the muscles of the abdomen, legs and arms, this powerful pose energizes your mental faculties, improves your memory, and is extremely beneficial for the lymphatic system. Inverted postures such as Wheel, Shoulderstand *(pp.52–53)* and Plough *(pp.114–15)* literally and figuratively "turn you upside down" in the sense that they give you a new perspective on life.

PREPARING FOR WHEEL

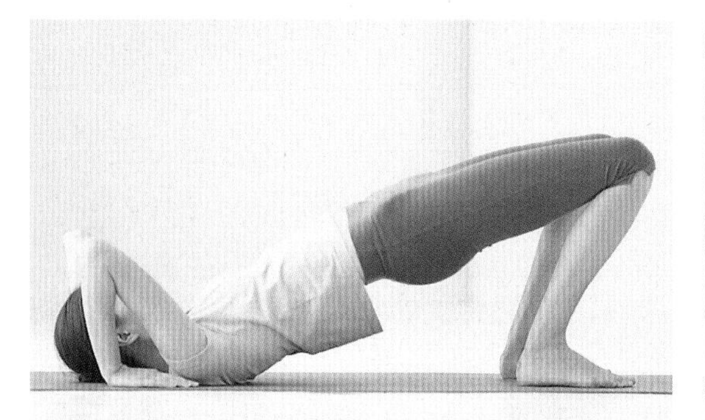

1 Lift up as high as possible in Bridge *(p.88)*, then bring your hands to the ground behind the shoulders. The palms should be flat on the ground with the fingers pointing towards the shoulders.

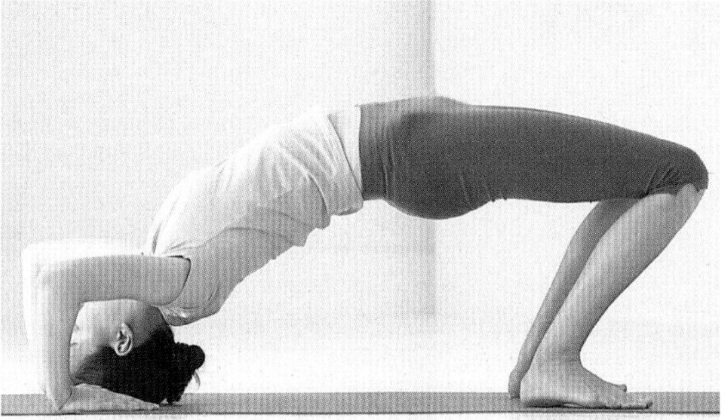

2 Arch your body further upwards as your arms and feet press the ground. Your neck will arch back as you bring the top of your head to the ground. Take a few deep breaths, then relax down slowly, releasing your neck carefully. Stay at this level as long as you like before trying the full pose.

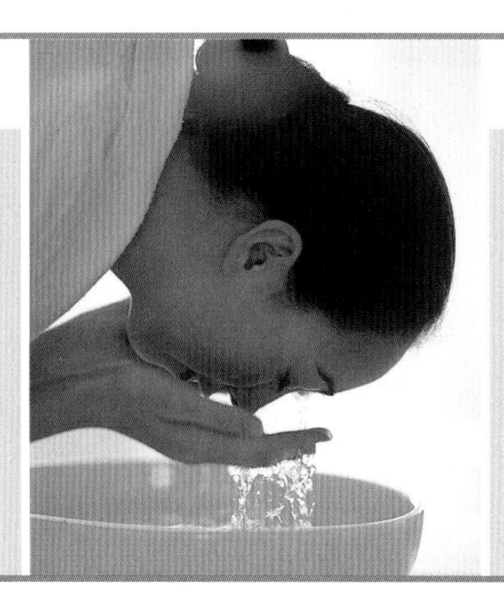

FOR ENERGY WHILE WORKING

In the fast-paced, complex lives we lead today, every woman is Superwoman. Most women push themselves to the point of overwork, and because they are women they are capable of doing just that. If you are a mother, you know exactly what I mean. There are always more demands on your time than you could possibly fulfill. It's just a fact of life. To energize your brain and soothe your eyes, or after hours sitting at a computer, splash cold water on your face and eyes and wet a paper towel to place at the back of your neck.

FULL WHEEL

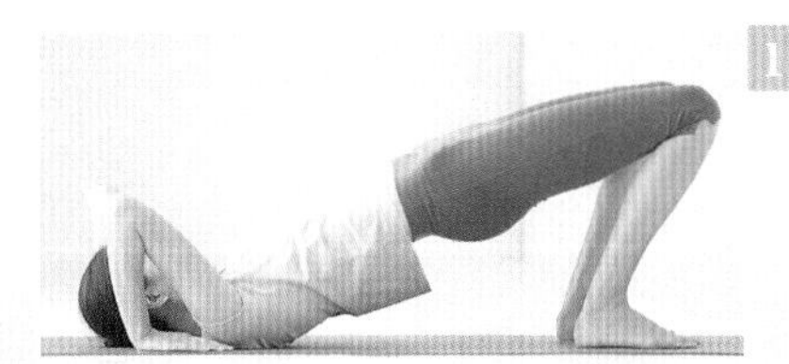

1 Lie on your back with your knees bent. Place the feet flat on the ground close to the buttocks. Bring your hands to the ground behind your shoulders, palms flat on the ground with the fingers pointing towards the shoulders.

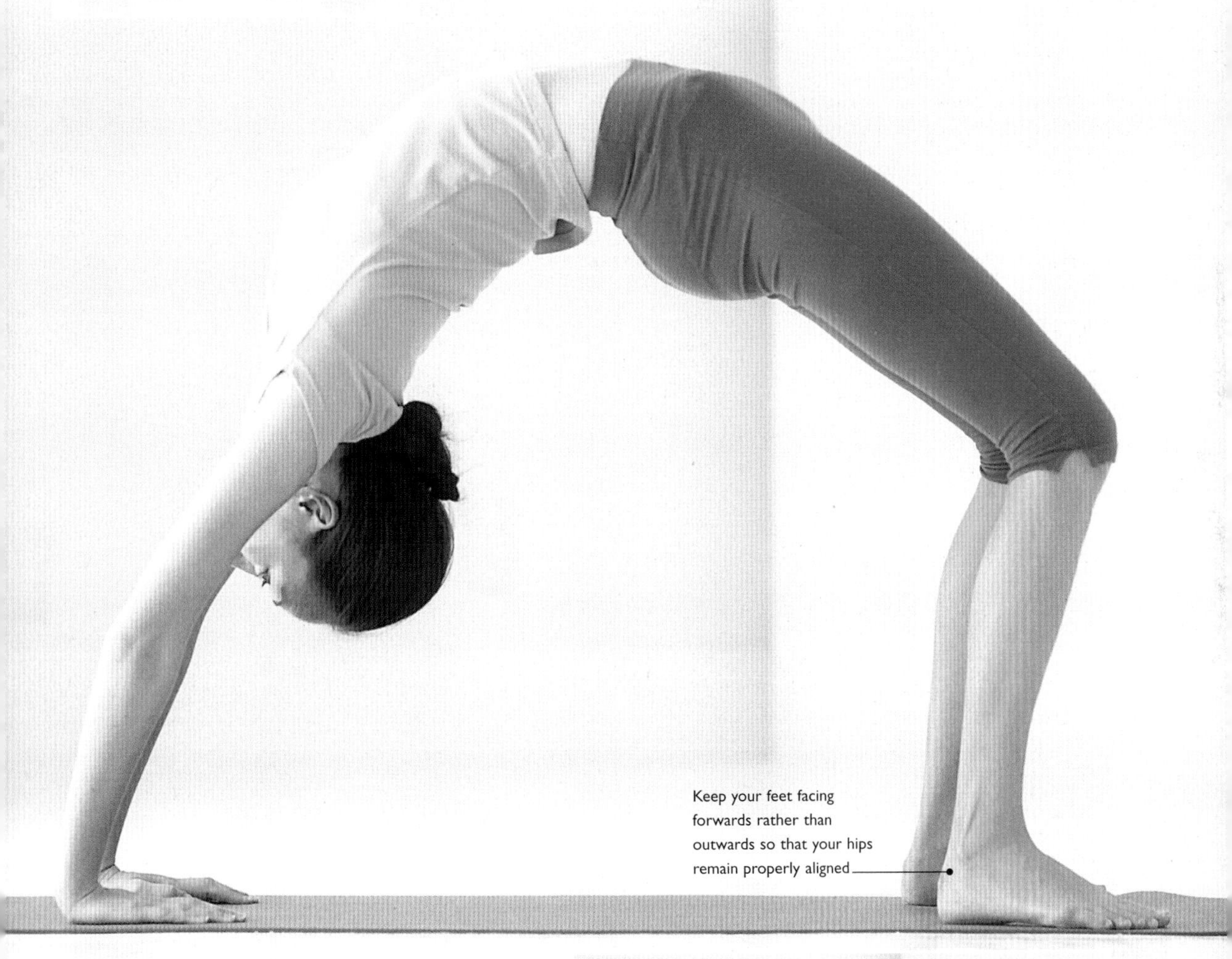

Keep your feet facing forwards rather than outwards so that your hips remain properly aligned

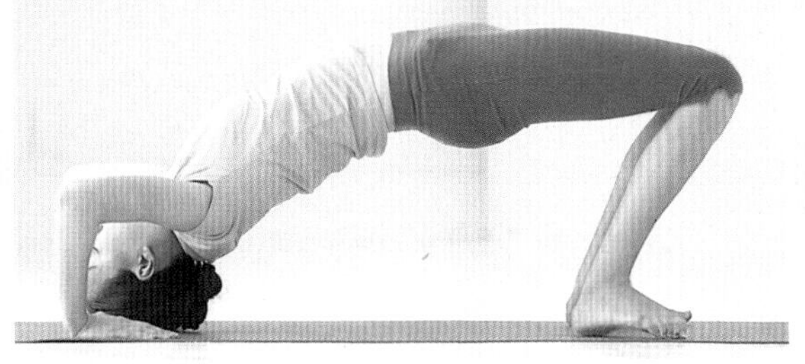

2 Inhale and lift your body upwards, straightening your elbows and arching your hips and chest up as high as possible. Allow your head to drop back. Do Breath of Fire or deep breathing *(p.24)* for between 30 seconds and 2 minutes.

3 Come down carefully and gently from the pose, starting with the upper body, and rest in counterpose *(p.89)*.

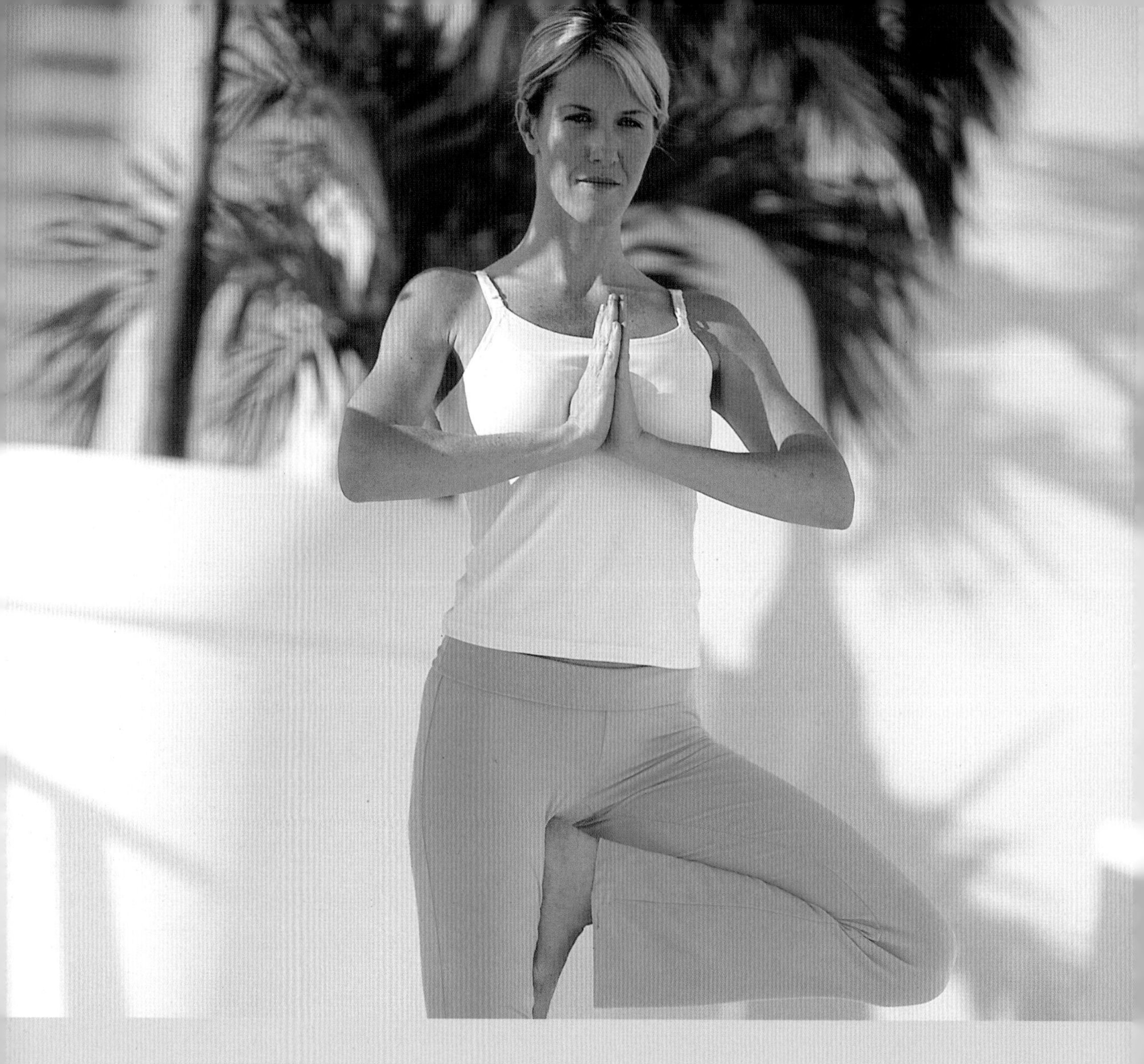

LIGHTENING UP

How do we develop the power to love ourselves as we are, and to change the things that we find no longer serve us? In yoga, often the answer is "navel power". In *Lightening Up* we'll work directly with this power source – the navel centre, third chakra energy. In the womb it was your original source of power through the nourishment you received from your mother. Now the navel centre is the seat of your physical wellbeing, and your ability to hold your intention and make it manifest.

Here you'll recharge your navel batteries, so to speak. This creates an internal heat, called tapas, that is self-empowering. The activated power is drawn upwards to the higher chakras with poses that lighten your heart and mind.

ALTERNATE LEG LIFTS

Leg raises aid the proper functioning of the intestines, and create an internal energy that activates the navel area. Coupled with strong, deep breaths, they revitalize the abdominal area and strengthen the back and thighs.

1

Lie on your back with your arms down at your sides, palms facing downwards.

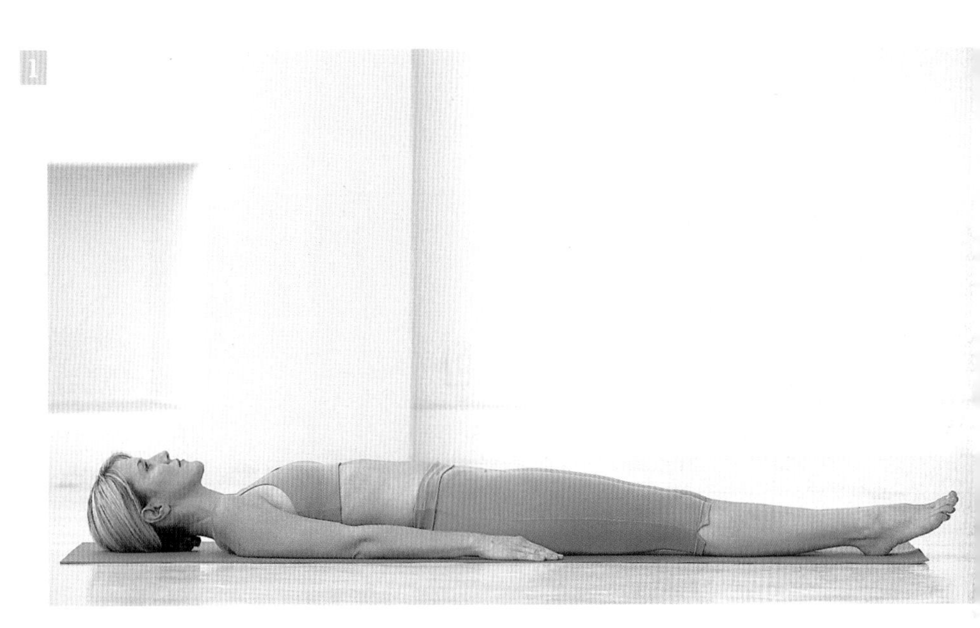

2

Inhale and lift your right leg straight up to a 90° angle, then exhale and lower it. Repeat with the left leg. Keep the knee straight but not locked and lift from the hip. Continue raising and lowering alternate legs with deep and powerful breaths for 2–4 minutes.

Do not over-lift the leg
The buttocks stay on the ground

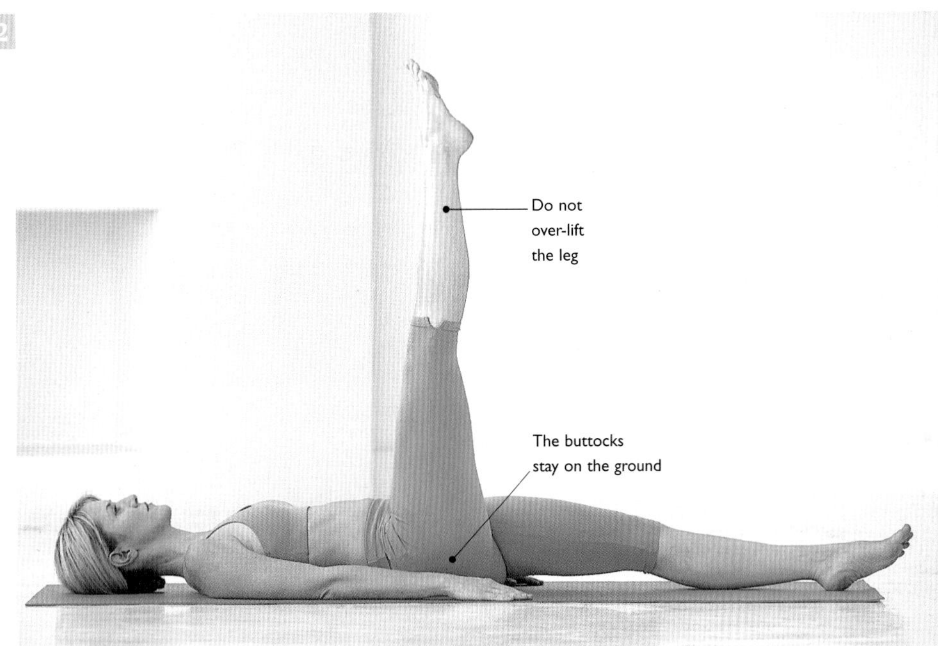

TREE

This balancing pose adjusts the vertebrae of the spine and promotes good posture. It refreshes and uplifts the mind. Beginners may want to practise standing with one shoulder next to a wall for support.

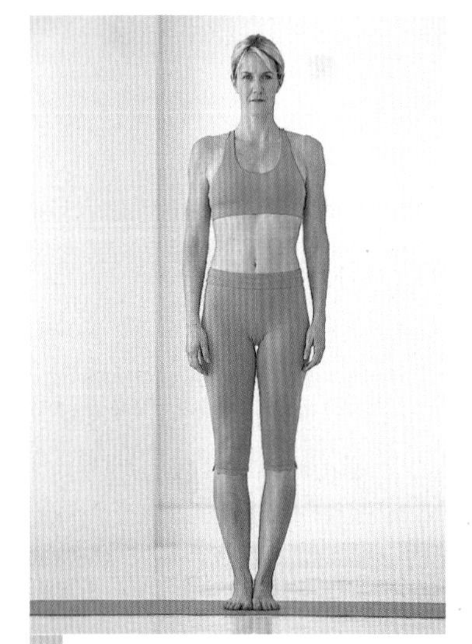

1 Stand tall on a firm surface with your feet close together and your arms at your sides.

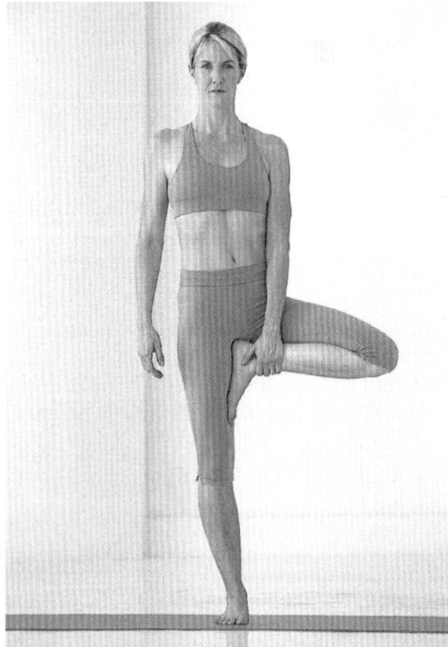

2 Place your left foot inside your right thigh. Ideally, it rests close to the top of the inner thigh, but can be placed towards the inside of the knee.

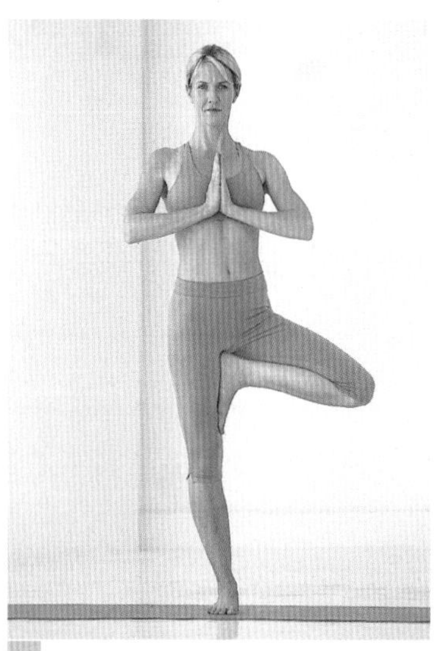

3 Steady yourself in this pose by focusing the eyes straight ahead. Breathe deeply and bring the palms together at the heart centre.

IRENE'S STORY (UK)

I have found yoga to be essential in helping me break addictive patterns. In my teenage years, I became dependent on food, romance, and recreational drugs to stave off my feelings of helplessness and boredom. My teenage years were spent in a daze. I turned to "treating" myself to rich foods, and my girlfriends and I basically formed our whole friendships around eating. I would develop obsessive crushes on boys at school, and all of my creative energy would be funnelled into making these hopeless relationships work.

After some time spent in this dark period, I gathered myself up and embarked on a healing journey. I sought help from many different therapists and healing processes, but nothing compared to my success with yoga. I noticed an almost immediate difference in my life after enrolling in my first yoga class, as though a fog was lifting, revealing a clear picture of my life – what it had been and what it could be.

I now teach yoga and meditation and practise it daily. I get high without drugs, and have recently graduated from college. I don't have severe food cravings, and my love relationships are healthy and mutually beneficial. Kundalini Yoga and meditation has helped me find my inner centre and my love for life.

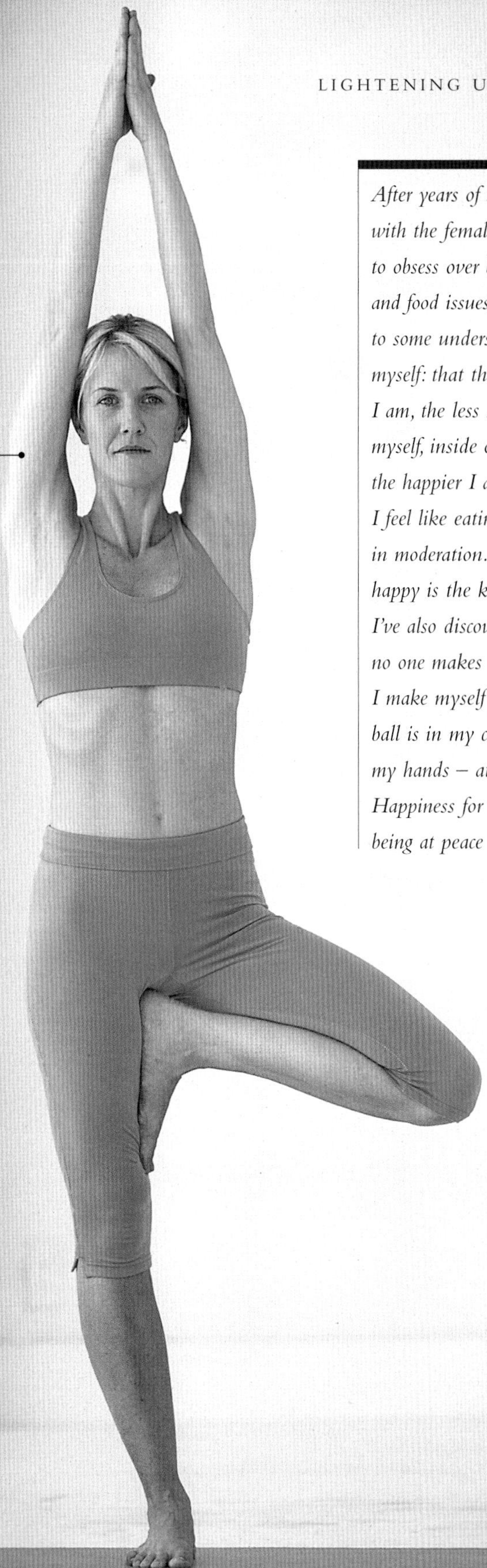

After years of struggling with the female inclination to obsess over body image and food issues, I have come to some understandings for myself: that the happier I am, the less I judge myself, inside or out; and the happier I am the more I feel like eating well and in moderation. So being happy is the key. What I've also discovered is that no one makes me happy – I make myself happy. The ball is in my court and in my hands – at all times. Happiness for me equals being at peace with myself.

Focus on the upwards stretch through the spine, rib cage, neck, and arms

4 When you feel ready, slowly inhale and stretch the palms up towards the sky, straightening the arms so that they are close to the sides of the head. Keep the spine straight and feel your whole body lift upwards. Continue in Tree pose for 1–3 minutes, then come out of the pose slowly and switch sides.

LIFT AND LAUGH

The angle of the first part of this exercise moves the activated navel energy into the heart and upper centres of the body. Belly laughing is good for the soul. It also improves digestion.

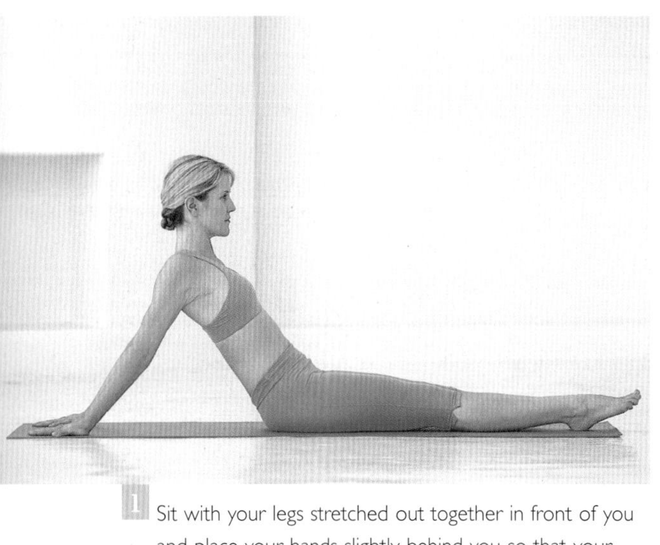

1 Sit with your legs stretched out together in front of you and place your hands slightly behind you so that your body is at a 45° angle to the ground.

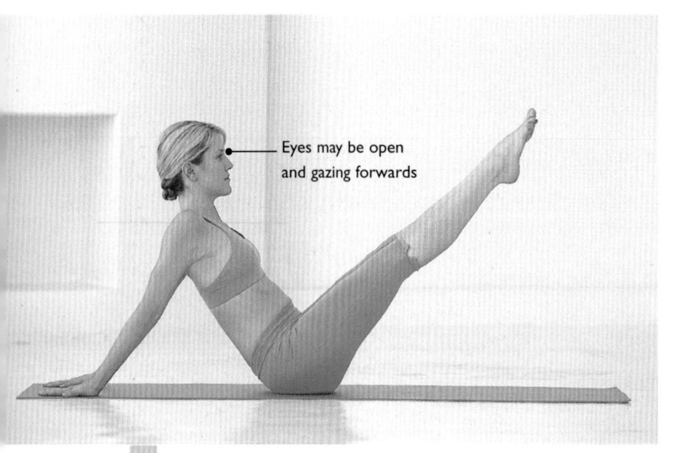

2 Point your toes and lean back slightly, keeping the back straight and the chest lifted. Lift your legs to a 60° angle and hold with Breath of Fire *(p.24)*. Continue for 1–2 minutes. Then inhale deeply, exhale, and hold the breath out. Apply Root Lock *(p.25)*. Then relax the breath, the lock, and the posture.

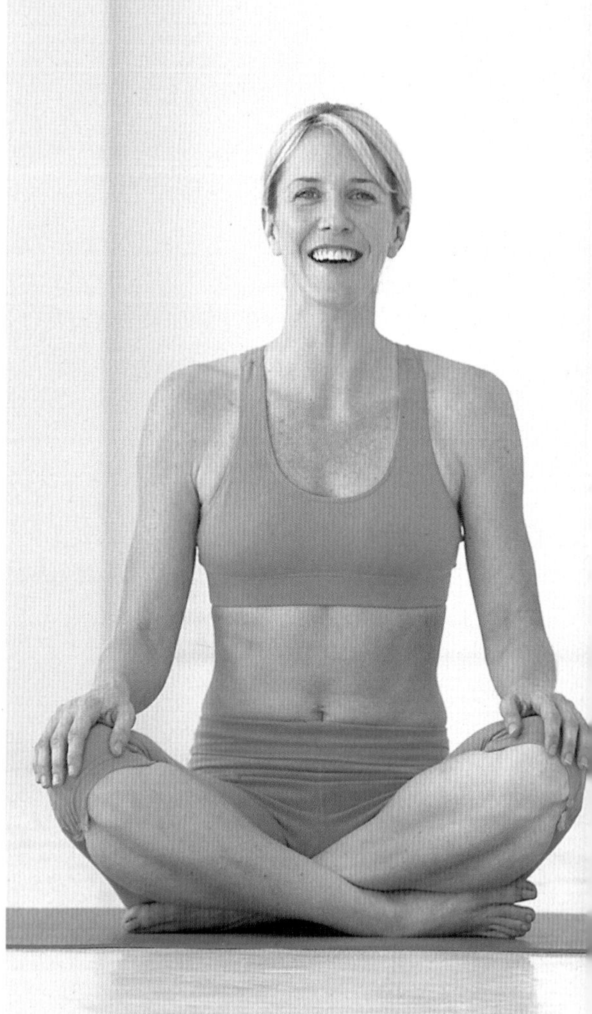

3 Immediately sit in Easy pose *(p.19)* and begin belly laughing. Use your navel and get loud! Enjoy even the ridiculousness of it.

SA TA NA MA MEDITATION

Sa Ta Na Ma *is one of the most well-practised meditations in the Kundalini tradition. It is a clearing house for unwanted thoughts and feelings, and is especially effective as part of your morning yoga practice or before bed for a restful sleep (see also* Music Resources, p.224*).*

Sit in Easy pose with a straight spine. Bring your hands to your knees. Your thumbs will sequentially press each finger as you chant the mantra: Sa *(Totality), press the thumb and index finger;* Ta *(Creation), press the thumb and middle finger;* Na *(Dissolution), press the thumb and ring finger;* Ma *(Regeneration), press the thumb and little finger. Continue pressing the fingers sequentially and chanting out loud for two minutes. This is the voice of the human. Then continue the finger movements, and begin whispering for two minutes. This is the voice of the beloved. Next chant silently, hearing the mantra internally while still moving the fingers for two minutes. This is the inner voice. Then reverse the process: two minutes of silent repetition, two minutes of whispering, and finally chanting out loud for two minutes. Work up to five minutes for each part of the meditation. As you repeat the mantra, imagine the sound of each syllable entering through the crown centre and going out through the sixth centre between the eyebrows. This energy flow strengthens the connection between different parts of the brain, clearing the subconscious mind and allowing access to the higher centres of the brain. Pressing the fingertips activates meridian points in the hands that also help energy flow to the brain centres.*

Dr. Dharma Singh Khalsa presents an experiment in his book, Meditation as Medicine, *in which a PET scan was done on a practitioner of this meditation. Different areas of the brain lit up as the fingers were pressed, demonstrating that the various finger movements have a direct impact upon brain function.*

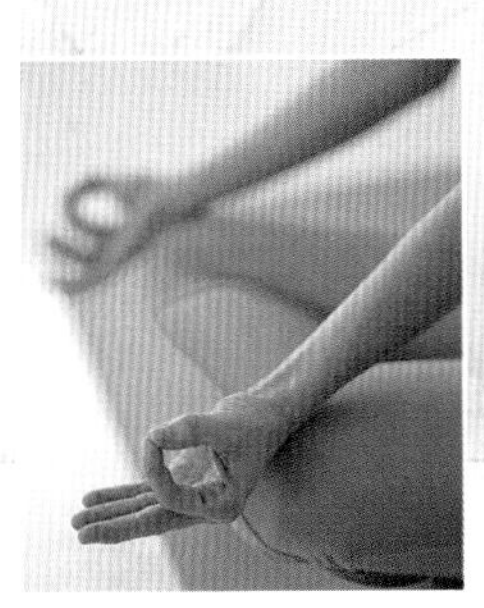

Sa: thumb, index finger

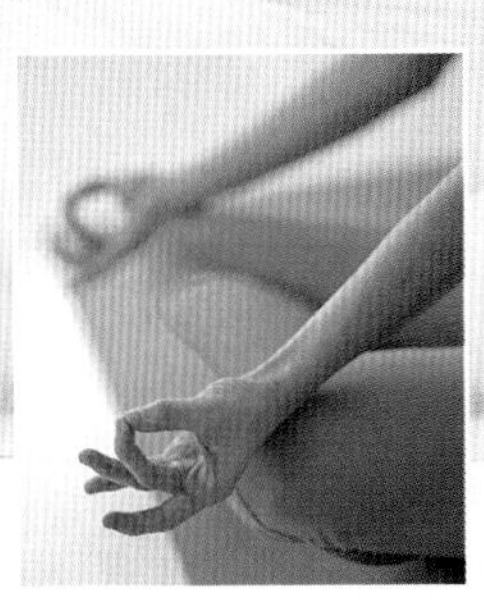

Ta: thumb, middle finger

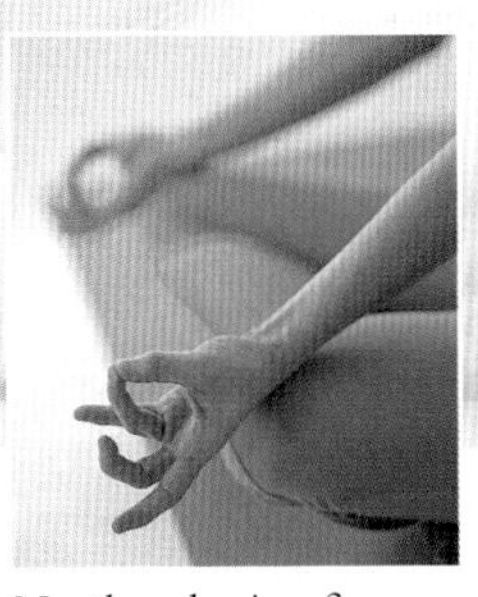

Na: thumb, ring finger

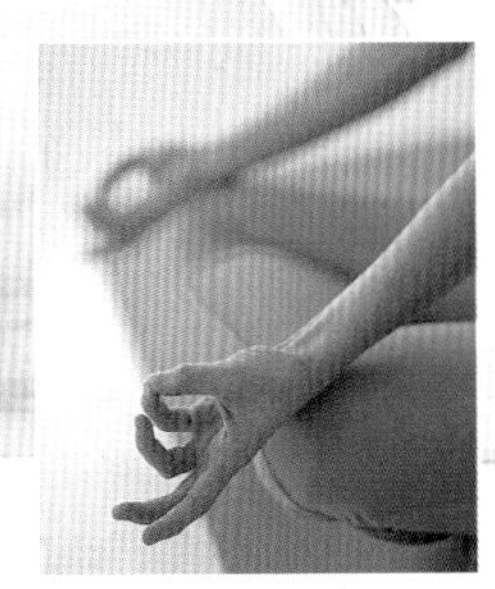

Ma: thumb, little finger

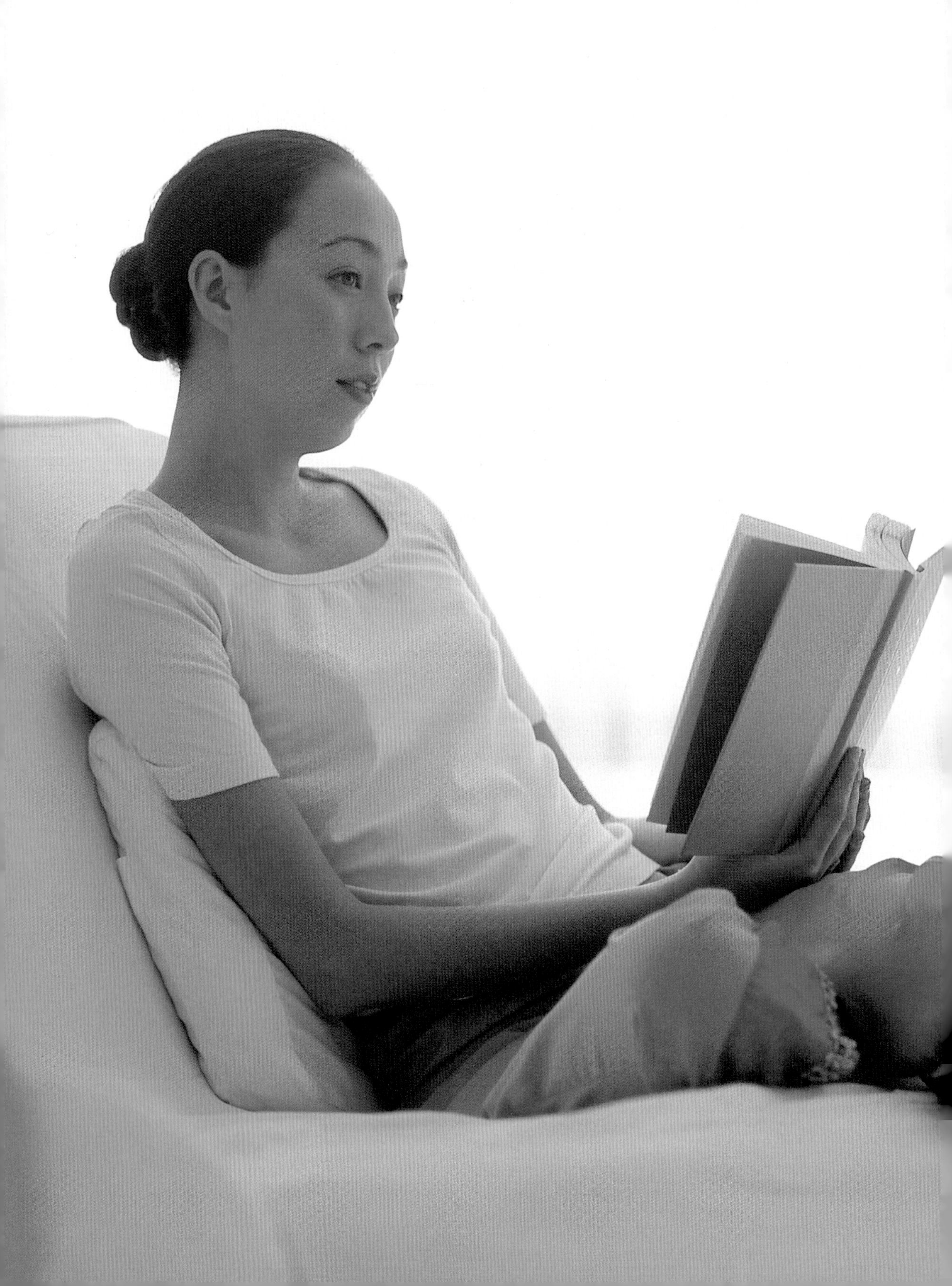

BALANCING

From the time she's young to the time she's a "wise woman", a woman's menstrual cycle profoundly affects her life. This one feature makes all the difference, on every level – mental, physical, and emotional. Each stage of life – from PMT to menopause – holds challenges and gifts.

Balance is the key to turning these challenges into gifts. In practising specific yoga exercises for dealing with PMT, mood swings, and menopausal symptoms, a balance comes into your life, a sense of wellbeing. No matter what your current phase of life, these chapters have something priceless to offer – an opportunity to experience calm in the midst of the storm.

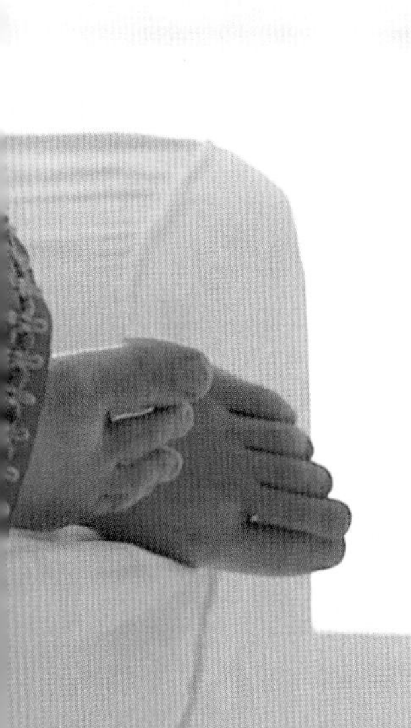

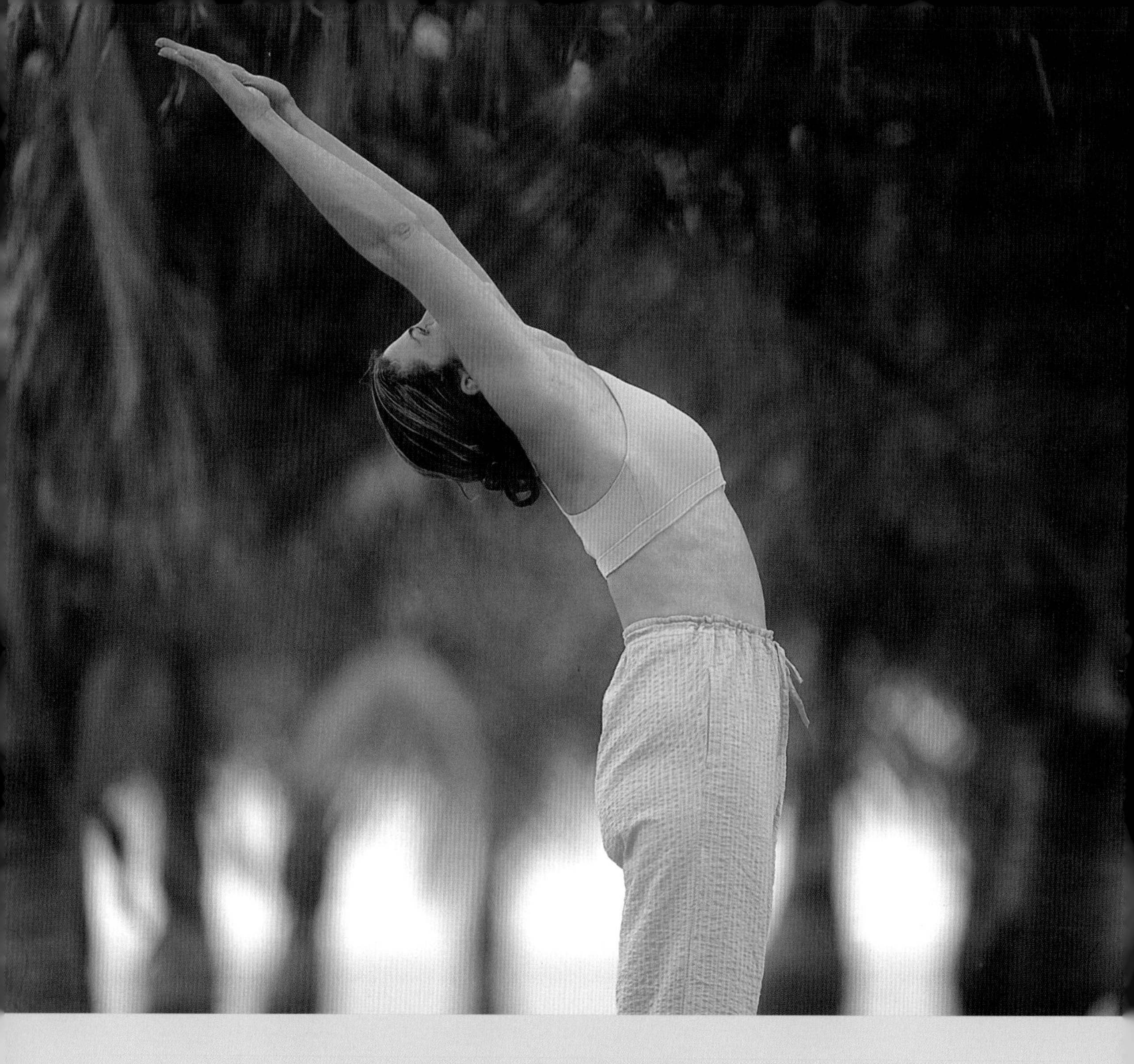

LEVELLING OUT

Whether it's our fluctuating hormones or just the sensitivity we women are born with, we tend towards highs and lows. We may overreact, take things too hard, project our own pain into situations, and just generally get out of balance. But what can seem like a curse can also be seen as a blessing. We are blessed to be aware, sensitive beings. Whether the issue is depression, extreme behaviour, or both alternately, the first step in evening out highs and lows is to pick up one foot and put it down. Then continue to place one foot in front of the other until you are standing on your yoga mat. Promptly sit down, tune in, and get ready to feel better with yoga and meditation for balance, clarity, and stability.

BALANCING POSES

The intricate connection between body, mind, and spirit is quite apparent in the practice of balancing poses. Working with them strengthens your focus and brings your mind to a neutral place. And the more focused and stable you are, the easier it is to remain steady in your practice.

TRIANGLE

This pose stretches the spine and spinal nerves laterally, helps to adjust the sacrum and lower back, and stretches the muscles and nerves in the legs and arms. It reduces stress and anxiety through its capacity to centre and balance you.

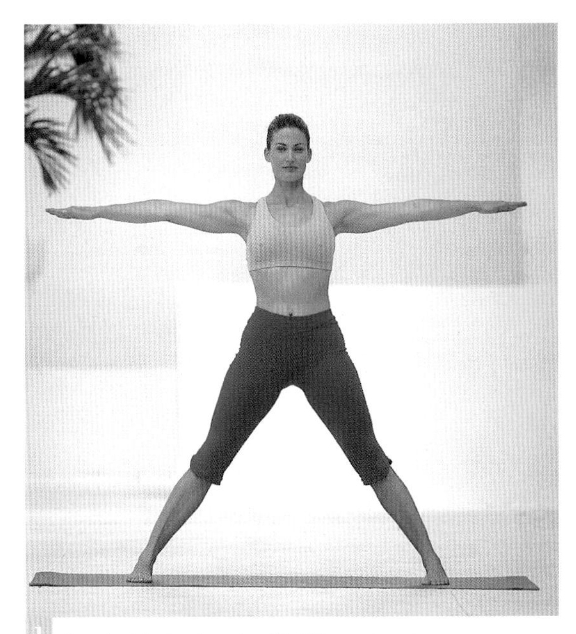

1 Stand with the feet 1m (3–4ft) apart and your arms raised so that they are straight out to the sides at shoulder level.

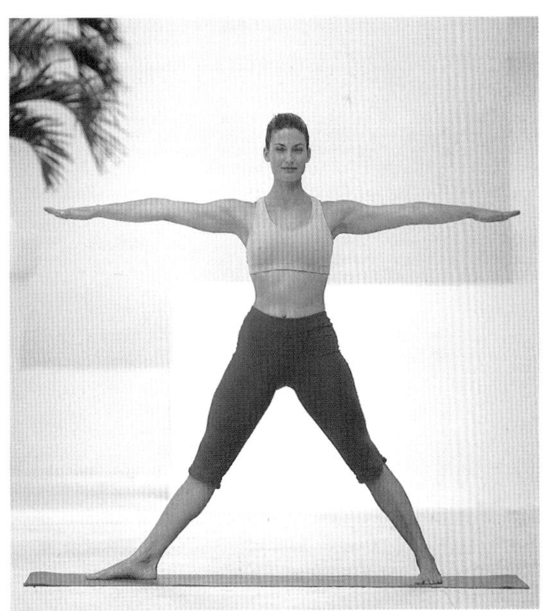

2 Pivot your right foot 90° to the right and turn your left foot in slightly by moving the heel outwards. Check your right heel is in line with the arch of your left foot and that your weight is evenly distributed. Keep your pelvis facing forwards and your shoulders relaxed, lift your chest, and breathe deeply a few times before continuing on with step 3.

TERRY'S STORY (USA)

I am a 21-year-old woman with a history of depression and anxiety disorder. A regular practice of Kundalini Yoga over the last half year has blessed me with the tools and resources I need to help me overcome my disorder. There was a time when I was so trapped in my mind and negative thoughts that I was totally cut off from my body and whole being. I would sometimes look at my hands and not recognize them, and self-destructive habits such as eating poorly were symptomatic of this separation.

In my experience, Kundalini Yoga has been the most effective form of therapy, allowing me to quite literally integrate my body, mind, and soul. I have confidence now, and it helps me get out of bed and look forward to each day. My daily practice of Sat Kriya has allowed me to work through a great deal of pain and fear, and has helped me to experience my authentic self. Simple things such as brushing my teeth and making myself something to eat are no longer difficult.

In the past I rarely felt comfortable in my skin, and my mind was a source of torment. I felt alienated from the world and God. My yoga practice has helped me shift to a more neutral and balanced outlook on life, and has given me a deep faith in the presence of God always with me and around me.

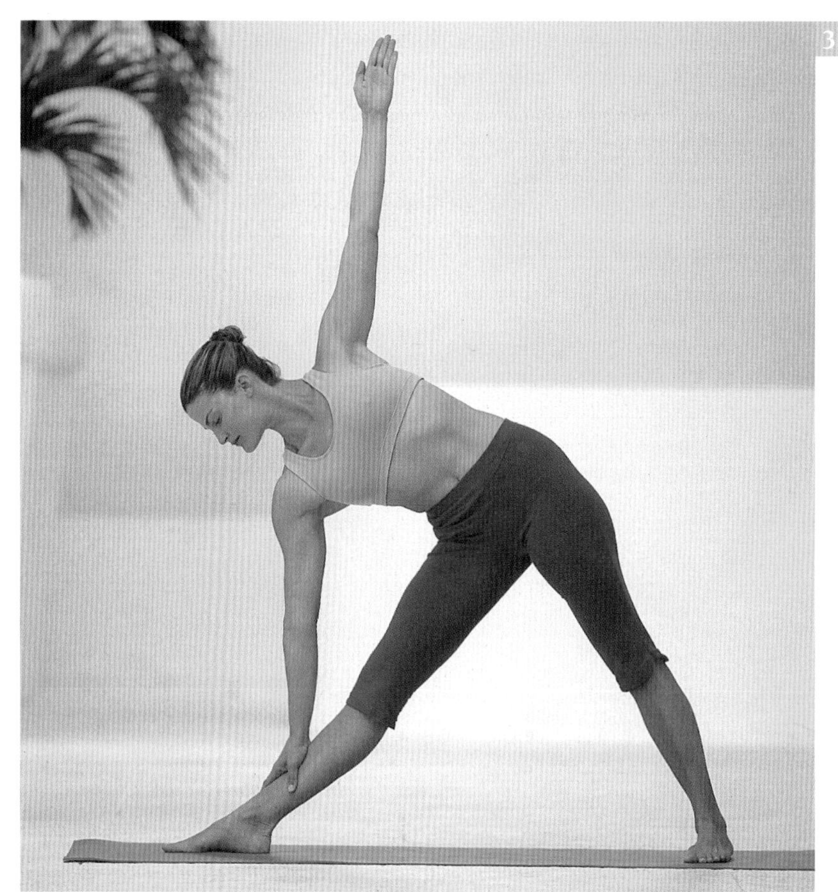

3 Inhale, lower your right arm, and bring it to rest on your shin. Extend your left arm up from the shoulder with the palm facing forwards. Exhale and shift your pelvis to the left while moving the shoulders towards the right, bringing the right shoulder out and over the right leg. Keep your chest and pelvis open and facing forwards. Take a few deep breaths.

4 Slide the hand down towards the ankle, as far as you can without rotating the left hip forwards. Fully extend both arms, keeping them in alignment with each other and straight out from the shoulders. Look up towards the extended arm, straight ahead, or down at the foot. Relax and breathe as you hold the position for 30 seconds to 1 minute.

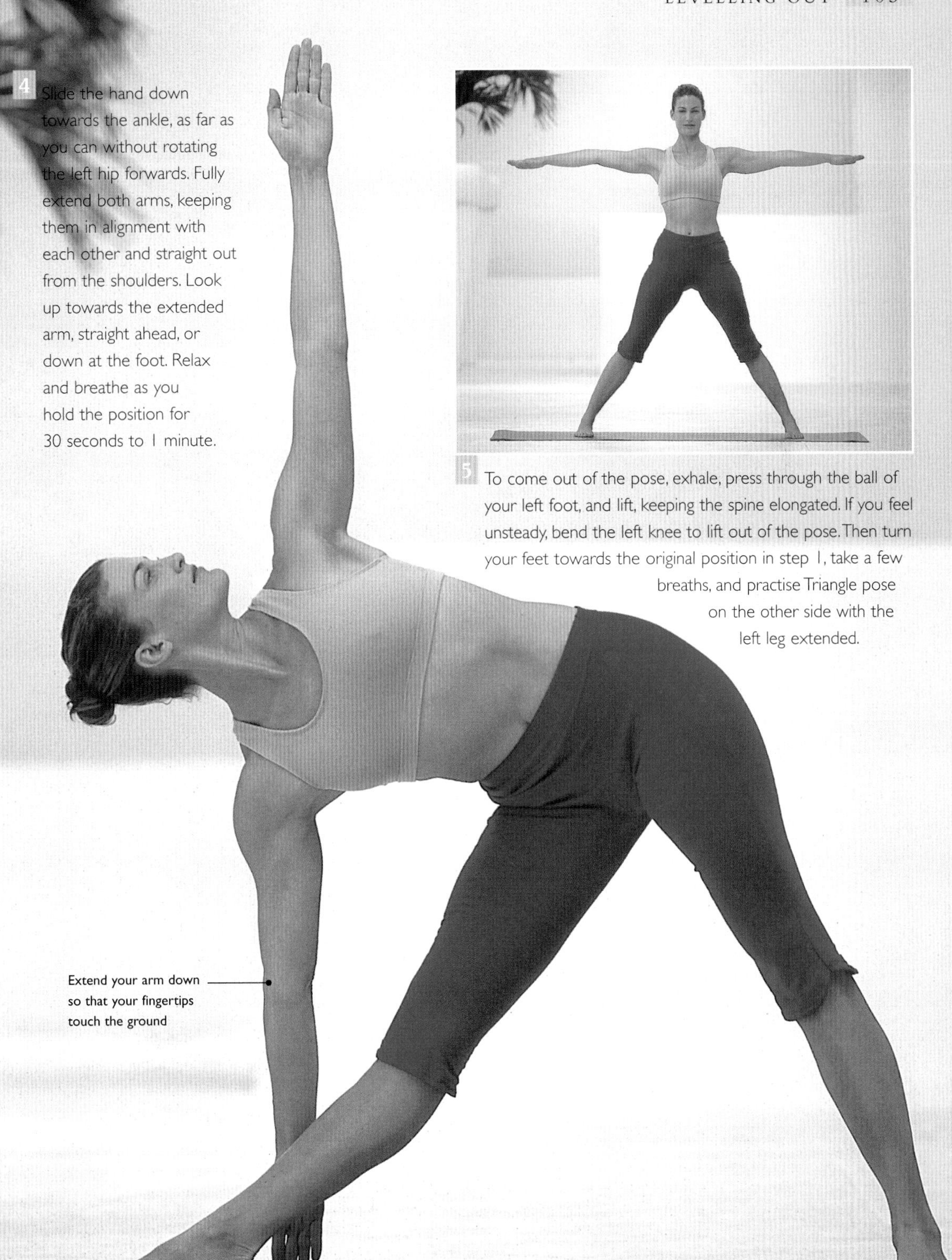

Extend your arm down so that your fingertips touch the ground

5 To come out of the pose, exhale, press through the ball of your left foot, and lift, keeping the spine elongated. If you feel unsteady, bend the left knee to lift out of the pose. Then turn your feet towards the original position in step 1, take a few breaths, and practise Triangle pose on the other side with the left leg extended.

CROW

This pose strengthens the arms, wrists, and shoulders and lubricates the joints, tendons, and ligaments of the upper body. The intense focus on balance strengthens the nervous system and gives excellent powers of concentration. Crow also encourages a feeling of inner balance and prepares the mind for meditation.

If you are new to Crow, put a folded blanket or firm pillow in front of your hands in case you tumble forwards.

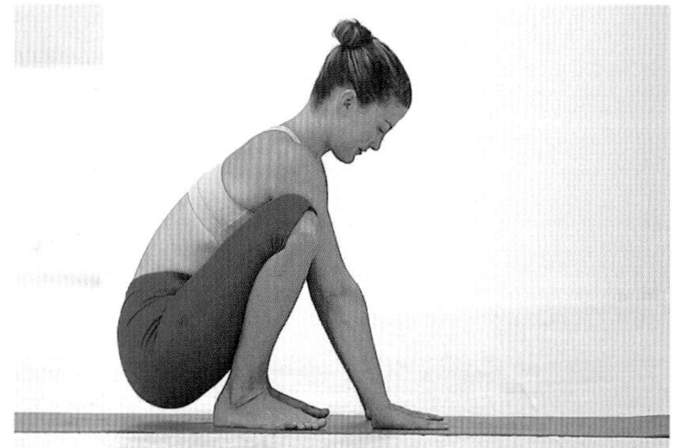

1 Come into a squatting position, with the feet flat on the ground and the arms between the knees. Place your palms flat on the ground and spread your fingers wide apart and turned slightly inwards, like the feet of a crow.

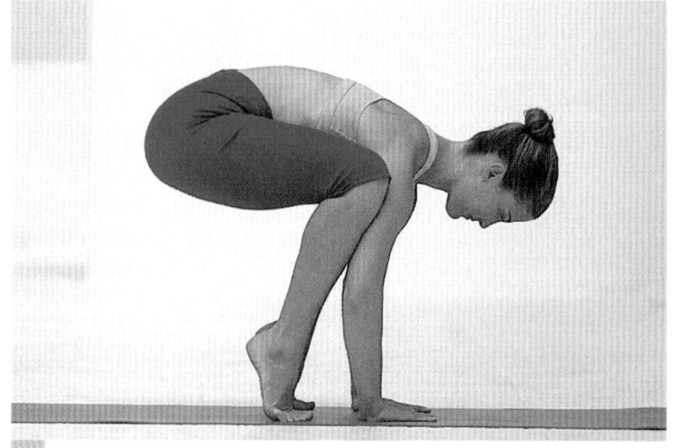

2 Bend your elbows outwards so that your upper arms can act as a support for your knees. Rise up onto the balls of your feet and rest your knees on each upper arm.

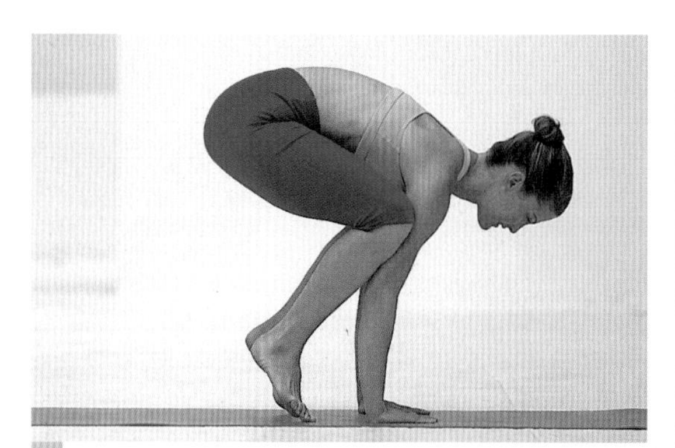

3 Keep your head facing forwards, with your eyes focused on a point a little way in front of you. Inhale deeply. Hold the breath as you gradually shift your weight forwards onto your hands so that your toes hardly touch the ground. Stay at this level until you can balance comfortably, or experiment by carefully lifting your toes off the ground for a few seconds at a time.

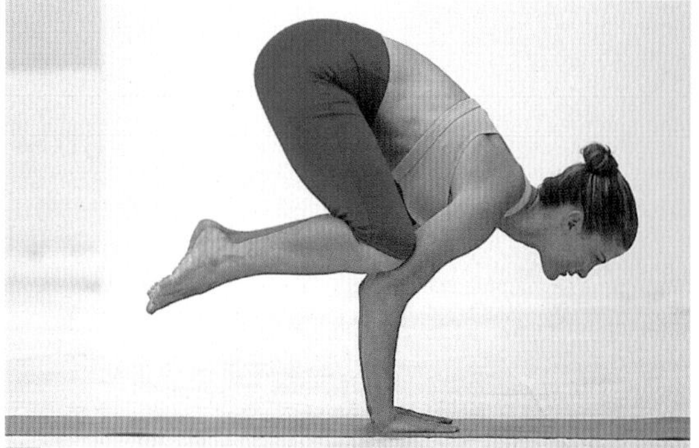

4 Keep your head up by focusing out in front of you and shift the balance of weight entirely onto the hands, slowly lifting the feet off the ground. If this proves difficult, try raising one foot and then the other. Ideally your knees are resting on the upper arms, and the lower legs are parallel to the ground with the feet relaxed. Breathe deeply and hold for as long as is comfortable.

YOGA FOR MENTAL AND EMOTIONAL BALANCE

This yoga set balances the pelvis and adjusts the navel area, which opens up nerve channels and builds pranic life energy. Strong backward bends and dynamic arm movements then encourage the pranic energy to flow through to higher chakras, activating the heart centre and bringing the mind into a state of equilibrium.

1 HIP CIRCLES

Hip circles bring flexibility to the pelvis since the lower spine and hips are adjusted and balanced in this movement. Mentally, this exercise gives you the spirit to keep going and not to give in.

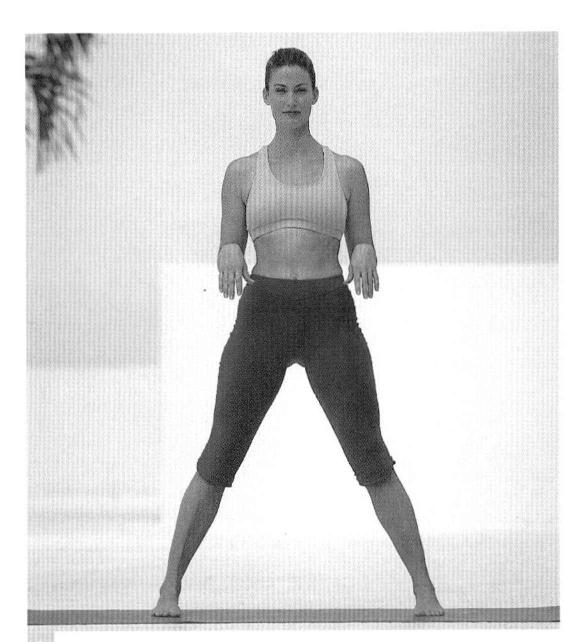

1 Stand tall, spreading the legs as wide apart as possible while maintaining your balance. Distribute your weight evenly across the soles of your feet. Keep your knees straight but not locked. Bring your elbows towards your sides, and bend them so that your forearms are more or less parallel to the ground and your hands are relaxed.

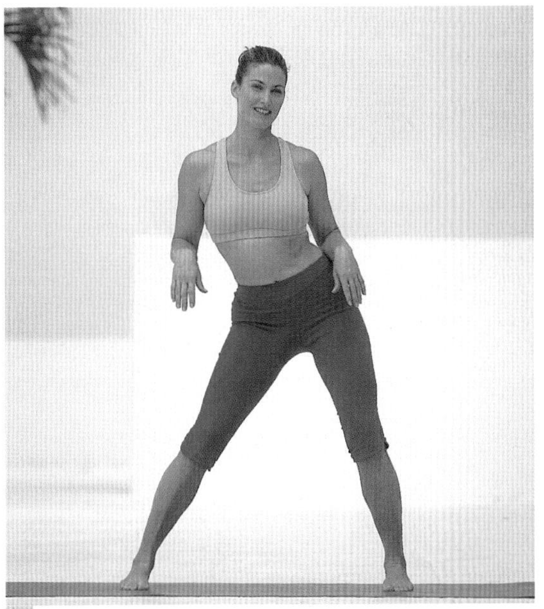

2 Begin to rotate your hips in large circles in one direction. Widen the circles as you continue for one minute. Breathe deeply as you circle. Then reverse the direction and repeat the movement for one more minute.

2 MIRACLE BEND

This pose activates the navel centre, which helps to give a woman the ability to find her inner security, balance her emotions, and release depression. It helps to process strong emotions and if practised with deep breathing, it can bring about a sense of calm.

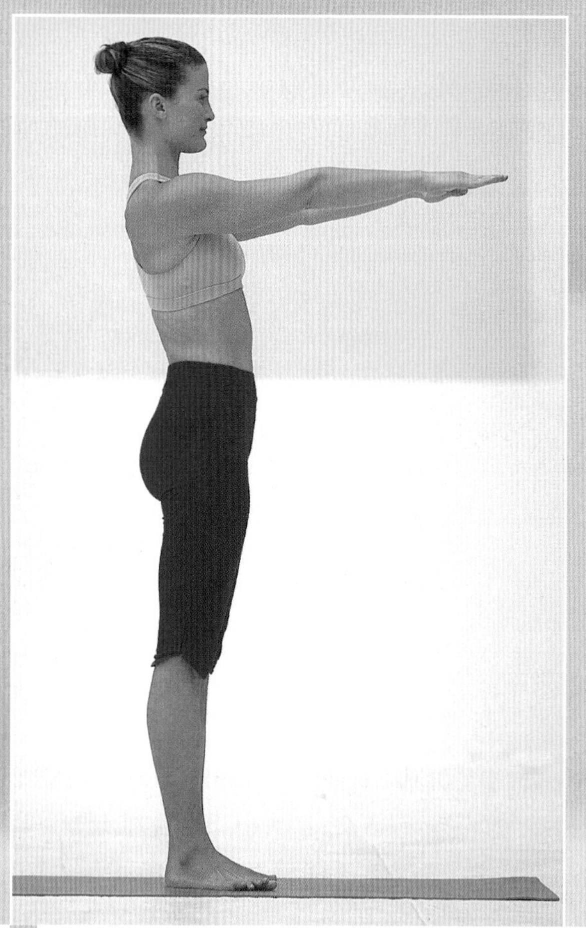

1 Stand with your heels together and your toes angled outwards for balance. Bring your arms straight out in front of you, with the hands close together and fingers straightened. The thumbs may be crossed over each other.

Use your breath and awareness to release tension in the upper back and neck

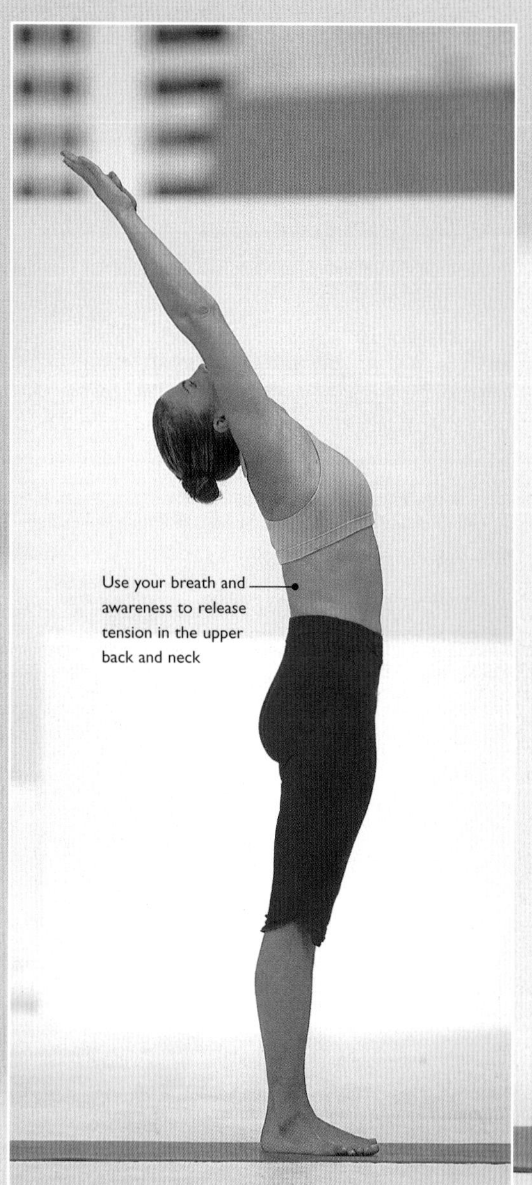

2 Begin to inhale deeply as you raise your extended arms upwards and backwards in a smooth, flowing motion. Your head and upper body follow your arms so that your arms, head, and upper body form an unbroken curve, lifted upwards and backwards as far as possible. Breathe deeply and slowly as you hold the position for 1–2 minutes.

Move as if in
slow motion
Take 30–45 seconds
to come fully forwards

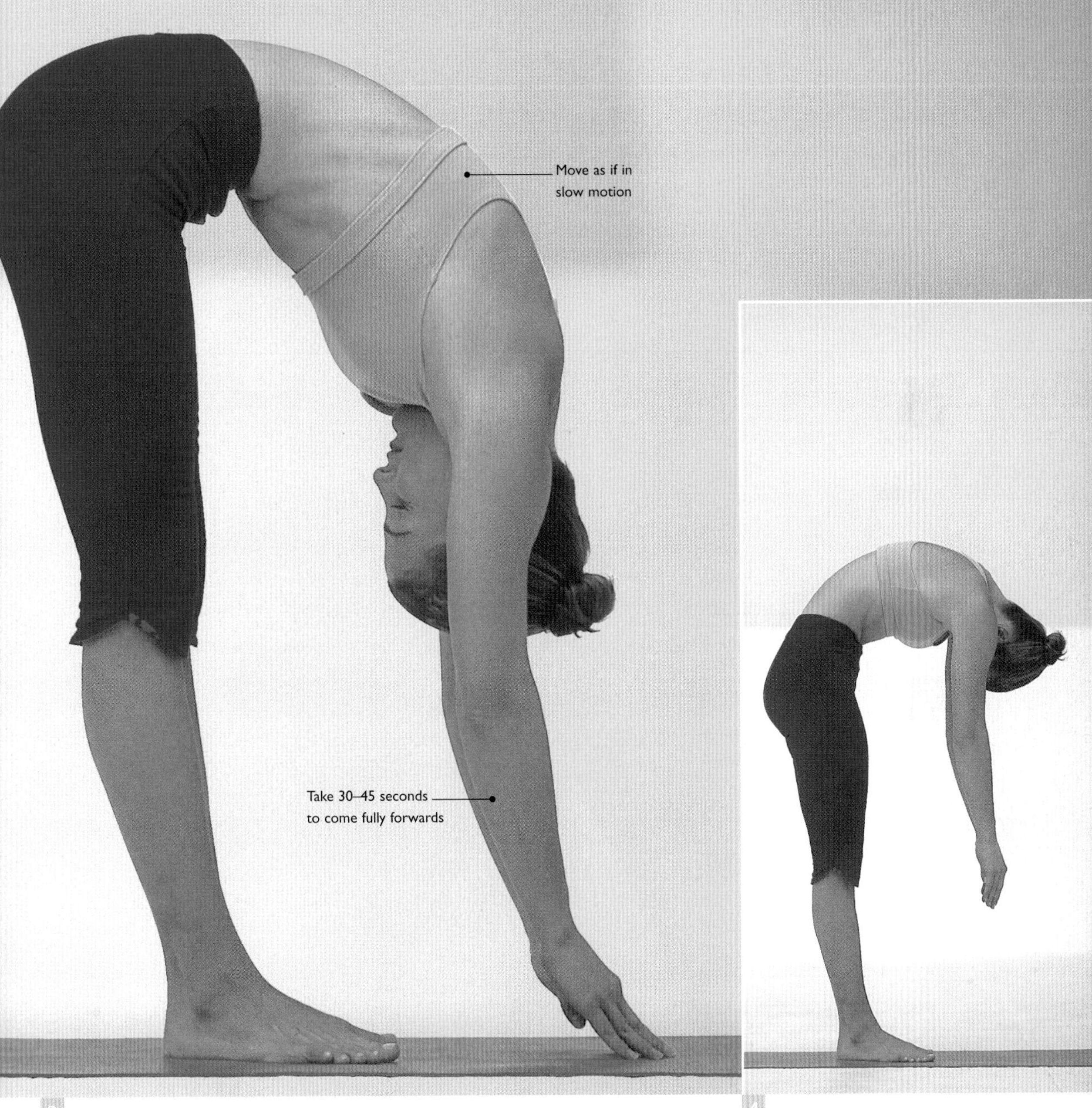

3 Exhale deeply and begin to slowly straighten your body and smoothly bend it forwards to your maximum capacity. Keep your arms and head moving together in an unbroken line. Then inhale, retain the breath within the rib cage, and for as long as possible begin to pump your navel, pressing it in towards your spine and releasing. Continue until you have to exhale, then do the same on the held exhalation. Inhale and continue this pumping pattern on the held inhalation and exhalation for 2 minutes.

4 Come out of the pose by rolling upwards at an unhurried pace while inhaling slowly and deeply. Uncurl one vertebra at a time in a slow, fluid motion.

3 ALTERNATE ARM CIRCLES

This exercise helps with stamina, clear thinking, and balance during menopause. Though there is no breathing pattern specified, you may want to inhale as you bend in one direction and exhale on the other.

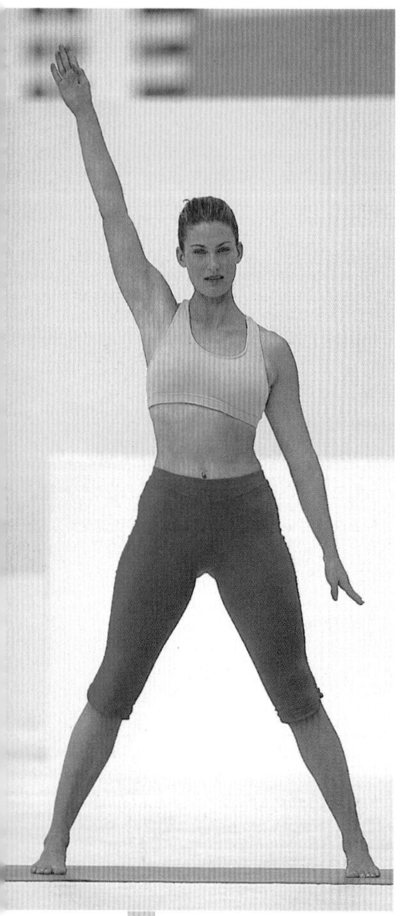

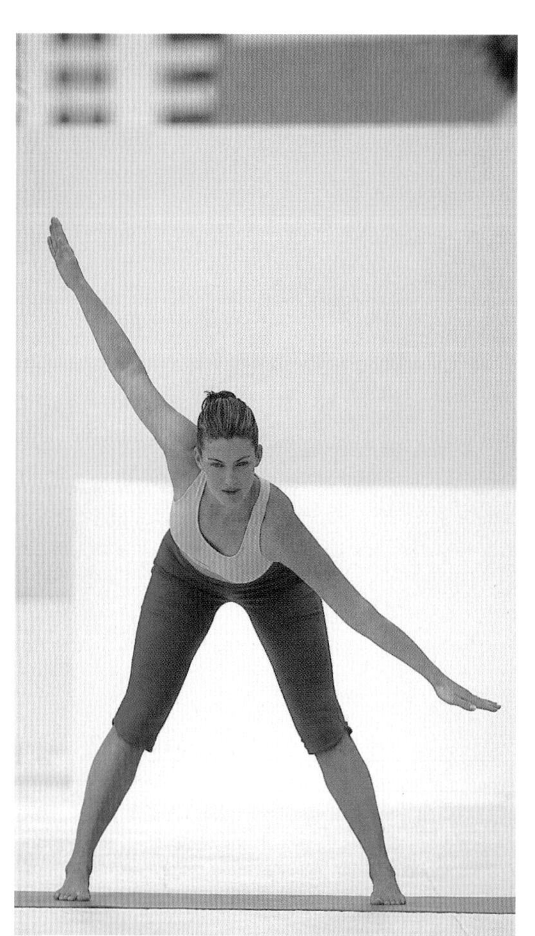

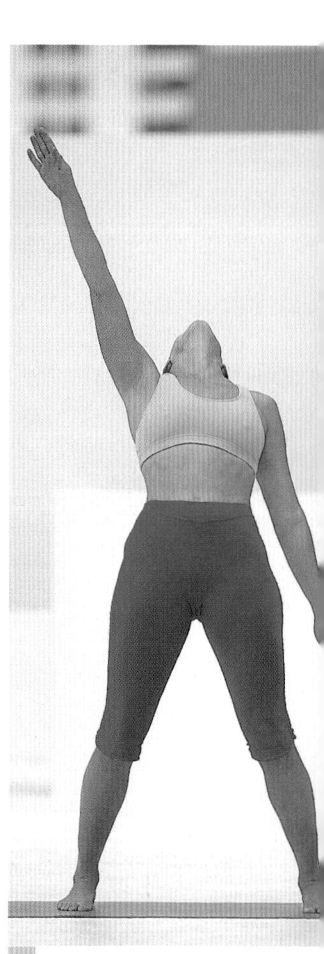

1 Stand with your feet 1m (3–4ft) apart. Straighten your arms and begin rotating them in backward circles, starting with one arm and then adding in the other. Your arms are positioned out to the sides as much as possible throughout.

2 Bend the torso forwards from the waist while continuing to move the arms in alternate circles. When you have bent forwards halfway, begin to straighten up again as you circle.

3 Without breaking the movement, bend back halfway, or as far as possible. The rhythm is around 15 seconds for a complete cycle of forward and backward bends. Keep circling the arms the entire time as you continue for 1–2 minutes.

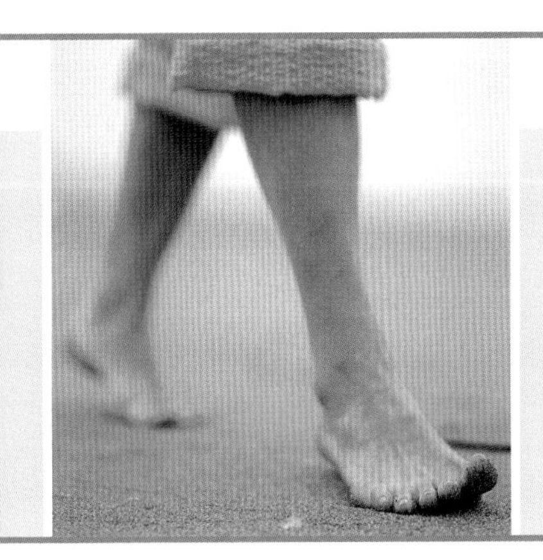

WALKING IN NATURE

Walking on the pads of your feet in natural environments opens the meridian points in the feet that connect to your spine, heart and lungs, and also helps to relax your mind. Let your feet feel the healing effects of surfaces such as soft sand and cool grass. Slightly rounded surfaces, for example, small, round bits of gravel or stone, are stimulating to the meridian points. Allow your feet to spread open as you walk in a rolling motion off the pads of your feet.

MEDITATION TO DEAL WITH LIFE

This meditation totally recharges you, and is an antidote to depression. It gives you the capacity and caliber to deal with life as it is. It strengthens your pranic life energy, your internal energy system for making optimum use of the vital life force of the breath. When the prana flows through the nadis, or energy pathways, the cells of the body come alive with vitality and toxins are released.

Sit in Easy pose (p.19) *with a straight spine. Extend your arms out straight in front of you, slightly below shoulder level and parallel to the ground. Close your right hand into a fist. Wrap your left hand around the right so that the fingers of the left hand are over the knuckles of the right fist. The heels of the hands touch each other. Straighten the thumbs, extending them up so that the sides are touching. Focus your eyes so that you gaze at your thumbs. Inhale for five seconds, then exhale for five seconds. Exhale completely and hold the breath out for 15 seconds. Then inhale and continue the pattern. Do not retain the inhalation; suspend the breath out of the body on the exhale only.*

Start with 3–5 minutes of this powerful breathing meditation. Build the time of this meditation gradually to 11 minutes. Eventually you can work up to holding the breath out longer, up to a maximum of a full minute, but always increase the time slowly and moderately according to your natural capability.

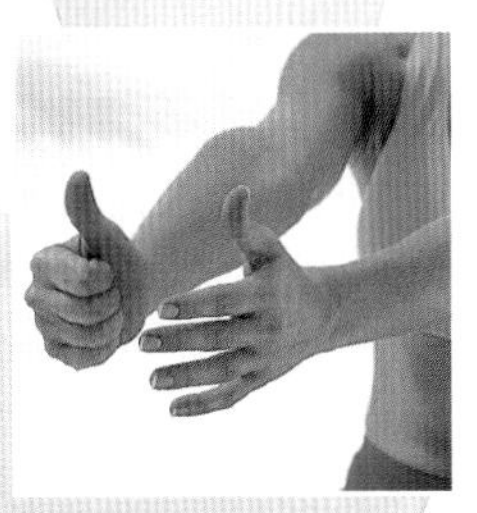

Wrap fingers around fist

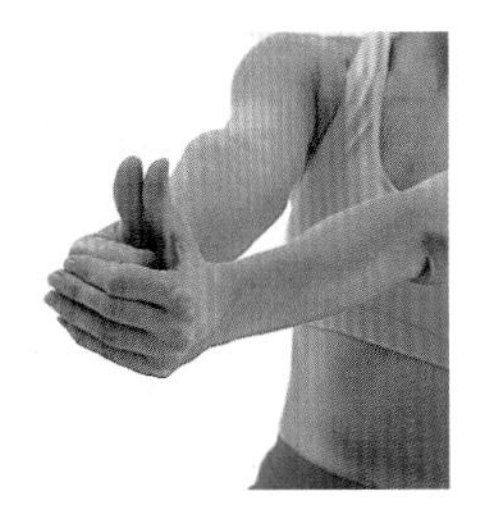

Thumbs should touch

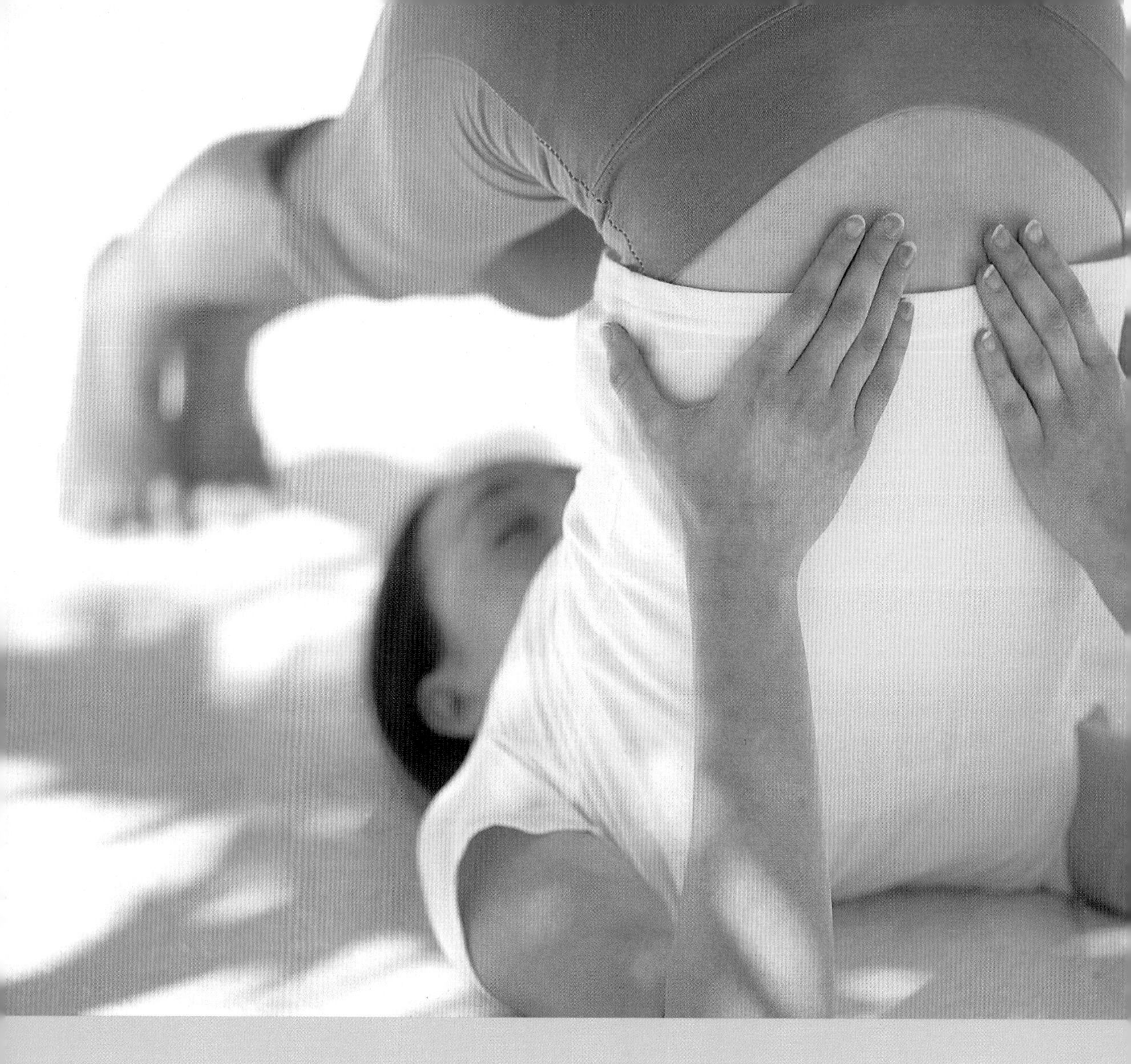

MONTHLY CYCLE

Throughout history, women have viewed the menstrual cycle as everything from an annoyance to "The Curse".

However, this special time is referred to as a woman's "moon cycle" in some indigenous cultures. Once a month a woman will set aside her usual roles of caregiver, counsellor, and innovator to enter a phase of self-nurturing retreat and inner communion with the "divine feminine" for the duration of her menstrual cycle.

Here you will have the same opportunity for meditative retreat using specially selected yoga exercises. You will also find yoga that strengthens your reproductive health so that you may enjoy being a woman in every way.

DURING A CYCLE

As we shed the old during menstruation and prepare for a new monthly cycle, we feel the instinct to let go to make room for the new. Folding the body forwards is a natural gesture of letting go and is usually accompanied by deep, extended exhalations. Allow the natural force of gravity to help you relax forwards in these poses especially for the menstrual cycle.

Gain energy and avoid cramping during the first few days of menstruation by eating a handful of unpeeled almonds, sautéed until slightly browned and with a little honey to taste.

FOLDED BUTTERFLY

This pose stretches and strengthens the lower back and hip areas. The forward stretch at the end is soothing to the ovaries and abdomen and helps to relieve lower back pain during menstruation.

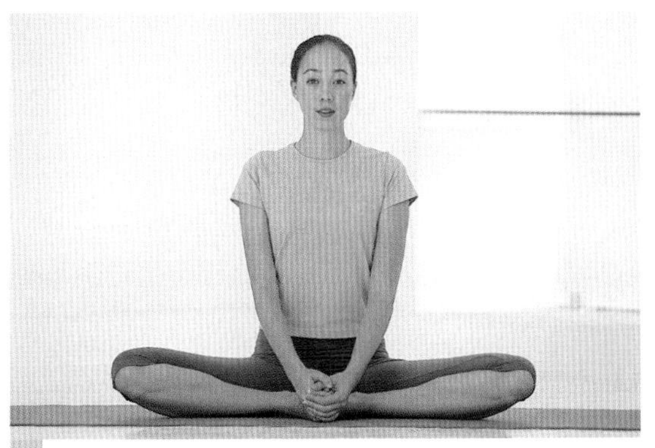

1 Sitting in Easy pose, bring the soles of the feet together in front of you, as close to your body as is comfortable.

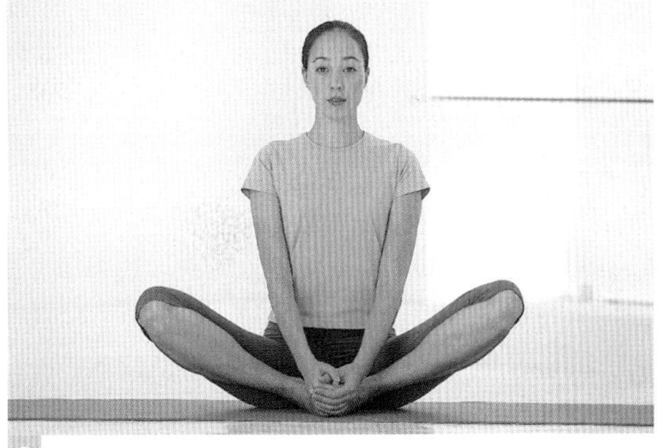

2 Hold onto your feet and flap your knees for 30 seconds to relax your hips.

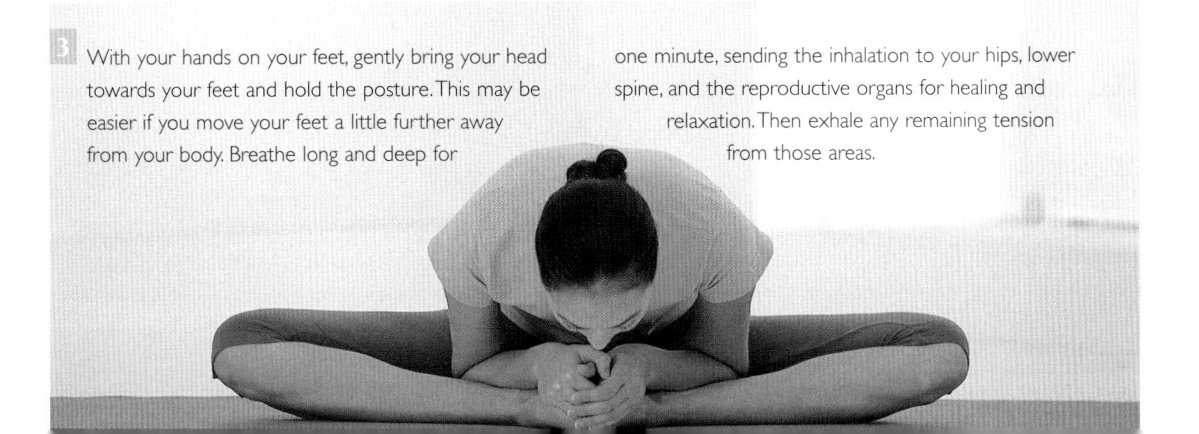

3 With your hands on your feet, gently bring your head towards your feet and hold the posture. This may be easier if you move your feet a little further away from your body. Breathe long and deep for one minute, sending the inhalation to your hips, lower spine, and the reproductive organs for healing and relaxation. Then exhale any remaining tension from those areas.

EXTENDED CHILD'S POSE

Extended Child's pose relieves tension from the ovaries and revitalizes the hormonal system, so it is excellent for the premenstrual time as well as during menstruation. Practising regular Child's pose is also excellent for releasing abdominal and reproductive tension.

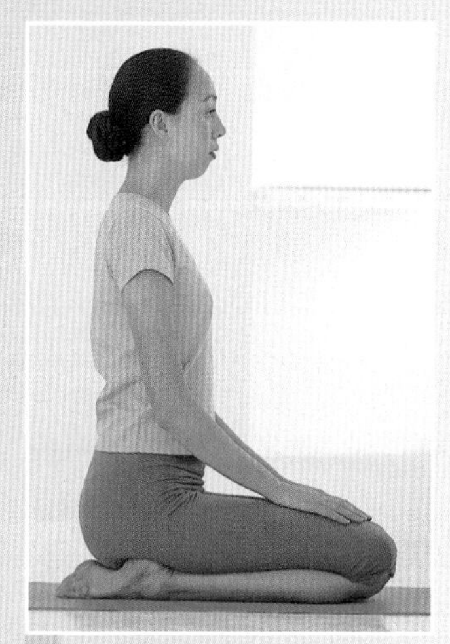

1 Sit on your heels in Rock pose *(p.20)* with your spine straight.

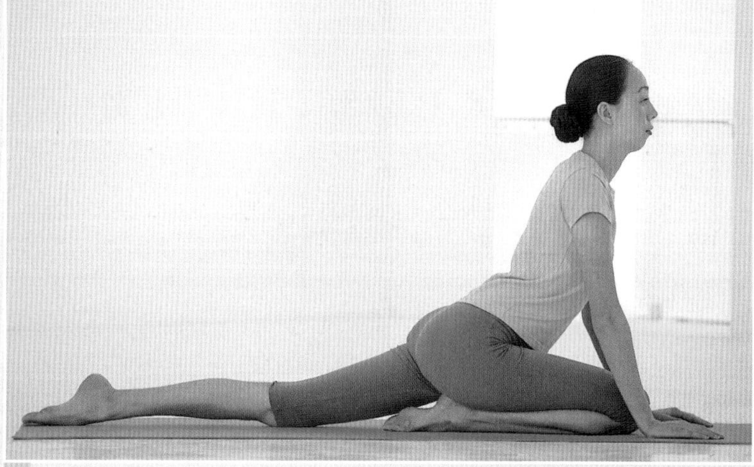

2 Place your hands on the ground in front of your knees. Shift your weight forwards onto your hands. Extend one leg straight out behind you, with the top of the foot resting on the ground.

Refrain from cold showers, Body Locks, inverted poses (like Shoulderstand), back-bending poses (like Bow), and abdominal poses (like Stretch) during a period. Do only light Breath of Fire.

3 Bring your forehead to the ground and relax your arms by your sides with your palms facing up. Allow your entire body to relax. Your hands will naturally curl slightly. Allow your shoulders to drop forwards. Feel your hips and buttocks relax and spread, and drop all tension from your straightened leg. Breathe long and deep for 1–3 minutes, then switch legs by supporting your body with your forearms as you sit up slowly and come back to position 1.

MARYANN'S STORY (USA)

It was always the same. About two and a half weeks into my menstrual cycle, I would wake up and feel a familiar sense of depression creeping in on me. I'd start to feel unsure of myself, and become anxious and a little irritable. As the days moved slowly on, the symptoms would increase in intensity. Some months were so bad that when it was finally over – the day my period arrived – I would feel as if I had finally crawled out of a dark hole.

Feeling that I could not continue to live in this way, I increased my exercise and calcium intake without a marked change. In desperation I sought the help of my doctor. I've never been comfortable taking medication, but I couldn't see another solution. I remember staring at the pills in my hands – their bright colours full of the promise of chasing away the dark moods. As I was due to start taking them at the beginning of my next cycle, I put them back in my medicine cabinet and left for my Hatha Yoga class, which I had started a few months before. It was day 22 and PMT was raging through my body. Yet as I rode home from my yoga class, I began to notice the familiar calmness I always felt afterwards. I wondered at the way yoga managed to reach through even the haze of PMT. I felt surprisingly good the next day, too. When I awoke the day after, and the familiar feelings began to return, I decided to pull out my mat and do some yoga. I continued to do yoga every morning through the rest of that cycle, and beyond.

I crawled out of my last dark PMT hole 11 months ago. I do yoga and a short meditation every day. I still experience mild symptoms of PMT, but I handle it differently. I notice that I lack confidence and am not very willing to start something new. But I have also learnt to sit with those feelings and take a break from chasing life. Even the migraine headaches I experienced at the end of my cycle are gone. Needless to say I am very grateful for yoga in my life.

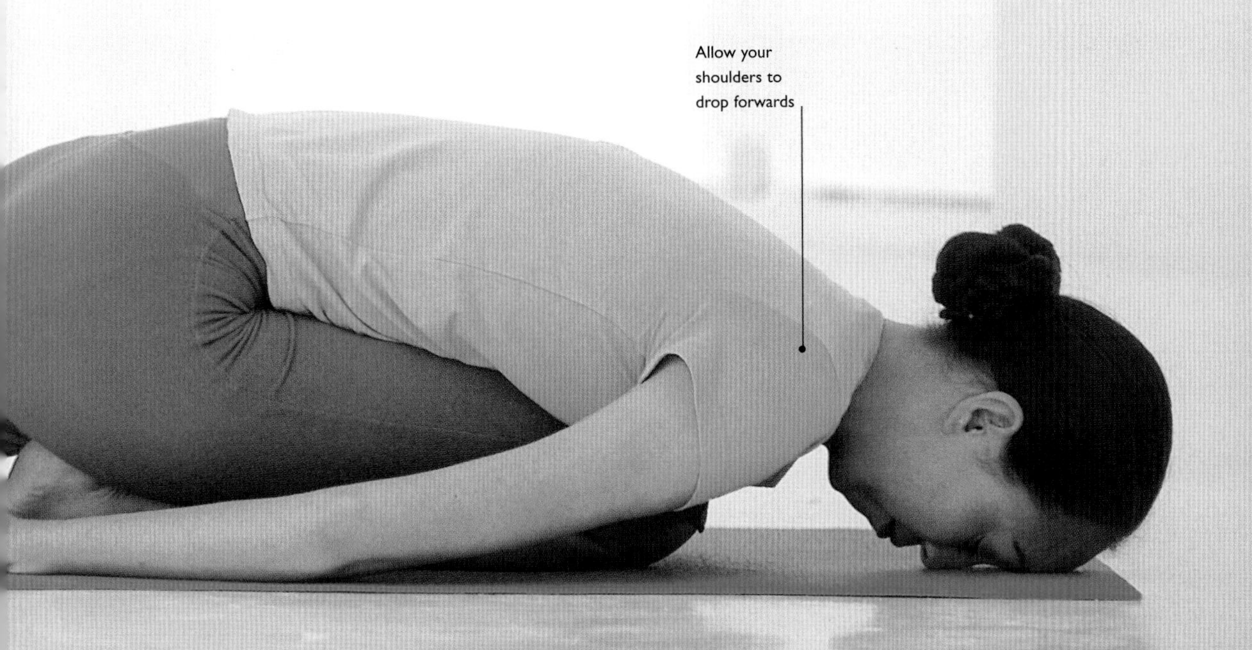

REPRODUCTIVE HEALTH

The following two poses build reproductive and hormonal health. Although they may not be comfortable to practise during menstruation, they can be practised at all other times of the month, either together or individually.

GINGER TEA

At once calming to the nerves and energizing to the body and mind, ginger tea is good at any time, and especially helpful for women during their monthly menses.

Boil 4–6 thin slices of fresh unpeeled ginger root in 450ml (¾ pint) water. Boil for about 20 minutes until the water is light brown in colour. Add a dash of fresh lemon juice and a little honey to taste, if liked.

PLOUGH

Plough is said to benefit the entire body, particularly thyroid function and circulation. The back, shoulder and arm muscles are stretched and strengthened, too. The pose provides an inverted gravitational pull that suspends and relaxes all your internal organs, including your reproductive organs. Afterwards, be sure to rest on your back for a minute or two with the legs out straight, or with a firm pillow under the knees. If your feet do not easily reach the ground in Plough, position yourself so that they rest against a wall. To relieve pressure from the neck, use a prop *(p.52)*.

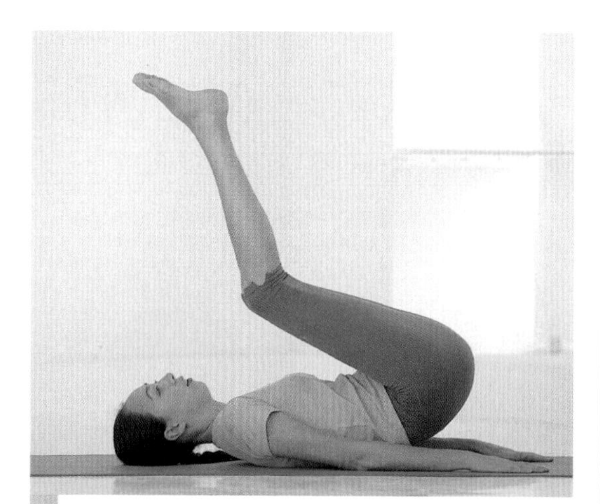

1 Lie on your back, your arms at your sides and palms facing downwards. Using your abdominal muscles and the pressure of your arms against the ground, raise your legs and buttocks up.

Move your hands further up your back to stretch more deeply

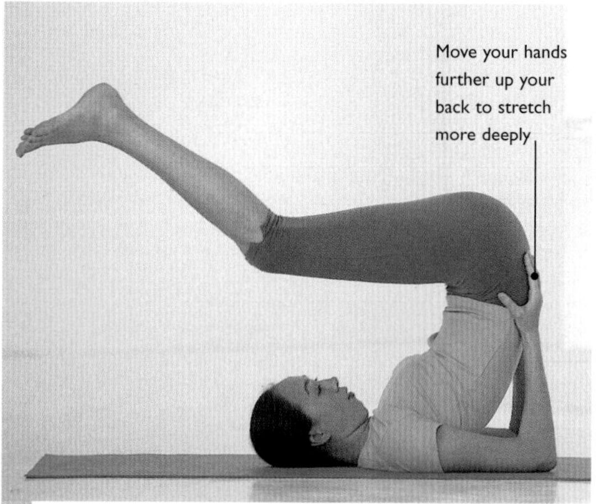

2 Lift your buttocks and lower back off the ground while supporting your back with your hands, which are positioned at the waist. Rest your elbows firmly on the ground. Bring your legs overhead as you come up onto your upper back and shoulders. Your chin will be close to your chest.

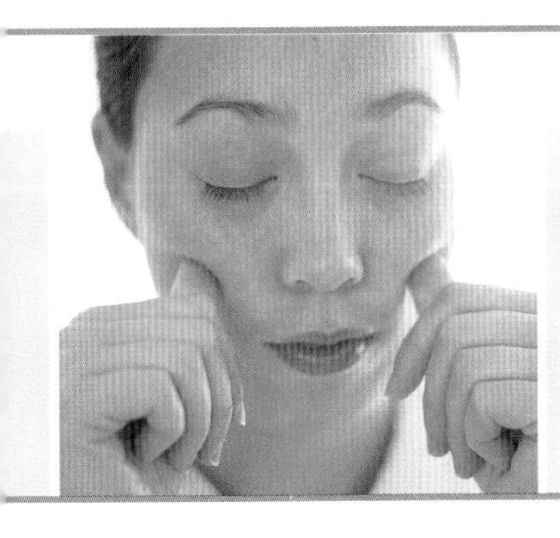

CHEEK PRESS

Using your thumbs, find the indentation directly under your cheekbones. Press strongly and hold in each position for three breaths. This releases facial tension. For a deeper release of tension, begin to press all along that ridge, massaging the muscle under the cheekbones from the inside area close to your nose to the outer edge where it meets your jaw.

3 Straighten your legs and, if possible without straining, bring your feet to the ground behind your head. Once you feel stable in this position, bring your hands to the ground beside you with your palms facing downwards. Relax and breathe for 1–3 minutes.

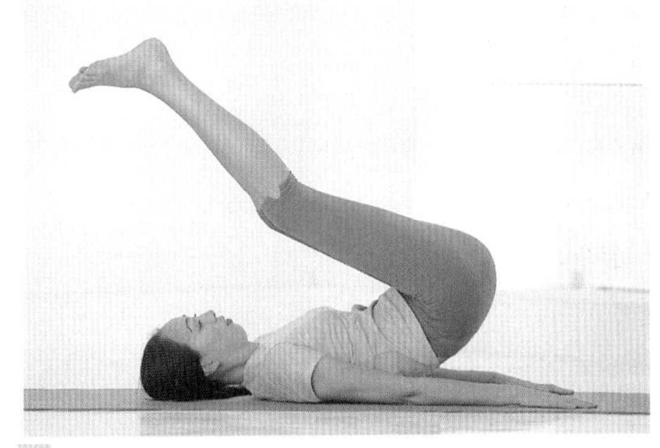

4 Roll out of this position slowly by exhaling and rolling your spine down, vertebra by vertebra, using your hands on the ground for support.

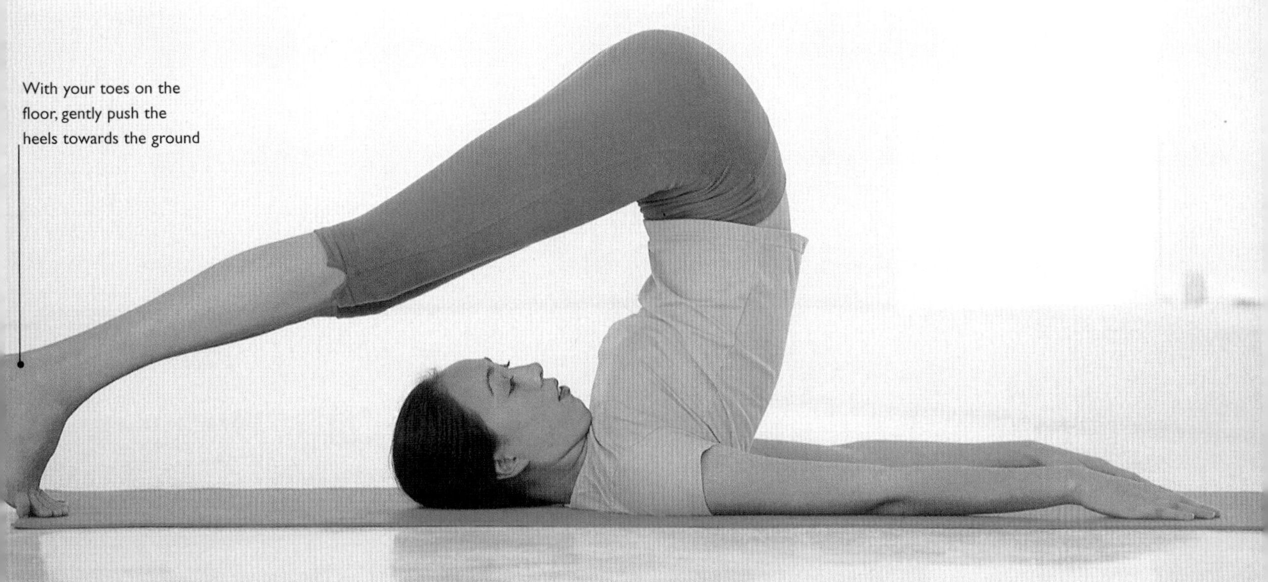

With your toes on the floor, gently push the heels towards the ground

COBRA

This pose increases flexibility and rejuvenates the spinal nerves. Combined with deep breathing or Breath of Fire *(p.24)*, it massages and expands the rib cage. Cobra is particularly helpful in relieving tension in the ovaries and uterus, often the cause of menstrual problems. Cobra stimulates the flow of pranic energy in the body and awakens the higher chakras.

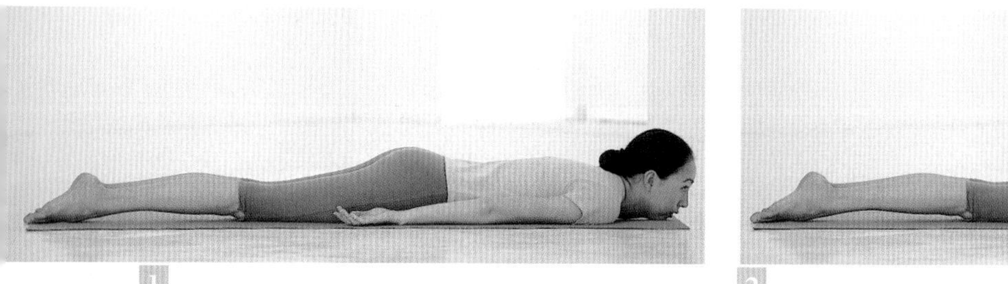

1 Lie down on your front with your arms resting at your sides and your chin on the ground. Take a deep breath.

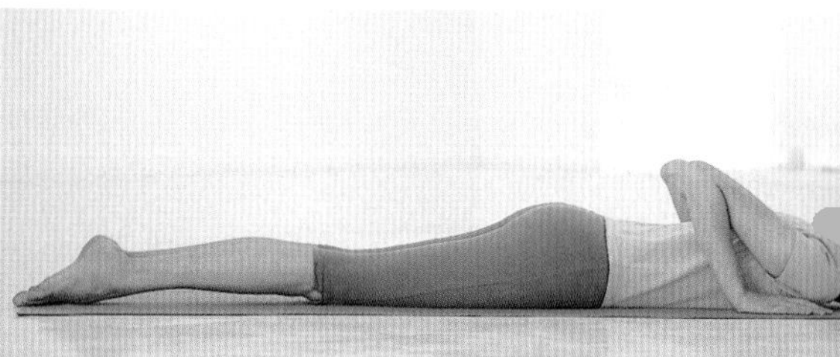

2 Keeping your lower body relaxed, place your hands on the ground under your shoulders to prepare for Cobra.

3 Lead with the head and chest and curve your spine up and back into Cobra as you inhale. Exhale and relax more deeply into Cobra. Continue holding the posture for 1–3 minutes with deep breathing or Breath of Fire. Then inhale deeply, exhale, and slowly lower the chest down, then the head. Rest for a few breaths with your arms at your sides and your head turned to one side.

Roll the body up into Cobra rather than using the arms to push the body up
Tuck the elbow into your sides bend them to k the shoulders relaxed downw

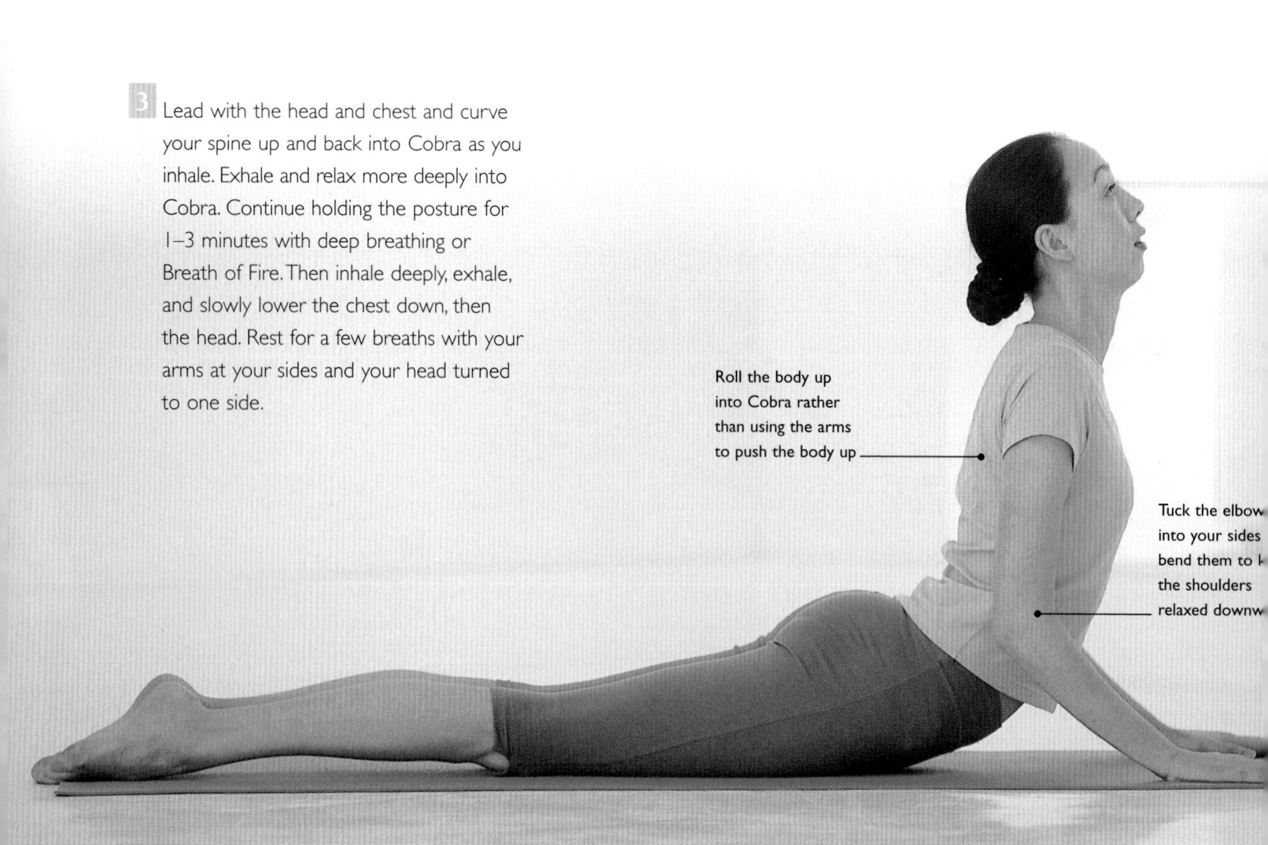

MEDITATION TO BALANCE THE MENSTRUAL CYCLE

An erratic menstrual cycle can be regulated through a steady practice of this meditation. Negative thought patterns are released, and in their place comes mental clarity, positivity, and a radiant aura. This breath meditation uses the "broken breath" technique. The inhalation is broken into four equal sections, while the exhale is one long breath. In yogic teachings this type of breathing pattern is used to heal oneself and break depression.

On a physical level, the positive attitude of this four-part breathing meditation rejuvenates the pituitary and pineal glands, which are crucial for the emotional and physical health and wellbeing of the whole person. All other body systems rely on the "ductless glands" of the endocrine system since they regulate the hormones that keep you young, healthy, and mentally stable.

1 *Sit in Easy pose with your hands resting on your knees, palms facing upwards. You will be breaking the inhalation into four equal parts. Each part will be a short "sniff", and you will feel your navel press slightly inwards on each of the sniffs if you are practising it correctly. On each sniff, press your thumb and one of your fingers as follows:*
On the first sniff, press your thumb and first finger as you meditate on the sound Sa.

On the second, press your thumb and second finger as you meditate on the sound Ta.

On the third, press your thumb and third finger as you meditate on the sound Na.

And on the fourth and final sniff, press your thumb and little finger as you meditate on the sound Ma.

2 *Then exhale in one long stroke. Continue with the four-part inhalation, meditating on* Sa Ta Na Ma *for three minutes.*

The length of time for this meditation may be increased by one minute daily, up to seven minutes, then practise for a week or more at seven minutes, then increase again by a minute per day. The maximum time for this powerful meditation is 31 minutes.

For a complete explanation of the Sa Ta Na Ma *meditation* *see page 97.*

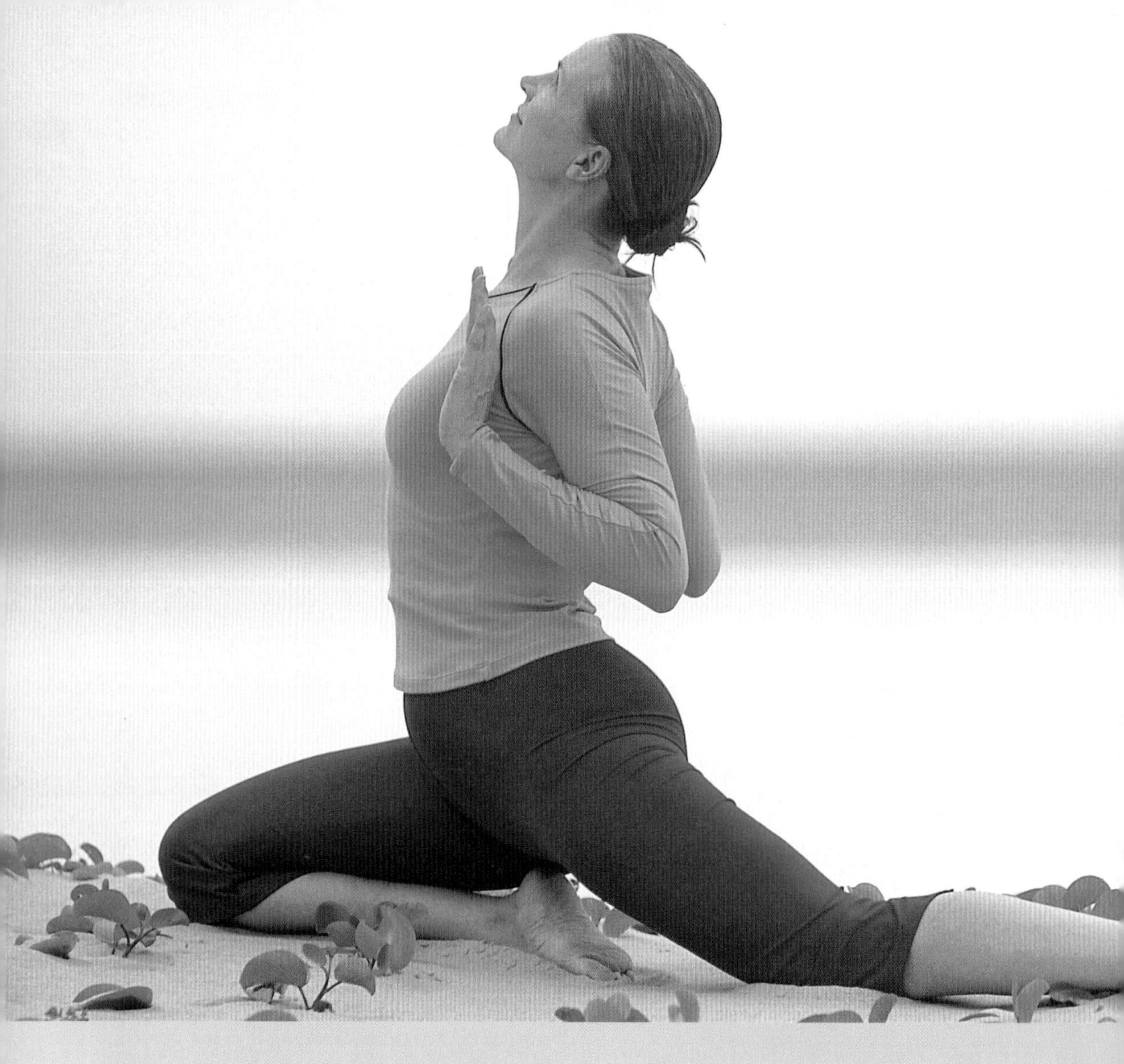

EASING INTO MENOPAUSE

With the right combination of attitude and holistic lifestyle – a healthy plant-based diet, daily yoga and meditation, supplements and herbs, (as well as hormone replacement therapy if needed) – menopause can be, dare I say it, a blessing! Hearing these words, those of you who are going through nightmarish symptoms of hot flushes, long nights of erratic sleep, and irritability bordering on rage, may be heading towards that point at this very moment!

Every woman's experience is unique; there are as many different stories about menopause as there are women. Still, a 1998 Gallup survey showed that more than half of American women between the ages of 50 and 65 felt happiest and most fulfilled at this stage of life.

I believe that once the physical and emotional challenges become manageable, many women make a miraculous discovery about menopause – that it heralds a new consciousness, a new way of looking at life, and even, if one is brave and bold, a new life itself. Menopause gives us cause to stop in our well-worn tracks and ask, "What am I all about? What do I really want? What calls to me?"

Dr Christiane Northrup draws upon her own personal experience in her book, *The Wisdom of Menopause*, which reveals the difficult and liberating process of life change that is initiated through menopause. These changes can be wonderfully life-affirming, a time of personal empowerment and positive energy. As Dr Northrup writes: *"Our brains are changing. A woman's thoughts, her ability to focus, and the amount of fuel going to the intuitive centres in the temporal lobes of her brain all are plugged into, and affected by, the circuits being rewired. After working with thousands of women who are going through this process, as well as experiencing it myself, I can say with great assurance that menopause is an exciting developmental stage – one that, when participated in consciously, holds enormous promise for transforming and healing our bodies, minds, and spirits at the deepest levels."*

Body, mind, and spirit is what yoga is all about. Although all yoga postures and exercises are helpful for smoothing out the rough edges of menopause, here the focus will particularly spotlight hormonal balance, supporting the nervous system, and reproductive health, and will end with a meditation to balance the emotions and bring the mind to a state of equilibrium and elevation.

AUDREY HEPBURN'S "BEAUTY TIPS"

✻ *For attractive lips, speak words of kindness.*

✻ *For lovely eyes, seek out the good in people.*

✻ *For a slim figure, share your food with the hungry.*

✻ *For beautiful hair, let a child run their fingers through it once a day.*

✻ *For poise, walk in the knowledge that you never walk alone.*

✻ *People, even more than things, have to be restored, revived, reclaimed and redeemed; never throw out anyone.*

✻ *Remember, if you ever need a helping hand, you'll find one at the end of each of your arms. As you grow older, you will discover that you have two hands, one for helping yourself, the other for helping others.*

✻ *The beauty of a woman is not in the clothes she wears, the figure that she carries, or the way she combs her hair. The beauty of a woman must be seen in her eyes, because that is the doorway to her heart, the place where love resides.*

✻ *The beauty of a woman is not in a facial mode, but the true beauty in a woman is reflected in her soul. It is the caring that she lovingly gives, and the passion that she shows.*

✻ *The beauty of a woman grows with the passing years.*

SUPPORT FOR GOOD MENOPAUSAL HEALTH

This group of poses can help to reduce many of the most common symptoms of menopause, such as hot flushes, mood swings, undue weight gain, or sleeplessness. They particularly rejuvenate the reproductive organs and stimulate the proper functioning of the endocrine system. They can each be practised with either deep breathing or Breath of Fire. Feel free to practise them together or individually.

BANANA SHAKE

Bananas, one of nature's perfect foods, are especially good for women as they contain potassium and magnesium – minerals that women thrive on. Freeze ripe bananas with or without skins until you need them. Run hot water over the skins first to remove them easily.

Blend together 2 frozen bananas and 300ml (½ pint) organic dairy or non-dairy milk until smooth and creamy.

FISH POSE

This pose opens the hips and pelvis and revitalizes the digestive and reproductive areas. If needed, place several folded blankets or a firm pillow or bolster behind your back before lying down. Be sure to support your neck with a rolled towel or small pillow.

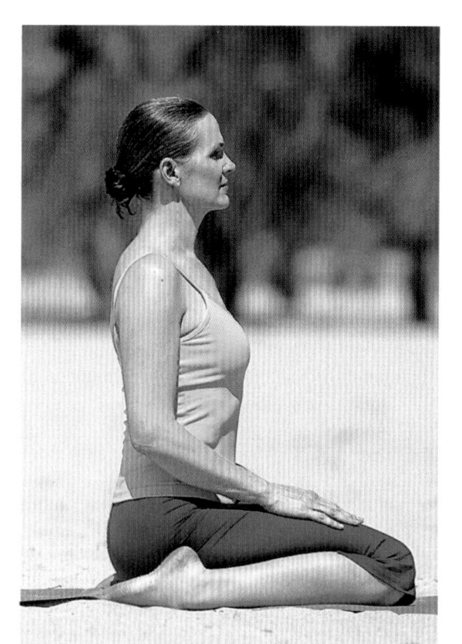

1 Sit between or on your heels. If your heels feel over-pressured, place a rolled towel or pillow between your thighs and calves.

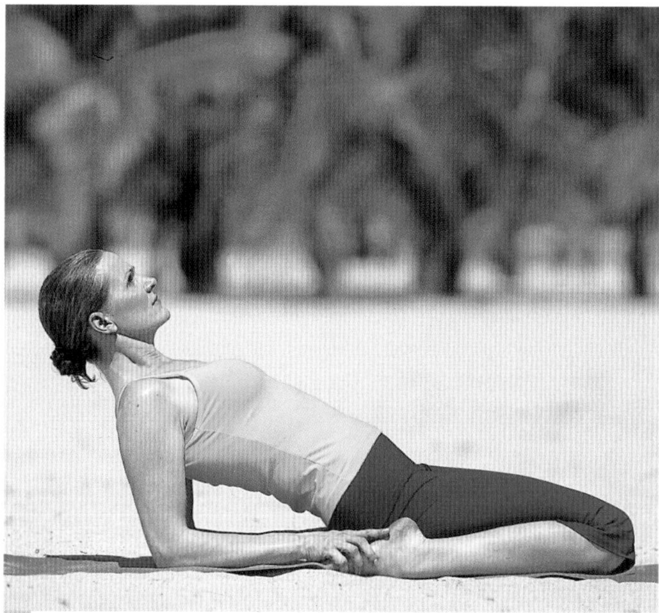

2 Bring your elbows down to the ground behind you, lean back, and ease yourself into a lying position, with your hands grasping the soles of your feet. Take care not to strain the neck.

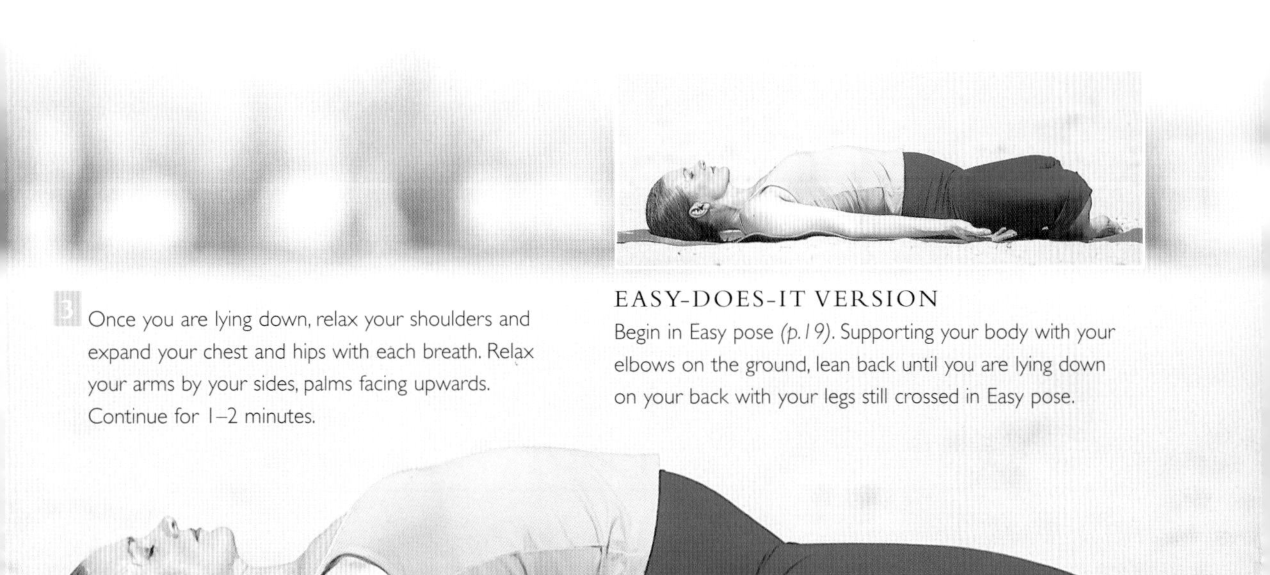

3 Once you are lying down, relax your shoulders and expand your chest and hips with each breath. Relax your arms by your sides, palms facing upwards. Continue for 1–2 minutes.

EASY-DOES-IT VERSION

Begin in Easy pose *(p.19)*. Supporting your body with your elbows on the ground, lean back until you are lying down on your back with your legs still crossed in Easy pose.

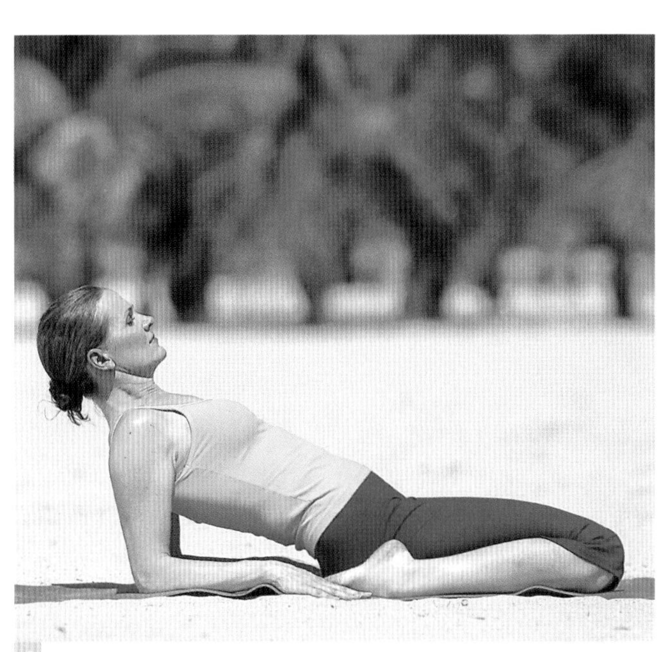

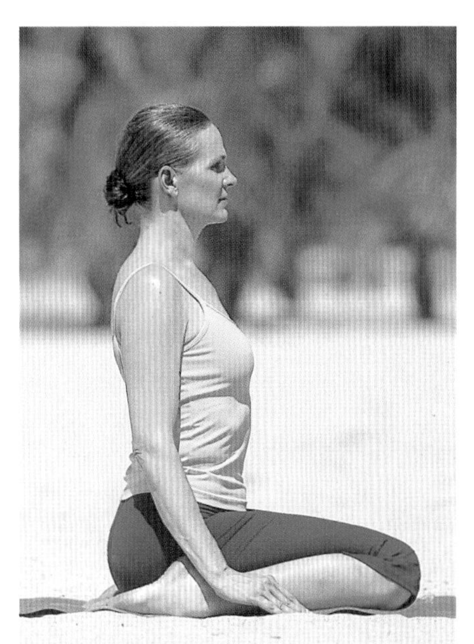

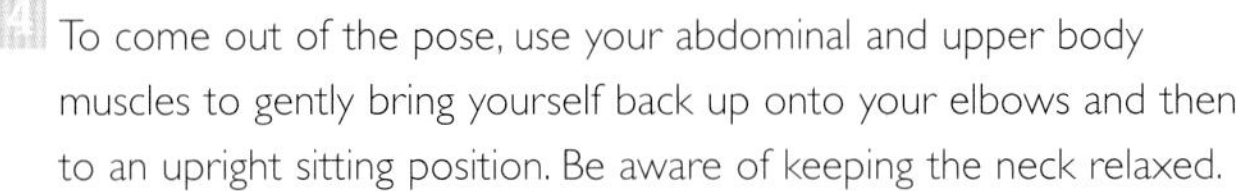

4 To come out of the pose, use your abdominal and upper body muscles to gently bring yourself back up onto your elbows and then to an upright sitting position. Be aware of keeping the neck relaxed.

5 Sit up straight and release your legs. Then stretch your legs out and enjoy a Forward Bend *(p.73)* for a few seconds.

DOWNWARD FACING DOG

With regular practice, Downward Facing Dog rejuvenates your whole body. An inverted pose, it allows for the reversed flow of gravity and increases the flow of blood to the head and heart. It reduces stiffness in the shoulders, legs, and heels, and makes the legs strong and agile for walking and running. If practised regularly, it can help check heavy menstrual flow and help prevent hot flushes during menopause. If you have low blood pressure, come out of the position gradually to avoid dizziness. This pose is easier to do on a non-slip mat.

Beginners may use a bolster to support the head. To facilitate this pose without strain to the legs and feet, use a prop such as a block of wood under each hand to shorten the distance between the hands and the feet.

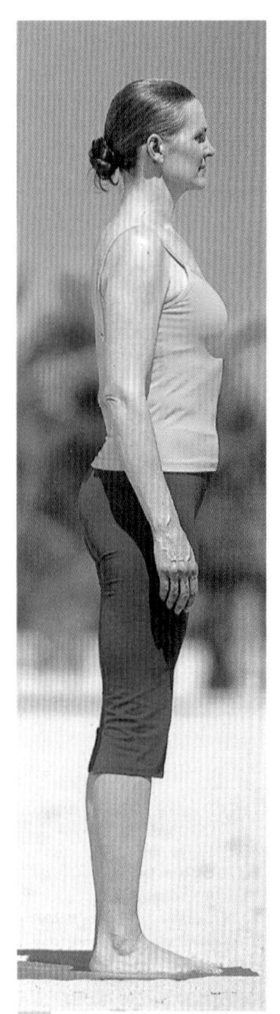

1 Stand up straight at the front edge of your mat, your arms at your sides.

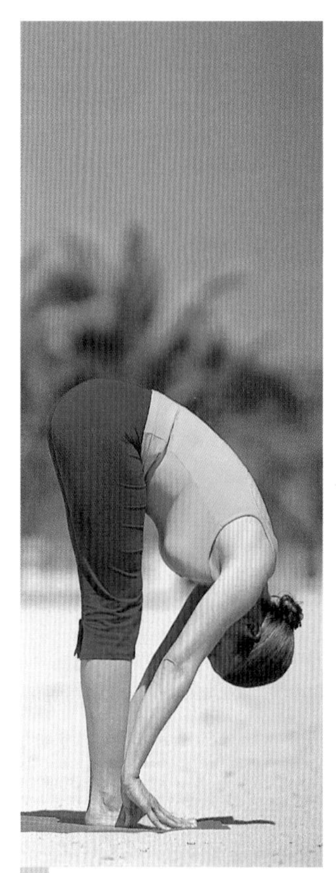

2 Exhale and bend over at the waist, placing your hands on the ground beside your feet. If your hands do not reach the ground easily, bend your knees.

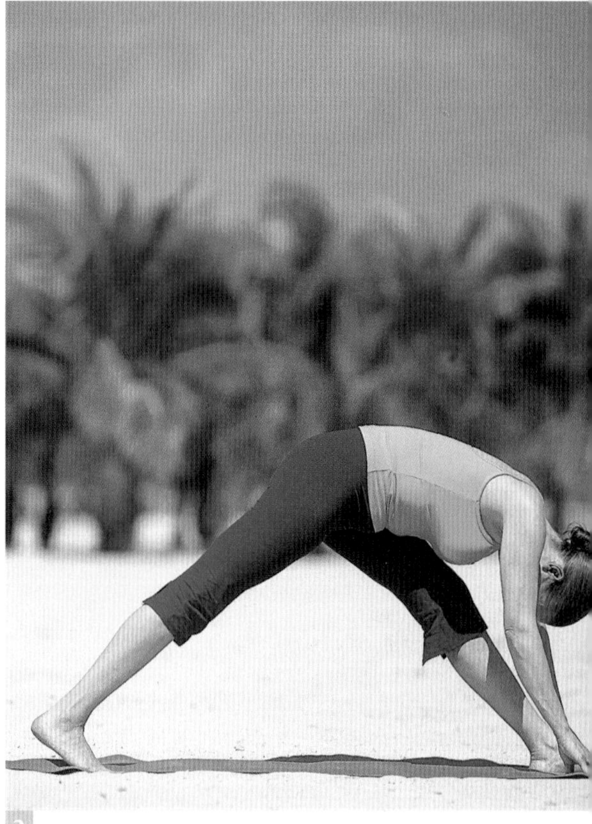

3 As you inhale, step back with one foot so that your foot is approximately 1m (3ft) away from your hands. Step back with the other foot so that it aligns with the first foot. Both hands and feet are now about 1m (3ft) apart.

Your head is pressed downwards, aligning with your arms
Your weight is evenly distributed between your hands and feet

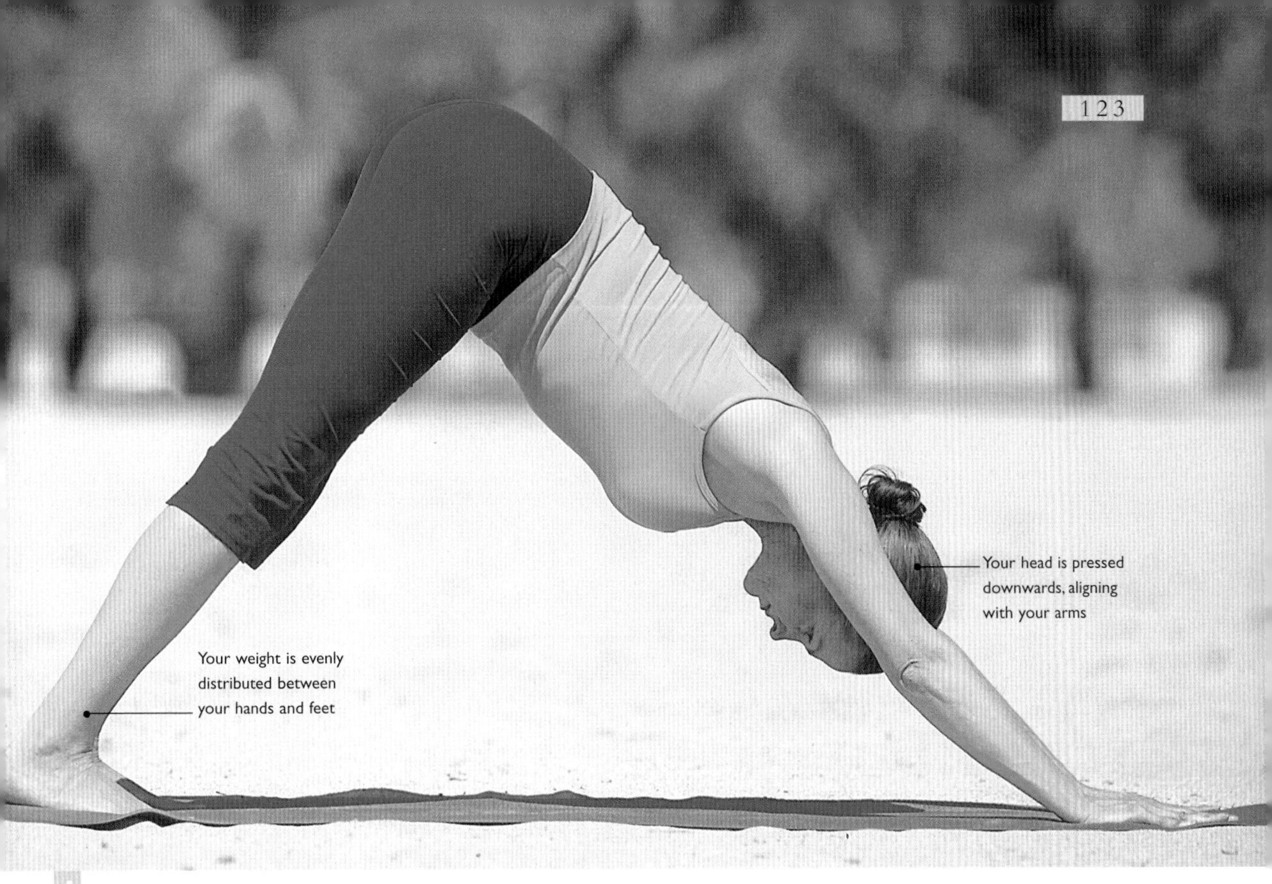

4 Position your right leg so that it is in line with your right arm, and your left leg is in line with your left arm. Stretch and open your fingers and toes. Feel the stretch from your palms to your heels. Move your torso towards your legs. Keep your hips lifted and stretched upwards and backwards. If possible, stretch your heels down to the ground. Slightly lower the crown of your head towards the ground. Continue stretching in this position for 1–2 minutes.

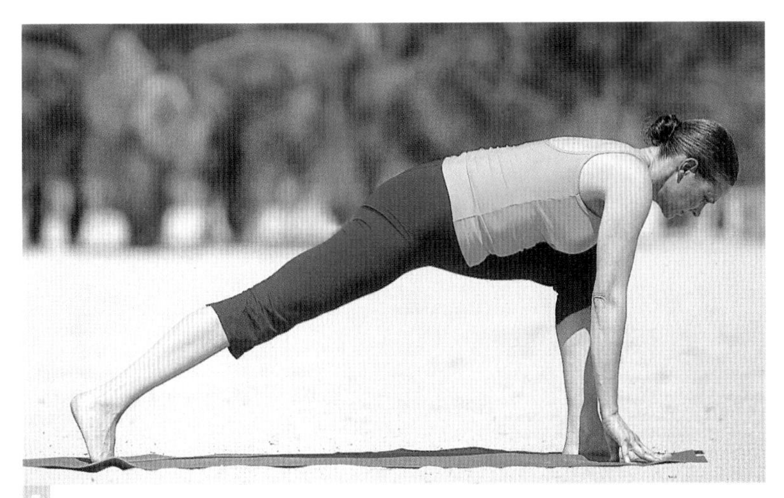

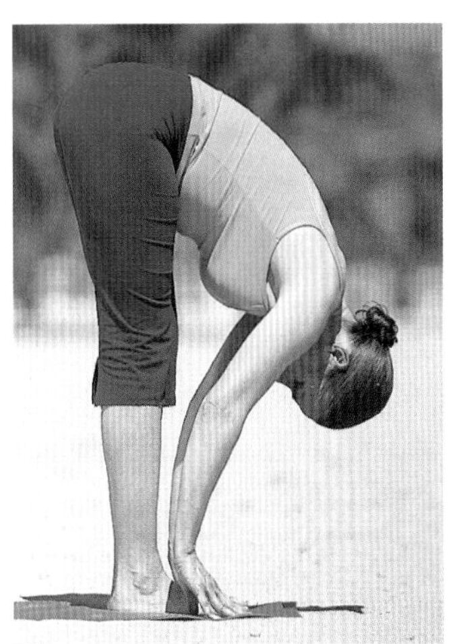

5 To come out of the pose, inhale as you bend one knee and step forwards, bringing the foot as close to the hands as possible. Continue to support yourself with your hands on the ground.

6 Step the other leg forward while exhaling, bringing both feet into alignment. Bend your knees slightly if necessary. Then inhale and stand up straight. You may like to repeat the pose on the other leg.

CHAIR

This is an excellent pose for bringing energy and improved blood circulation to the ovaries, uterus, and pelvic area. It strengthens the leg muscles and opens the hips. It helps activate the energy of the first three chakras *(p. 15)* and circulates that energy into the solar plexus (emotional balance) and heart (compassion, selfless service) chakras. If your heels do not reach the floor comfortably, roll or fold a towel or blanket to place under your heels while in this position.

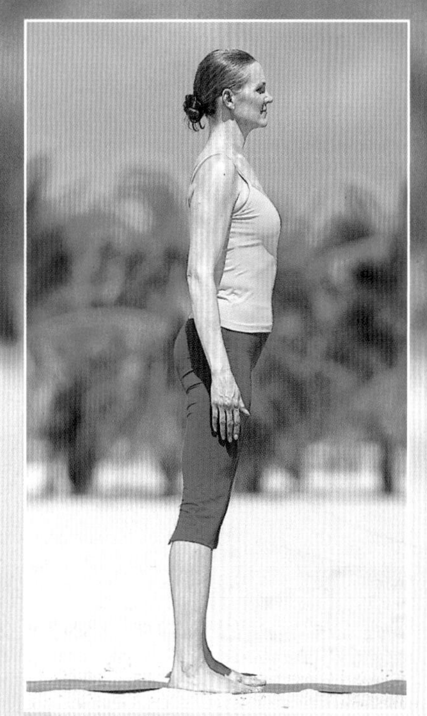

1 Stand up straight with your feet about 60cm (24in) apart, parallel to each other and facing forwards. Inhale deeply.

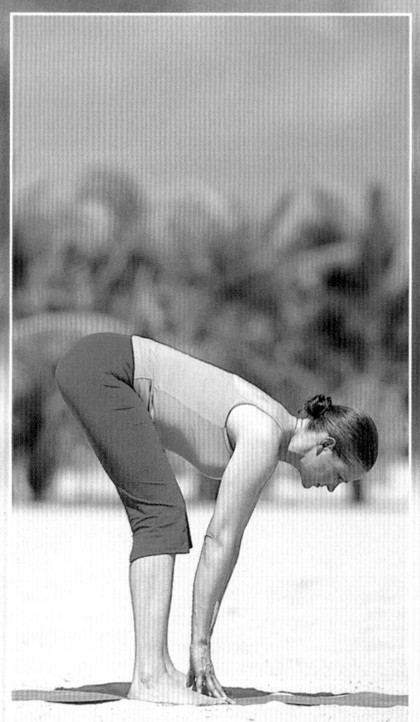

2 Exhale as you bend forwards, keeping the back straight and your head facing forwards. Bend your knees so that your hands reach the floor. Your arms will be close to the inside of your bent knees.

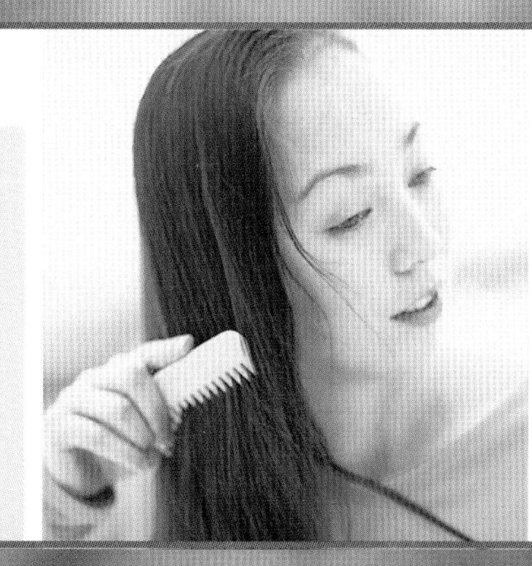

COMBING HAIR

According to the yogic understanding of the human body, hair is the antennae of pranic energy. Uncut hair collects pure protein at its root, which supports the brain, especially when coiled at the highest chakra, the crown centre. When the hair on the head is combed with a wooden comb, it neutralizes static electricity. The wooden comb massages and stimulates the scalp while absorbing excess oils on the surface of the scalp.

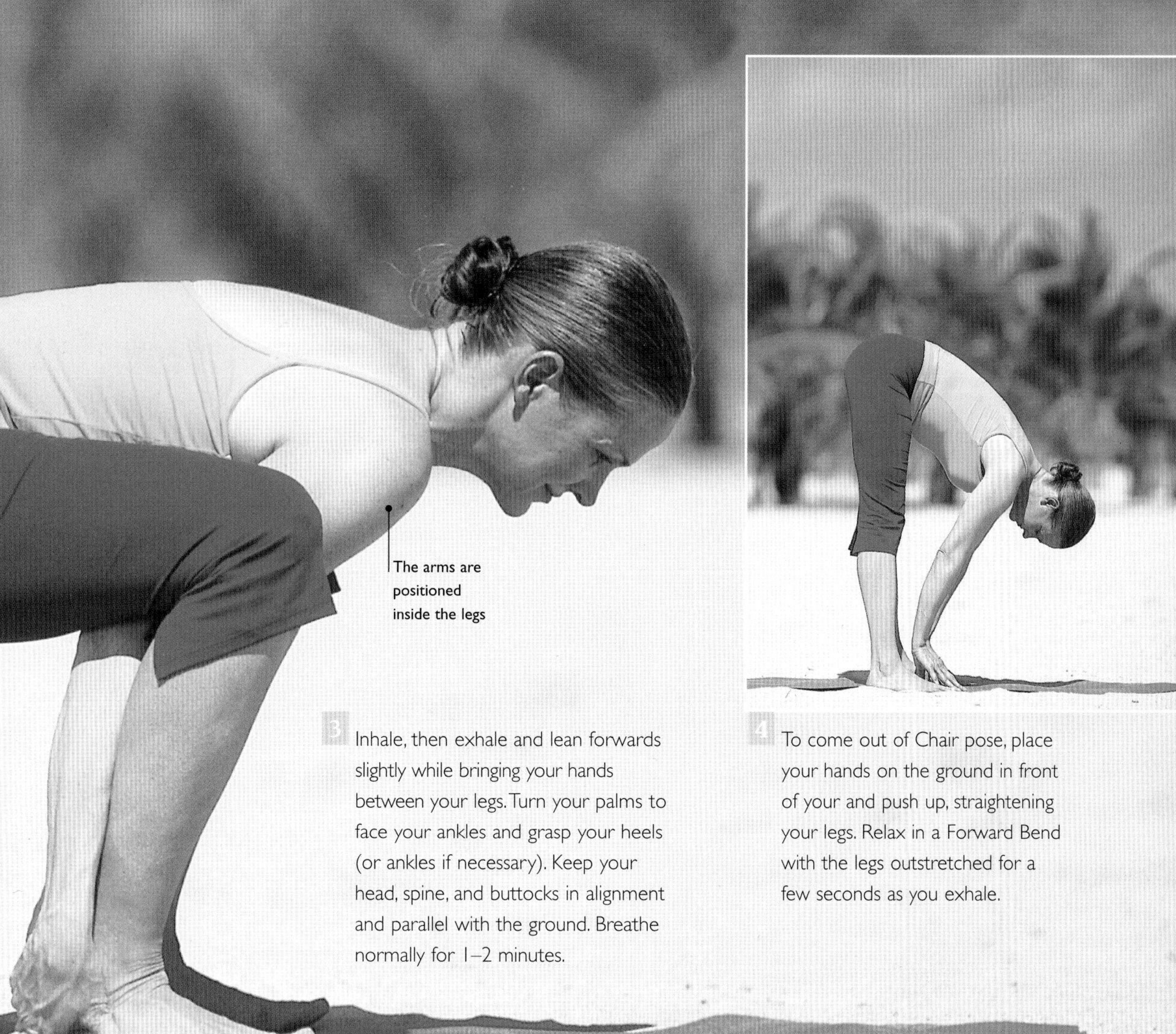

3 Inhale, then exhale and lean forwards slightly while bringing your hands between your legs. Turn your palms to face your ankles and grasp your heels (or ankles if necessary). Keep your head, spine, and buttocks in alignment and parallel with the ground. Breathe normally for 1–2 minutes.

4 To come out of Chair pose, place your hands on the ground in front of your and push up, straightening your legs. Relax in a Forward Bend with the legs outstretched for a few seconds as you exhale.

PIGEON

Pigeon pose increases flexibility in the hips and groin and stretches the thigh muscles. It expands the chest, strengthens the lungs, and facilitates deep breathing. This pose strengthens the back muscles and revitalizes the kidneys and the entire endocrine system.

A healthy, balanced endocrine (hormone) system means a well-integrated connection between mind, body, and emotions.

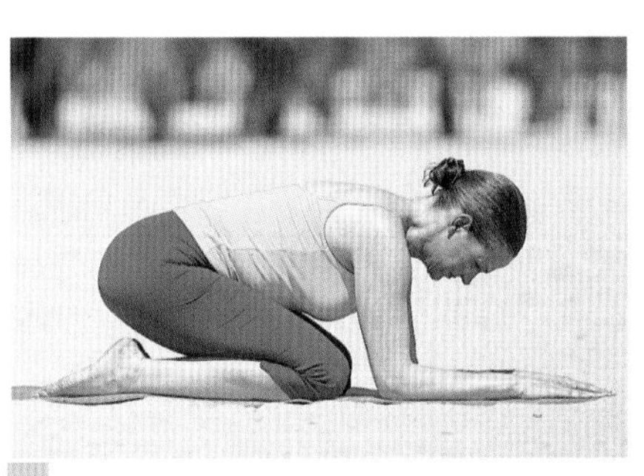

1 Begin by sitting on your heels and bringing your forearms to the ground with the palms facing downwards.

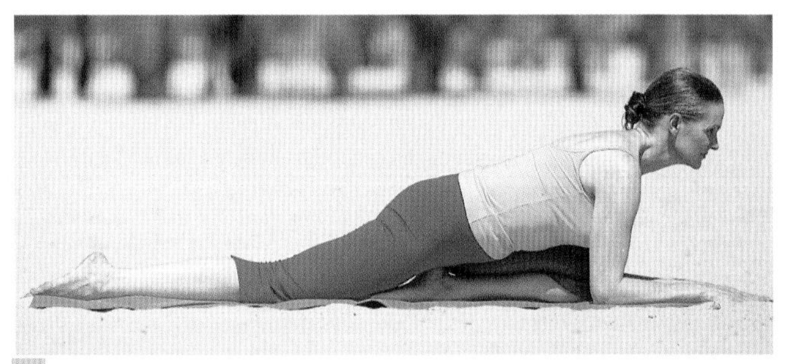

2 Slide your left knee forward between your elbows and your right leg straight out behind you. Square your hips to the front, and lie the right foot flat on the ground. Lower your left hip towards the ground. If this is uncomfortable or feels unsteady, place a blanket under your left hip to support it. If needed, stay in this position, or go on to step 3.

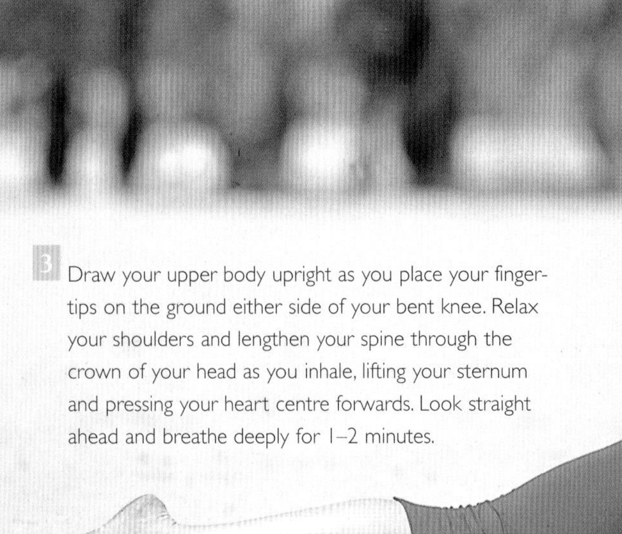

3 Draw your upper body upright as you place your finger-tips on the ground either side of your bent knee. Relax your shoulders and lengthen your spine through the crown of your head as you inhale, lifting your sternum and pressing your heart centre forwards. Look straight ahead and breathe deeply for 1–2 minutes.

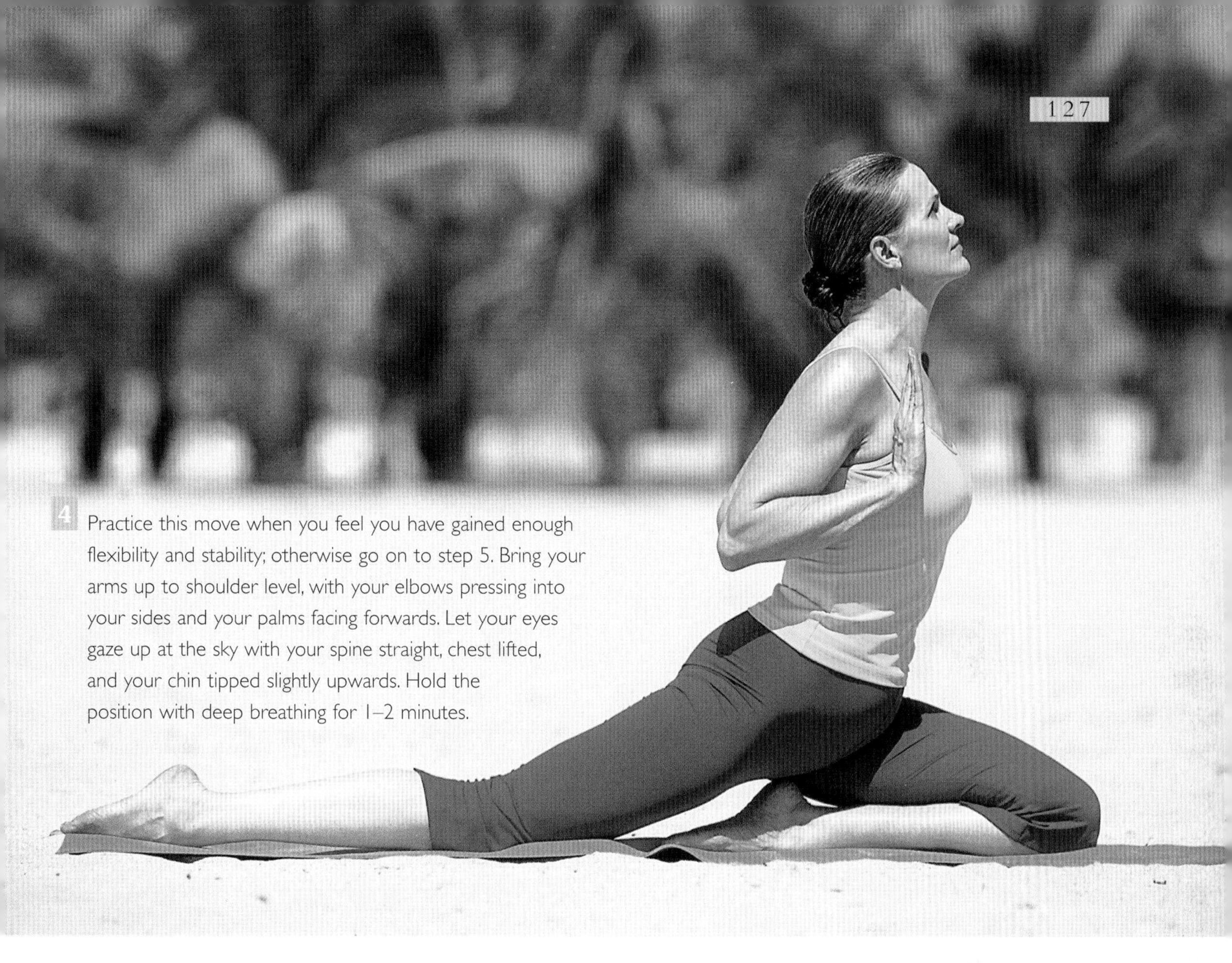

4 Practice this move when you feel you have gained enough flexibility and stability; otherwise go on to step 5. Bring your arms up to shoulder level, with your elbows pressing into your sides and your palms facing forwards. Let your eyes gaze up at the sky with your spine straight, chest lifted, and your chin tipped slightly upwards. Hold the position with deep breathing for 1–2 minutes.

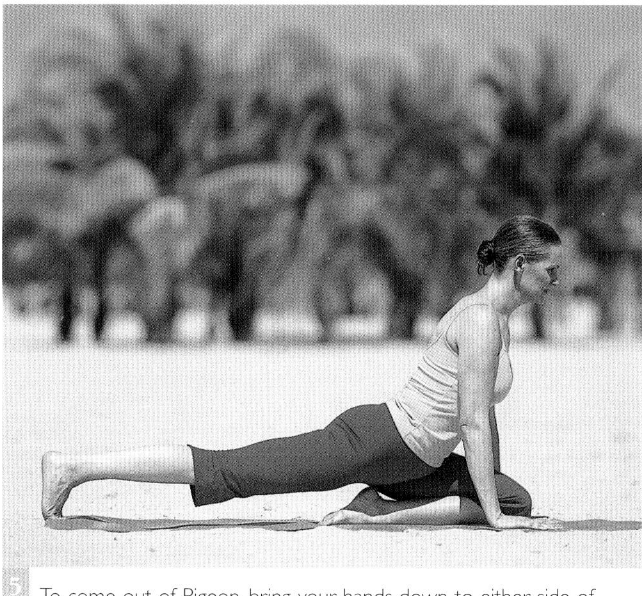

5 To come out of Pigeon, bring your hands down to either side of your front knee. Press your hands into the ground and lower your torso forwards slightly as you lift your hips away from the ground.

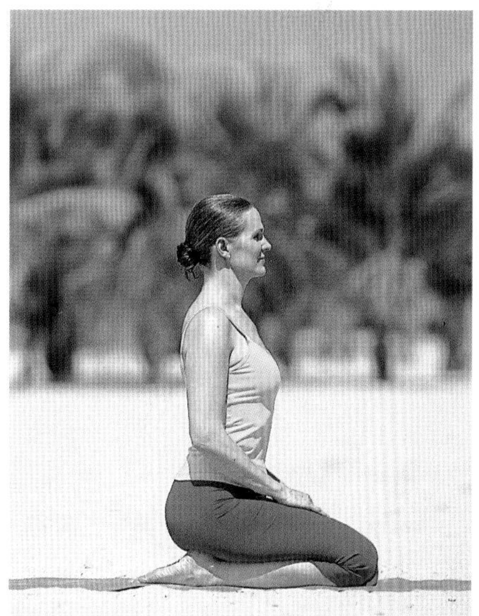

6 Bring your right knee forwards so that you finish by sitting in Rock pose *(p.20)*. Then repeat the pose with your left leg extended and the right leg bent.

FRONT LUNGE

Calming and soothing to the nervous system, Front Lunge dispels fatigue and refreshes the brain. The leg muscles are toned and strengthened. This pose can be helpful in relieving depression and stress-related headaches and migraines. If you have low blood pressure, come out of the pose gradually to avoid dizziness. Front Lunge is best done on a non-slip mat. Keep your eyes open to maintain your balance.

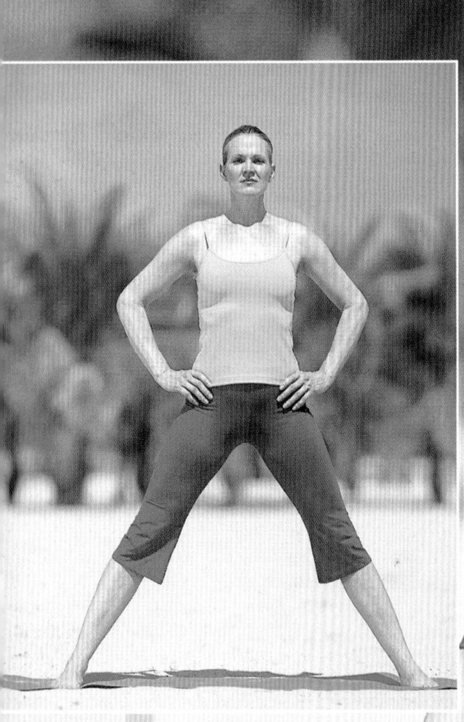

1 Stand straight with your feet straddled about 1.2m (4ft) apart. Place your hands on your hips and inhale.

2 As you start to exhale, bring your body forwards until it is parallel to the ground. Keep your back straight, your head facing forwards, and your chin up. Use your abdominal muscles to support your spine in this position.

GURUFATHA'S STORY (USA)

I have been battling menopause for years. It started innocently enough with irregular periods, then progressed to sleeplessness, foggy brain, and feelings of instability – then to excessive bleeding and a barrage of hot flushes, as many as 20–50 a day. Sometimes it has felt like I am inhabiting an alien body.

The excessive bleeding was taken care of through surgery, leaving me with all the other symptoms to deal with. Sometimes the natural supplements and creams have worked, but not on a consistent basis. However, yoga is the one thing that has helped me stay sane, flexible, and hopeful through this stage of life. If I practise yoga consistently and exercise strongly every day, there is a noticeable difference in my overall energy. Yoga exercises that work on stretching my entire body and strengthening my abdominal area have been especially helpful. Sometimes I can almost feel the endorphins in my body releasing during yoga, sending a wave of relaxation and peace throughout my raging body and mind. I do 11 minutes of Sat Kriya a day, done rhythmically and slowly, making sure to pull a complete Root Lock with each repetition. I also find that taking three deep breaths – slowed down to one breath per minute – really calms me down. I am then able to step out of the battle and be more accepting of the change my body is going through. My yoga and meditation practice continues to replace pain with peace, and allows me to look at my "womanly" body and say "wow" instead of "yikes"!

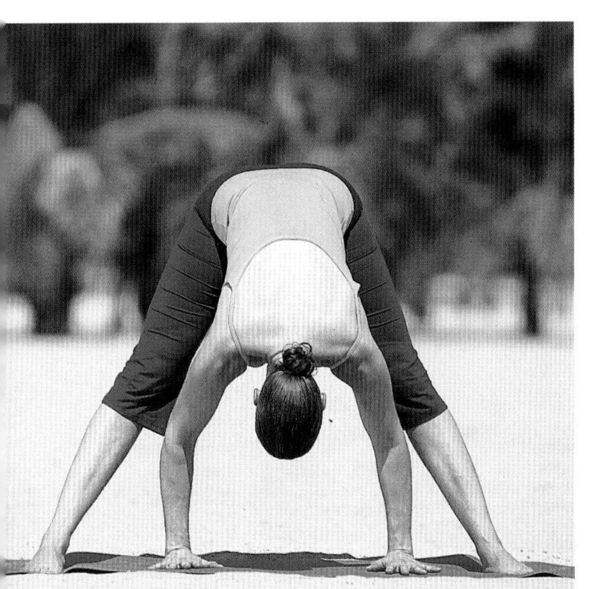

3 Place your hands on the ground in front of you, fingers spread and arms about shoulder-width apart. Press your hips upwards and backwards, moving your weight slightly towards your heels. Take a few breaths in this position.

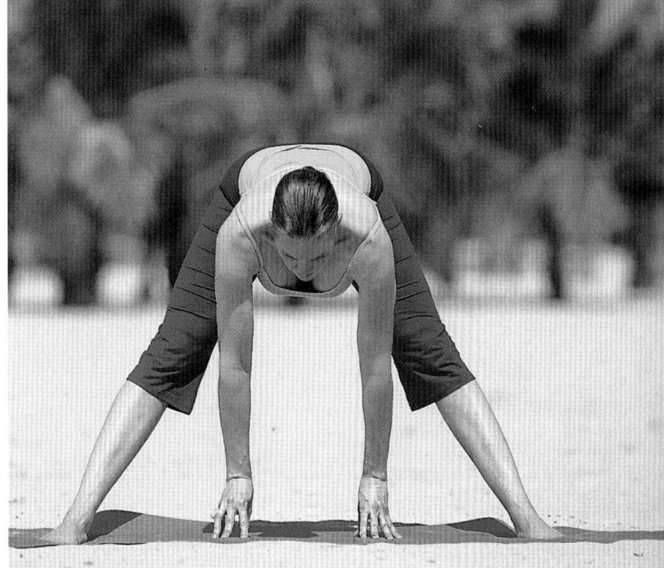

4 Move your hands closer to your body, with the fingertips touching the ground. Lift your chin and lengthen your spine as you flatten you back, inhale, and then exhale. Continue on to step 5.

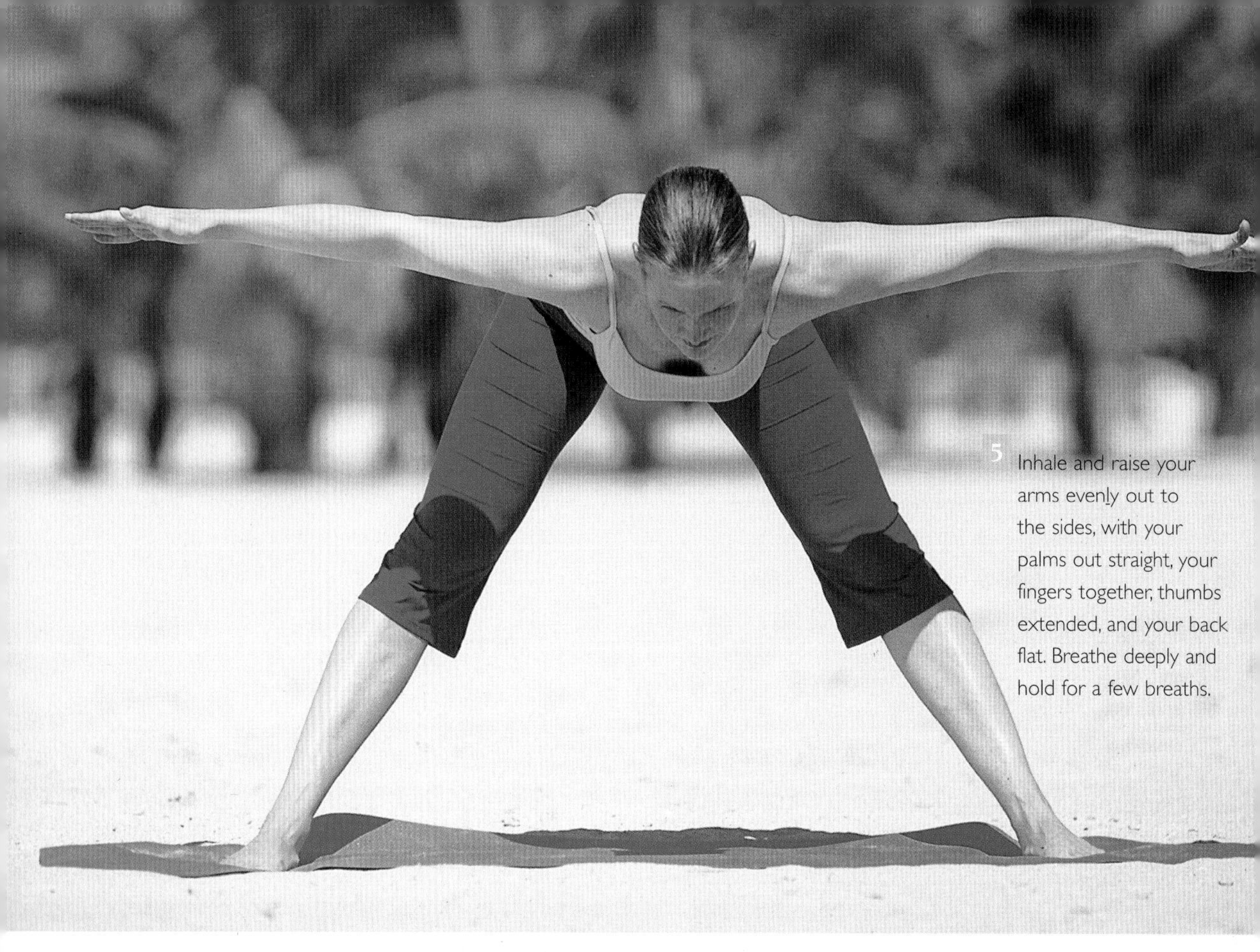

5 Inhale and raise your arms evenly out to the sides, with your palms out straight, your fingers together, thumbs extended, and your back flat. Breathe deeply and hold for a few breaths.

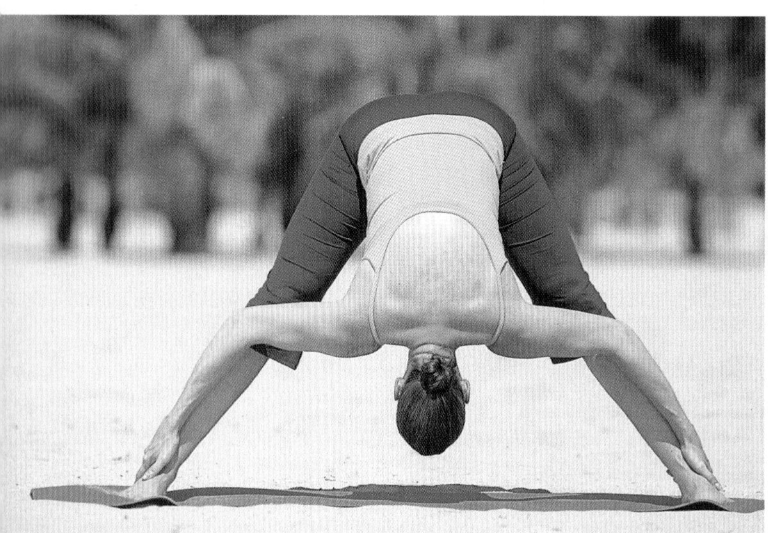

6 Relax your head and upper body downwards while exhaling slowly, bringing your arms down and clasping your ankles or heels, whichever you can reach comfortably. Lengthen your spine and stretch your head towards the ground. Breathe normally and hold for a few breaths.

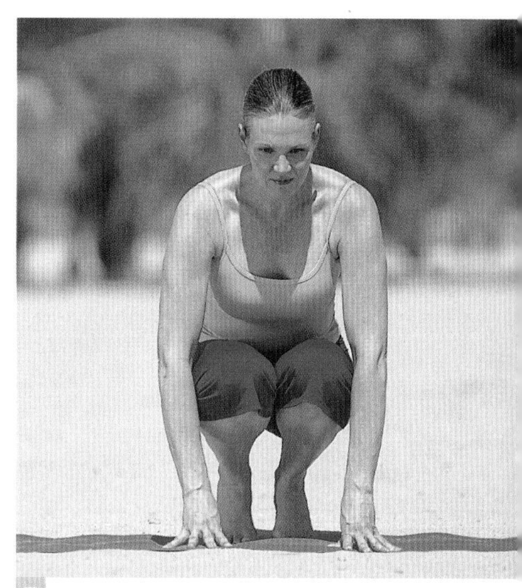

7 To come out of the pose, bring your hands to the ground in front of you, bend your elbows and knees slightly, and with a small jump bring your legs back together as you inhale. Bend your knees in a squatting position, then stand up.

MEDITATION FOR EMOTIONAL BALANCE

This meditation is very good for women, and is essential for those times when one is worried, upset, doesn't know what to do, or is on the verge of rage.

Before practising this meditation, drink a glass of pure water, preferably at room temperature. Emotions and the need for water are intricately connected. When there is an imbalance of water in the system and the kidneys are pressurized, there is a tendency towards anxiety and upset behaviour. From a scientific point of view, water is the medium that increases electrical potential across cell membranes, which is essential for the proper functioning of the nervous system.

The combination of drinking water, followed by applying pressure at the armpits with the raised shoulders and a Neck Lock, creates a tight lock on the entire upper body. Combined with a natural slowing of the breathing rate, this locked posture forms an automatic "brake" that is applied to the brain. The brain cannot continue its previous pattern of thinking, and within a short amount of time a balance is restored. Those with high blood pressure, a neck injury, or heart disease should consult with their GP before practising this meditation.

1 *Sit in Easy pose. If necessary, place a firm pillow, bolster, or thick blanket under your buttocks to allow the knees to relax down so that you are comfortable. Straighten the spine and relax the shoulders. Keep the chest lifted throughout the meditation. Place your arms across your chest and lock your hands under your armpits with the palms open and against the body. The thumbs may be outside the armpits. Close your eyes.*

2 *Raise your shoulders up towards your ear lobes as far as possible and hold them there. Apply a Neck Lock by contracting back on the neck and throat. The chin is pulled back towards the neck without tipping the head forwards. If you are doing it correctly, you will feel that the cervical vertebrae are in alignment with the spine. Stay alert throughout the meditation to maintain the Neck Lock and raised shoulders, which are the essential components of the "brake" you are applying to the brain. Your breath will automatically become slower.*

Begin with three minutes of practice, gradually increasing the time to 11 minutes.

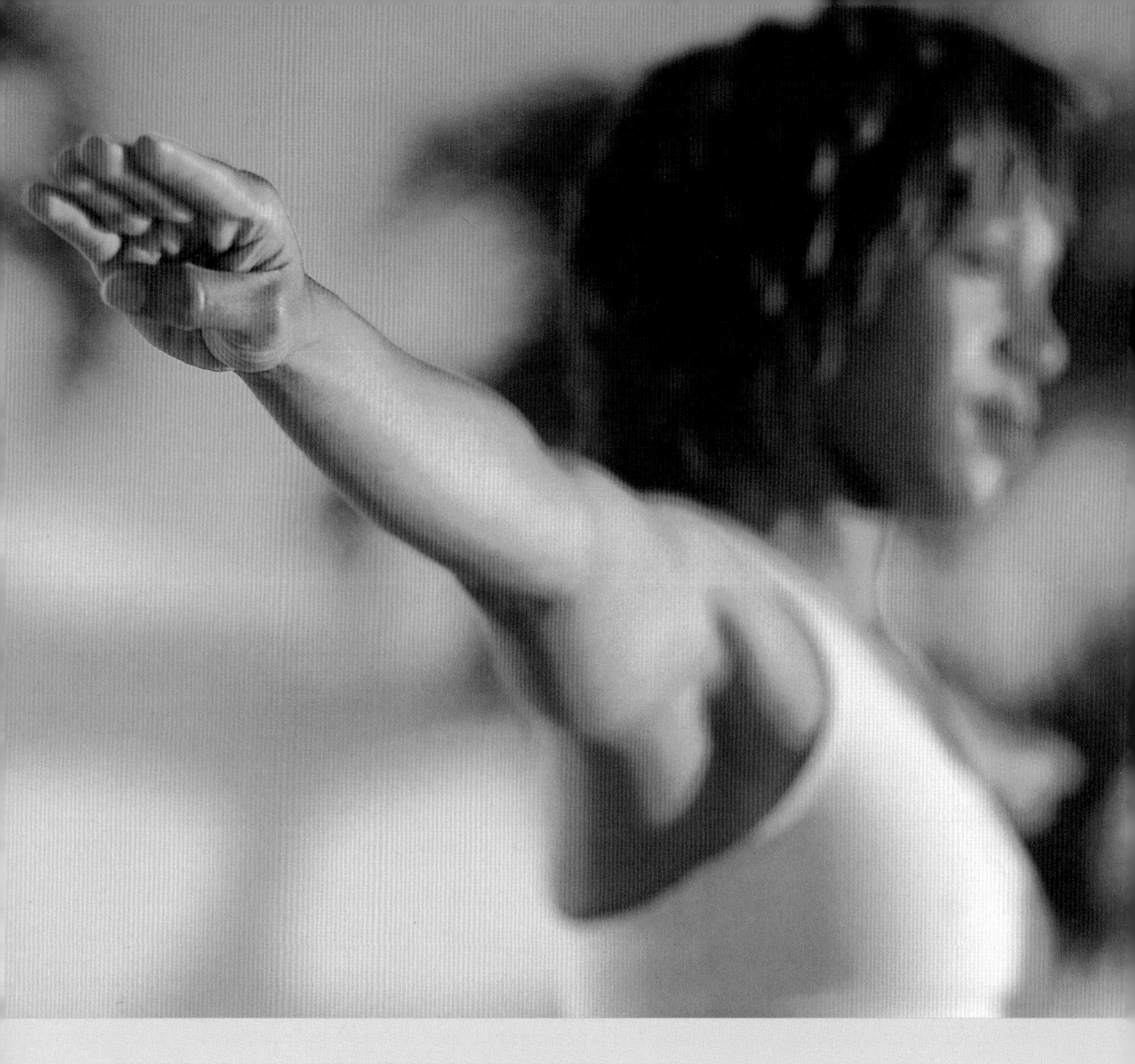

BREAST CARE

Among the women who come to my yoga classes are typically one or two breast cancer survivors, and often at least one woman who is in the midst of dealing with breast cancer. Keeping our breasts healthy is one of the most important things we can do. One of the best ways is to activate the lymphatic system, which, in addition to helping your body fight infection, removes potentially harmful materials from the body's tissues and cells. Lymph flow is dependent upon muscle contractions, which massage the outside of the lymphatic vessels, and breathing, which pulls lymph along with each inhalation. With its sensitivity to breathing and movement, it is easy to see how the lymph system responds so positively to yoga practice.

HEALTHY BREASTS

The following simple yoga exercises stimulate the circulation of blood and vital energy through the lymphatic system. Feel free to practise these exercises and postures individually or as a set. The first two, Diagonal Stretch and Reach for Health, can be done either sitting on the ground or on a chair with the spine straight and the feet flat on the ground.

The endocrine system, which includes hormones and glands, is balanced through yoga. This is important with regard to the breasts since oestrogen must be in balance with its partner hormone, progesterone, in order to function properly.

DIAGONAL STRETCH

In this exercise the lymphatic system is activated by vigorous movement and powerful breathing. The pad at the base of the little finger is a reflex point that empowers the communication centre of the brain.

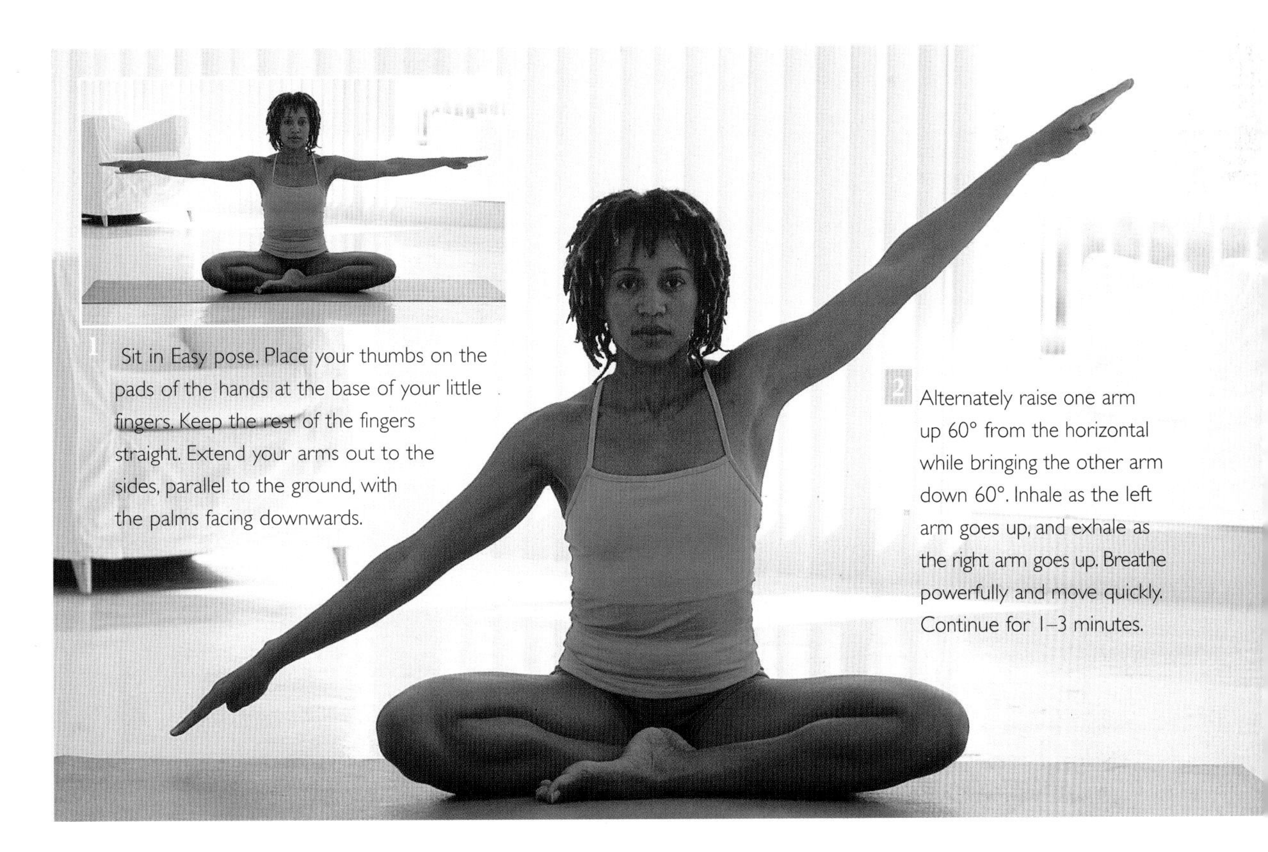

1 Sit in Easy pose. Place your thumbs on the pads of the hands at the base of your little fingers. Keep the rest of the fingers straight. Extend your arms out to the sides, parallel to the ground, with the palms facing downwards.

2 Alternately raise one arm up 60° from the horizontal while bringing the other arm down 60°. Inhale as the left arm goes up, and exhale as the right arm goes up. Breathe powerfully and move quickly. Continue for 1–3 minutes.

REACH FOR HEALTH

In this exercise the powerful movement of the arms, coupled with the forceful breath, is similar to a martial arts exercise. The "snapping back" movement activates the lymph and breast tissue.

Other yoga postures that benefit the lymph/breast area are Bow, Cobra, and Shoulderstand.

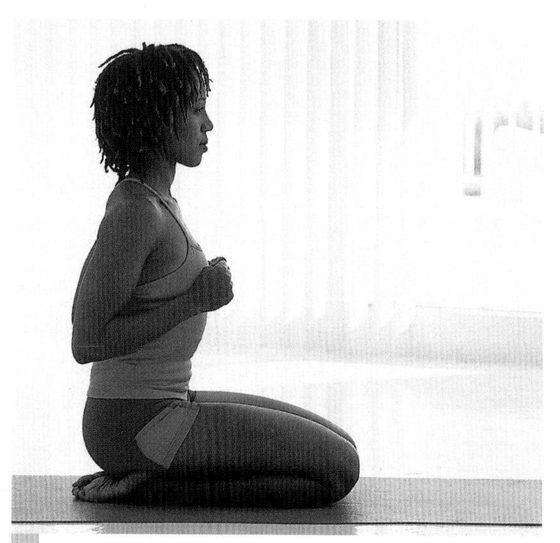

1 Sit on your heels. If you need to take pressure off the knee joints, place a firm pillow between your buttocks and legs. Make your hands into fists with your thumbs tucked inside. Bring your hands to chest level with your arms by your side, elbows pulled back.

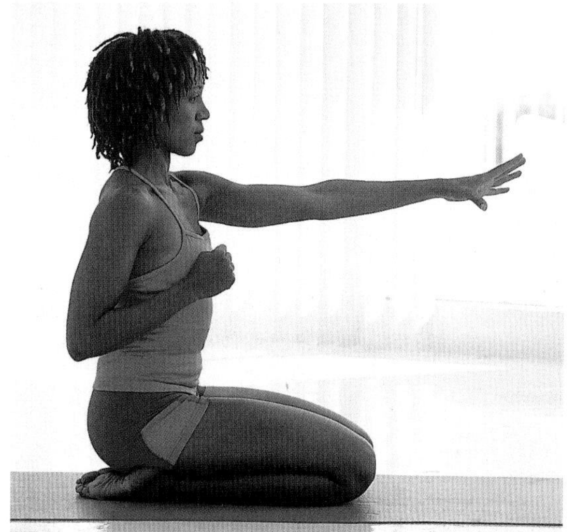

2 Powerfully extend one arm forwards on a deep inhale. As your arm extends its full length, open your fingers as though you were grasping something. Then close them quickly, again with the thumb inside, and snap the arm back powerfully to the side of your body as you exhale strongly. Repeat with the other arm and continue for 1–2 minutes.

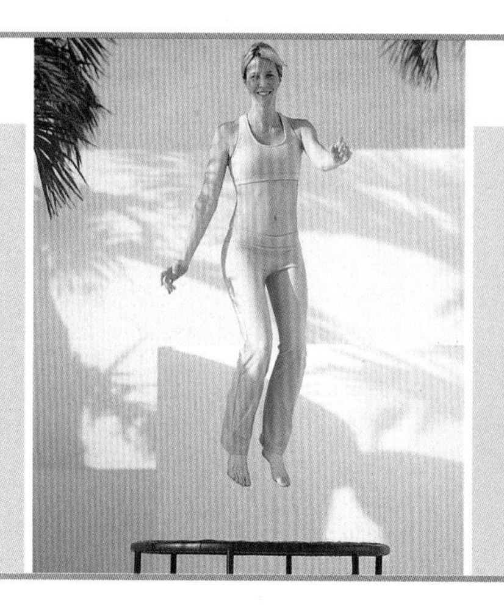

JUMP FOR HEALTH

Jumping on a rebounder, or mini trampoline, greatly improves the circulation of lymphatic fluid within the body. This improves the body's cancer-fighting ability as well. To help your lymph system, jump and jog while moving your arms up and down and in circles. Music that uplifts you and is lively will give you a rhythm to rebound to, and singing along will expand your lung capacity and just generally help you feel wonderfully alive. (See also *Music Resources*, p.224, for suggestions of suitable music.)

FROG POSE

This exercise increases the flow of energy to the body and mind. Internal heat (called tapas) and energy move from the pelvic area upwards through the heart centre and balance your hormones.

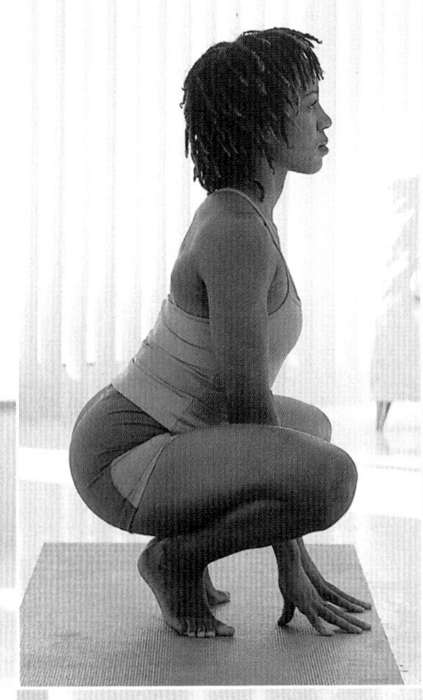

1 While standing, bring your heels close together, or touching, and turn your feet slightly outwards. Squat down keeping your heels off the ground and bringing your fingertips to the ground with arms inside your spread knees. Straighten your spine as much as possible in this squatting position.

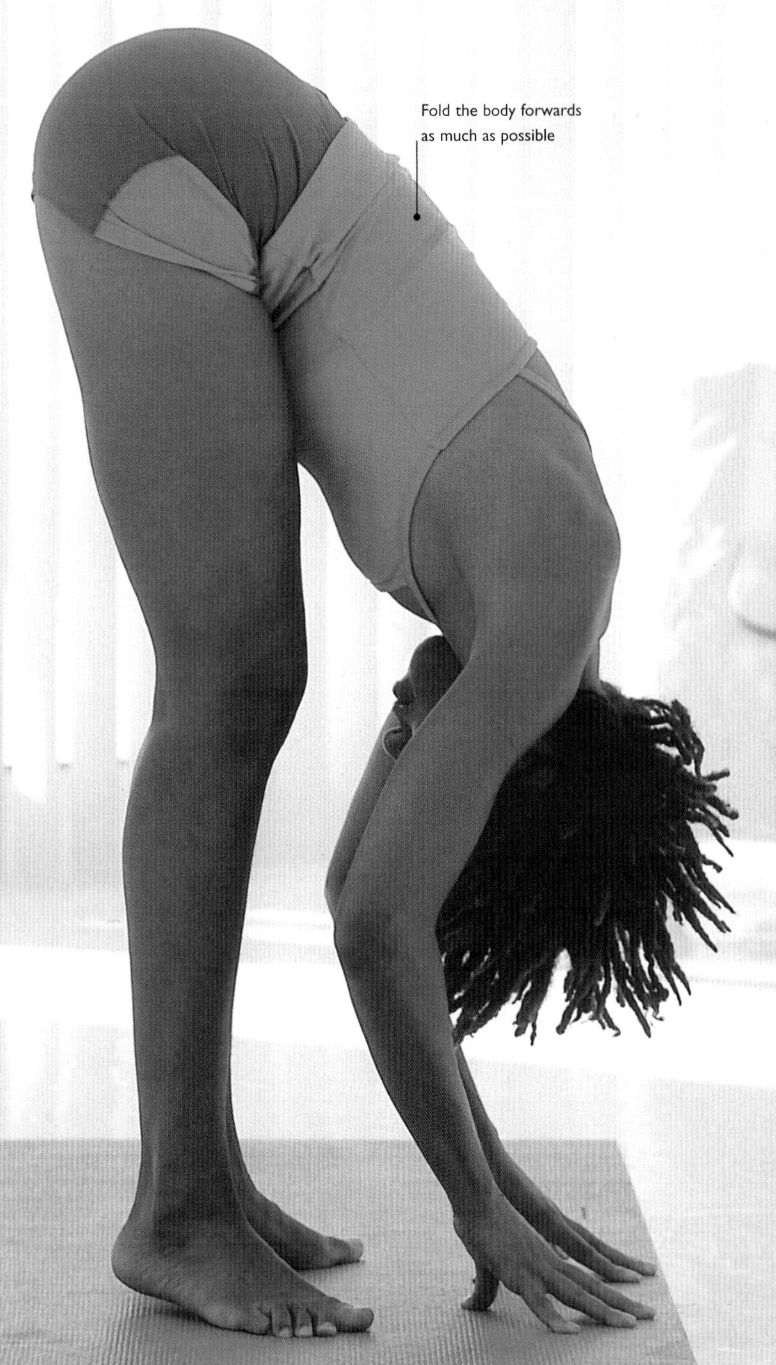

Fold the body forwards as much as possible

2 Inhale and straighten the legs, bringing the head as close to the knees as you can. The fingertips remain on the ground, and the heels stay slightly off the ground. Exhale and return to squatting position. Continue for one minute. Then relax.

ONE-LEGGED BOW

This exercise stretches and increases circulation under the arms where the lymph system is active. One-Legged Bow pose also stimulates the endocrine system.

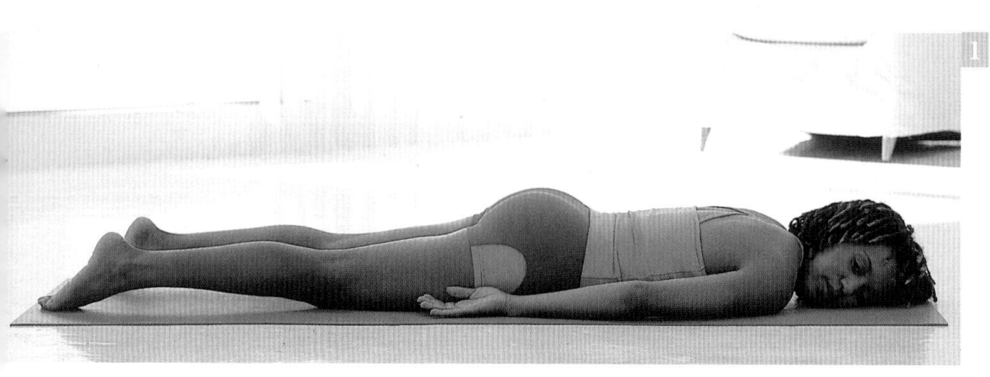

1 Lie down on your front with your arms resting at your sides, and your feet slightly apart.

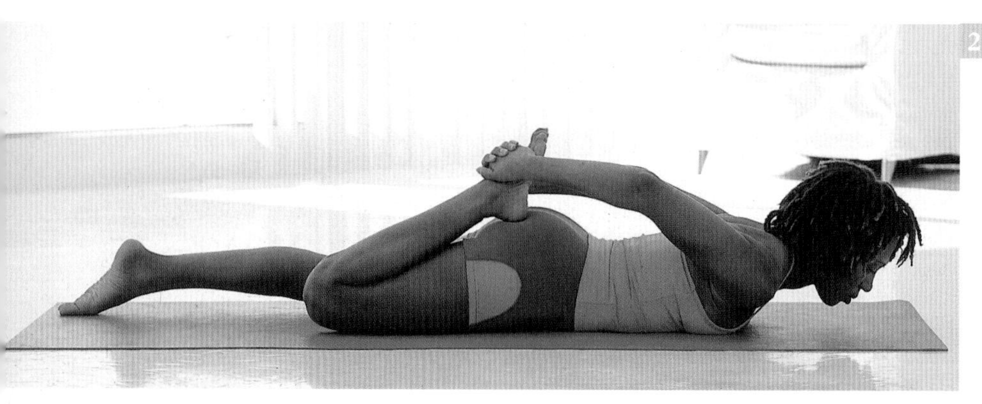

2 Bend one leg towards your head and grasp the foot with hands interlaced, or one hand on top of the other. If you cannot reach the ankle, loop a belt round the ankle and grasp either end of the belt.

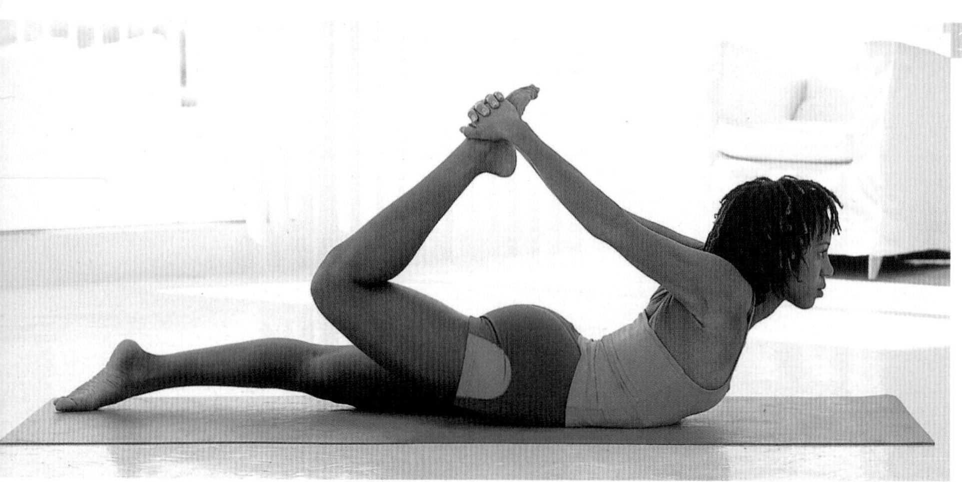

3 Create a tension between the arms and the leg and arch the body up in One-Legged Bow pose.

MARCIA'S STORY (MEXICO)

In 1995 I was diagnosed with fibrocystic breasts, which means that I had a lump in my breast. The lump was benign, but the doctor said that this condition can indicate a higher-than-normal chance of developing breast cancer later on. So I considered this to be a "wake-up call" from God.

I cut out foods that clog my system, such as an overabundance of meat, wheat, dairy products, refined foods, and fats, and instead I chose to eat fruits, legumes, vegetables, and whole grains. Caffeine had to go, and was replaced by the energy I felt with starting a daily yoga practice. Fibrocystic breasts are often characterized by a sluggish thyroid, and mine was no exception, so I began focusing on yoga poses that help the thyroid, such as Plough and Shoulderstand. To keep my lymph moving, I exercised my upper body, flapped my arms, rocked in Bow pose and breathed as though my life depended on it, for I felt very clearly that it did! Within a year, the lump was gone, and I was gratefully established in my new, health-giving way of life.

4 Inhale as you lift yourself higher and rock back onto your pelvis, arching your upper spine, expanding your chest, and lifting your head.

Elbows are straight
Your left leg remains relaxed on the ground

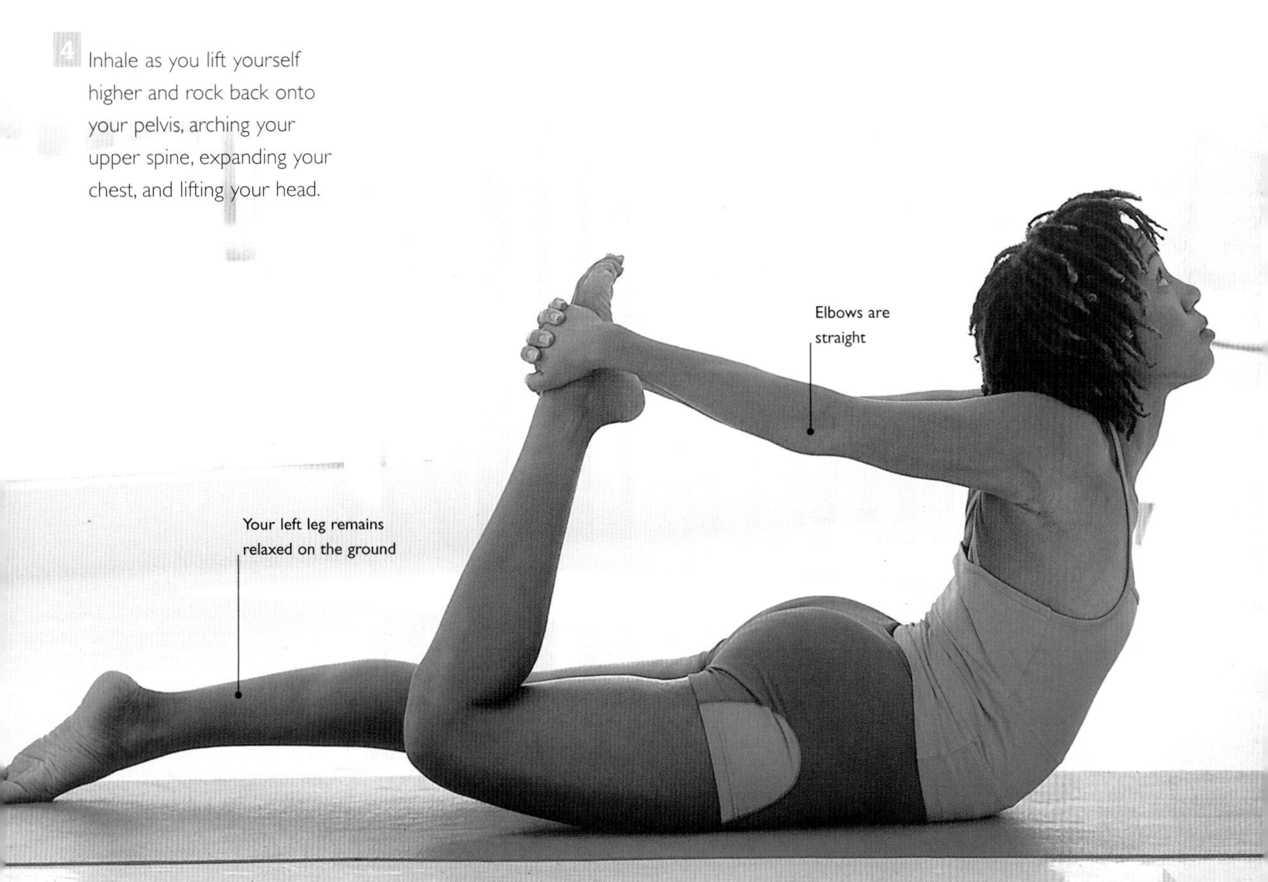

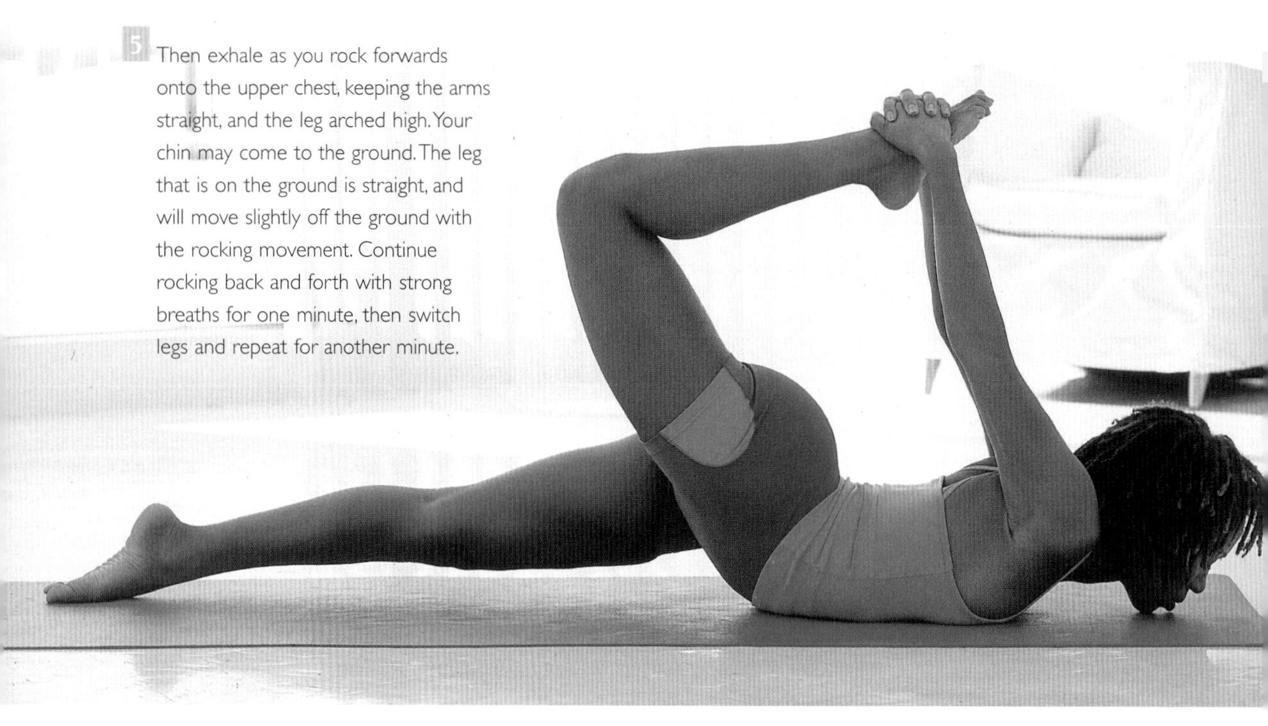

5 Then exhale as you rock forwards onto the upper chest, keeping the arms straight, and the leg arched high. Your chin may come to the ground. The leg that is on the ground is straight, and will move slightly off the ground with the rocking movement. Continue rocking back and forth with strong breaths for one minute, then switch legs and repeat for another minute.

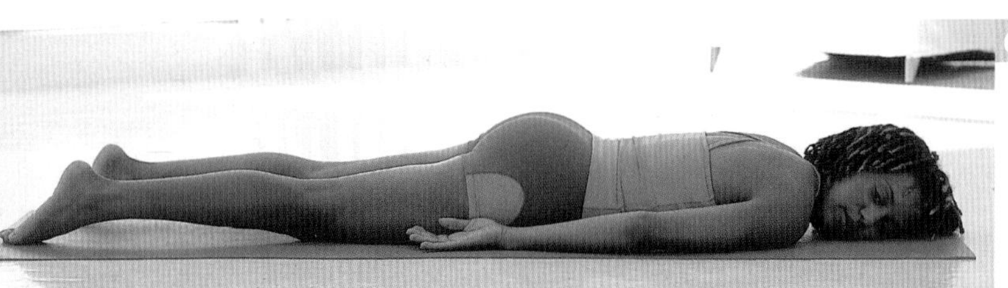

6 Rest for at least 20 seconds with the head turned to one side and your arms relaxed by your sides, palms facing up.

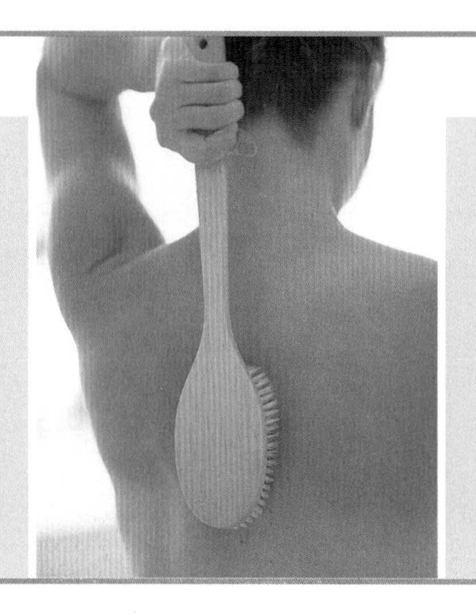

DRY BRUSH MASSAGE

One third of the body's impurities are eliminated through the skin; dry brush massage stimulates the lymphatic system to expel toxins through the skin, and allows it to breathe more efficiently. Using a long-handled natural bristle brush or loofah mitt, start with the soles of your feet, and then move upwards. Brush with as much pressure as is comfortable until your skin feels pleasantly warm. Continue for about five minutes. The face and ears can be brushed with a soft facial brush. Follow with a brief cold shower (p.33) *or contrast shower (alternating warm and cold water) to increase the cleansing effects.*

BEAUTIFUL BREASTS

Our breasts don't have to sag with the passage of time if we know what to do to keep the supporting muscles strong. Just think how much healthier your breasts can be when they are able to support themselves with their own muscles rather than relying on "supportive" but tight bras, which can seriously constrict your vital circulation. Here are a few exercises to keep your breasts firm and lovely.

In his book, Breast Health: A Ten Point Prevention Program, *Dr Charles Simone outlines a plan for breast care: optimize nutrition, take antioxidant supplements, avoid tobacco and alcohol. Exercise, minimize stress, become spiritually involved, and increase your awareness of your sexuality. Have regular physical examinations from the age of 35.*

PALM PRESS

This strengthens the muscles of the breasts, chest, and upper arms. Press with as much pressure as you can manage. In maintaining this lifted posture throughout the day, you will notice that it also uplifts your mind.

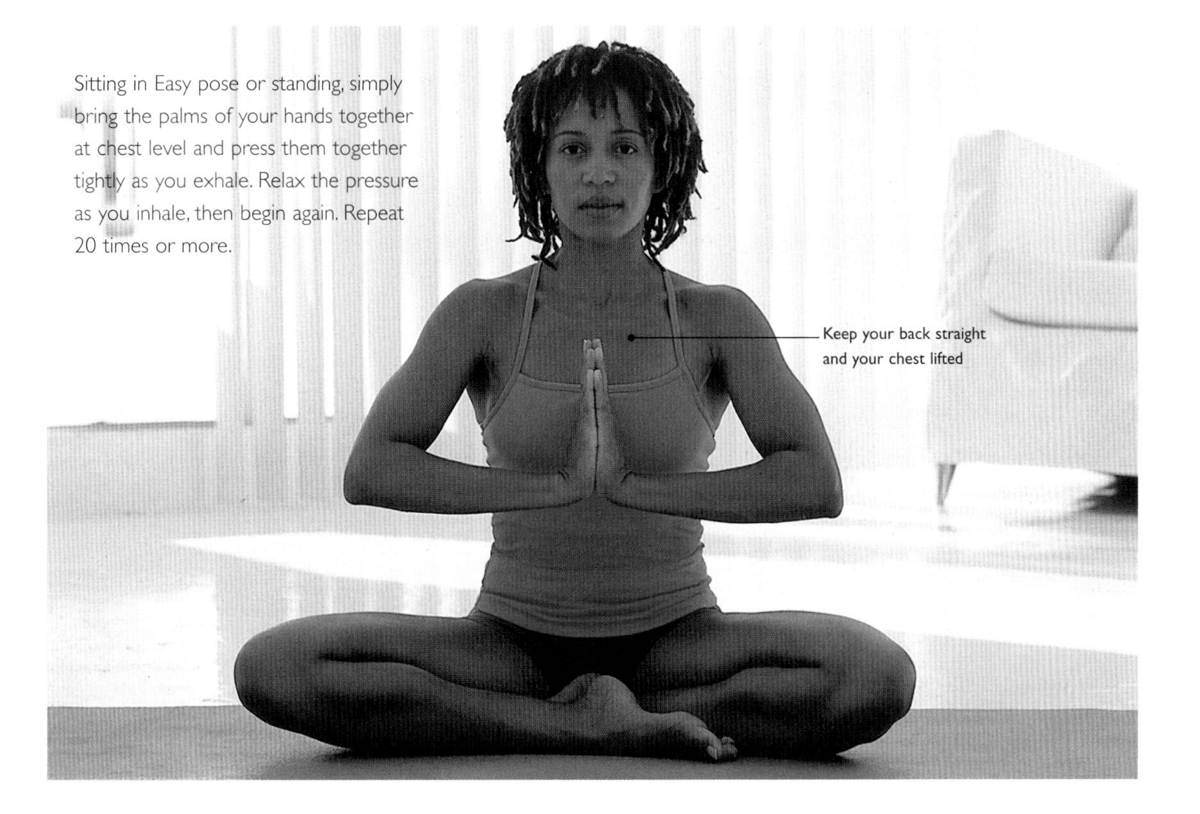

Sitting in Easy pose or standing, simply bring the palms of your hands together at chest level and press them together tightly as you exhale. Relax the pressure as you inhale, then begin again. Repeat 20 times or more.

ARM PRESS

This exercise strengthens the muscles around the breasts and the sides of the body. It also strengthens the nervous system. Press with the maximum amount of pressure for the most benefit, and repeat as often as you remember throughout the day.

Sitting in Easy pose or standing, place your palms and forearms together slightly above chest level. Lift your elbows a few centimetres away from your body. Press the entire length of the palms and forearms together on the exhale. Inhale and release the press. Repeat 20 times or more.

TOFU SPREAD

This delicious spread includes turmeric – a golden spice known to have antioxidant and anti-inflammatory properties.

Steam 450g (1lb) tofu for 5 minutes. Squeeze out excess water and mash. Add grated carrots, diced celery and dill pickles. Mix a dressing of eggless, sugarless mayonnaise, ½–1tsp turmeric, a little mustard, a dash of lemon juice, salt, pepper, dill weed, and sea kelp (good for the thyroid) and add to the tofu. Serve on bread or crackers.

WALL PRESS

This strengthens and tones the muscles of the chest and upper back. It is also beneficial for the abdominal and leg muscles, especially the calves and Achilles tendon in the heels. The inward-facing hand positions provide optimal benefit to the muscles around the breasts.

For good breast health, yogic teachings say that breasts should be kneaded like bread. Do it yourself or get your partner involved!

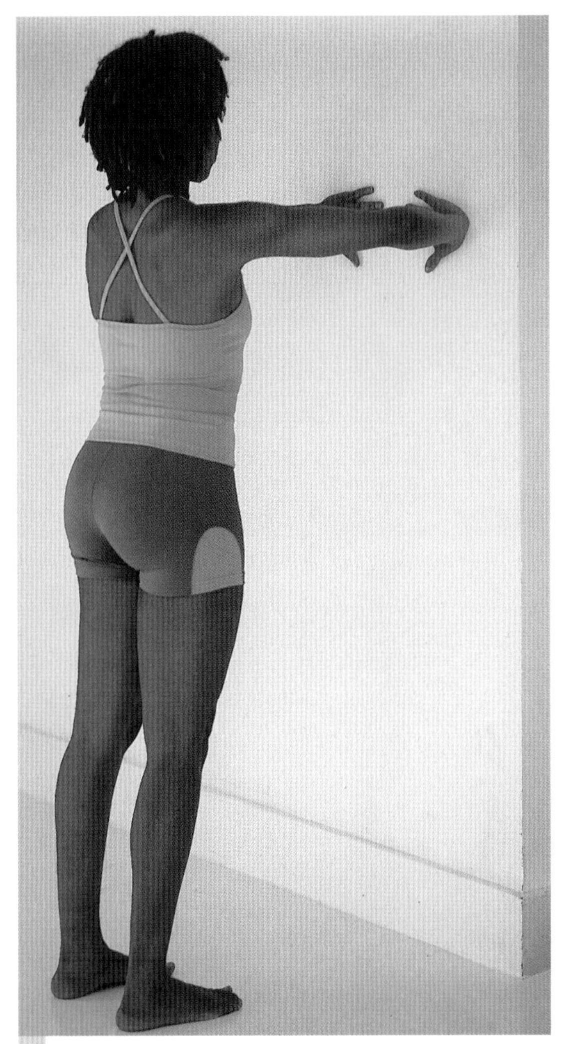

1 Stand with your feet on the floor 45–60cm (24–28in) away from the wall. Place your hands on the wall about shoulder-width apart, with the arms positioned so that the elbows are facing outwards and the fingers of each hand face inwards toward each other. Inhale.

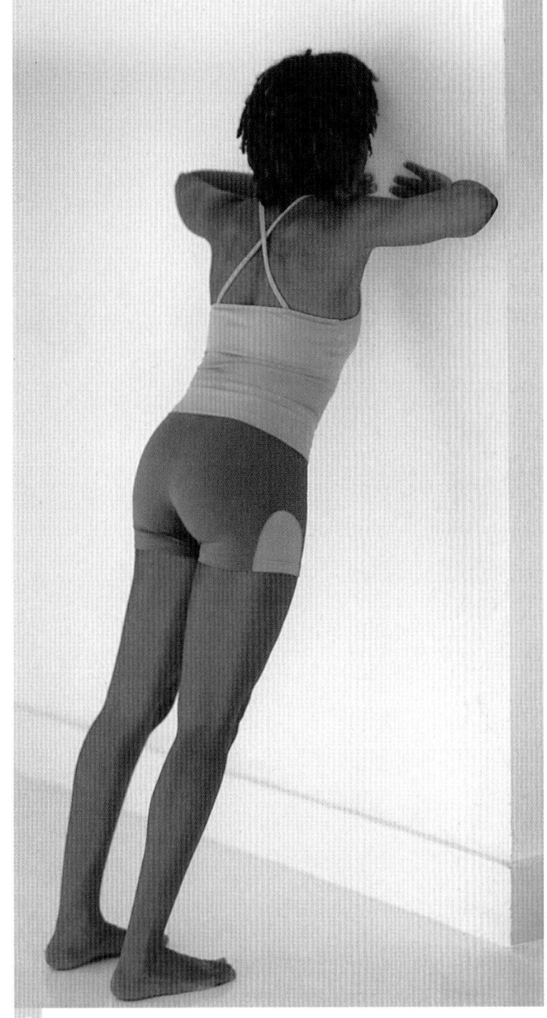

2 As you exhale, bend your elbows and bring your nose towards the wall. On the inhalation return to the original position. Bend only the elbows, keeping the legs straight. Continue for 10–20 repetitions.

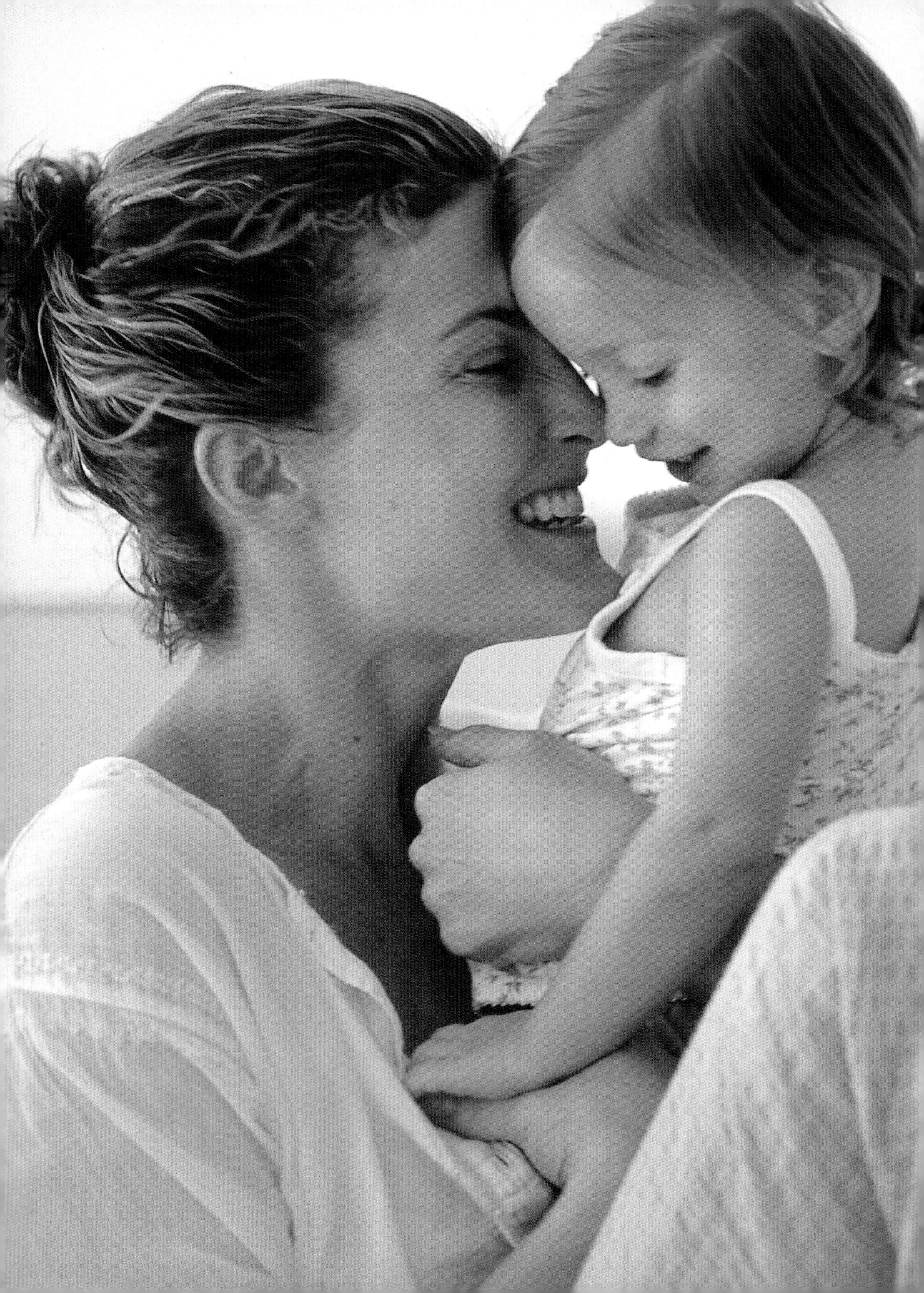

LOVING & MOTHERING

Loving starts with yourself, as does mothering. You've got to have something before you have anything to give. In this section you'll find yoga to empower your womanly spirit, which knows how to bend without breaking in the face of life's challenges. Quite often, our biggest challenges are about how we relate to and care for those we love most – our partners and our children – which can often bring out painful emotions. The yoga here not only helps you gain perspective and balance with strong emotional ties, but also helps to free up your ability to create the family life you want, and have fun in the meantime.

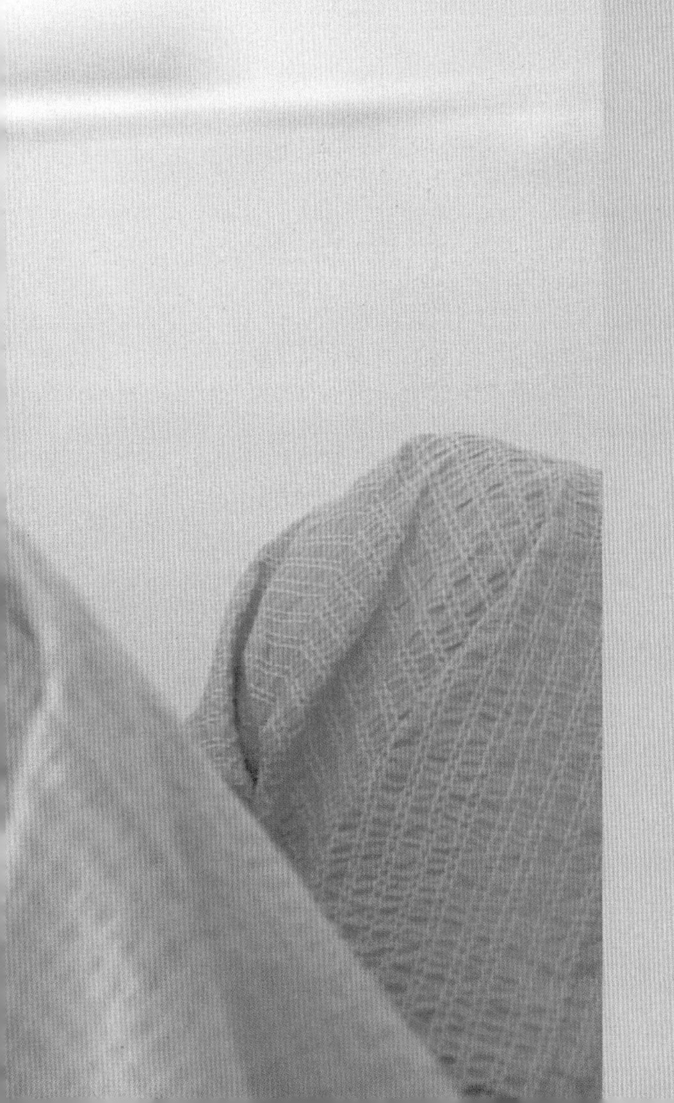

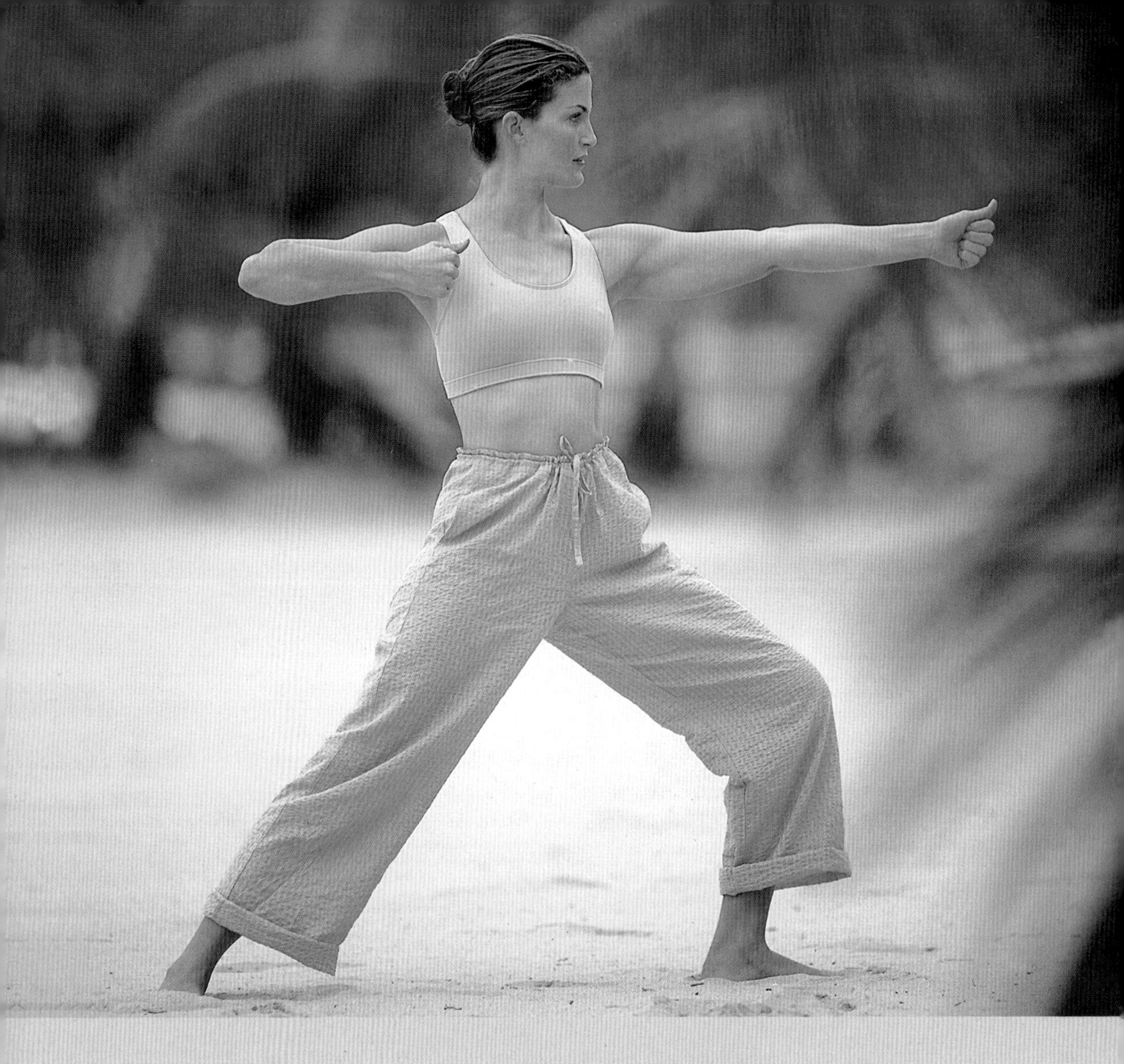

SELF-EMPOWERMENT

Ancient yogic wisdom speaks of the mythological figure Shakti, the divine feminine, as the creative power and principle of existence itself. Without Shakti nothing can manifest or bloom. Woman is said to be made in the image of Shakti. She represents that same creative energy on the earth. Simply put, woman equals power.

This chapter contains yoga and meditation to empower you in every way, including the ability to create a life of prosperity. True prosperity translates into every area of your life: physically, you are robust and healthy; spiritually, you enjoy life and share your abundance with others; and materially, you are successful and have the resources you need.

SET FOR SHAKTI ENERGY

This is an aerobic workout on every level: mind, body, and spirit. It strengthens the endocrine, immune, and nervous systems, empowers your sense of self, and helps you feel light and blissful. Meditation afterwards is effortless. As you chant, the tongue strikes the upper palate, stimulating the hypothalamus – a network of nerves in the brain that monitors hormone levels and controls hunger, thirst, and body temperature.

Each part of this set consists of eight movements coordinated with eight repetitions of the mantra Har *(the Infinite). Roll the "r" off the roof of your mouth so that* Har *sounds like "hudah". The set consists of 11 continuous exercises which are repeated. Start with 5–10 rounds and work up to as many as you can do without overexerting yourself.*

1 OVERHEAD CLAP

This pose stretches the spine and stimulates the meridian points in the hands, which activate brain clarity. The lymphatic areas of the arms and chest are stimulated, promoting good breast health.

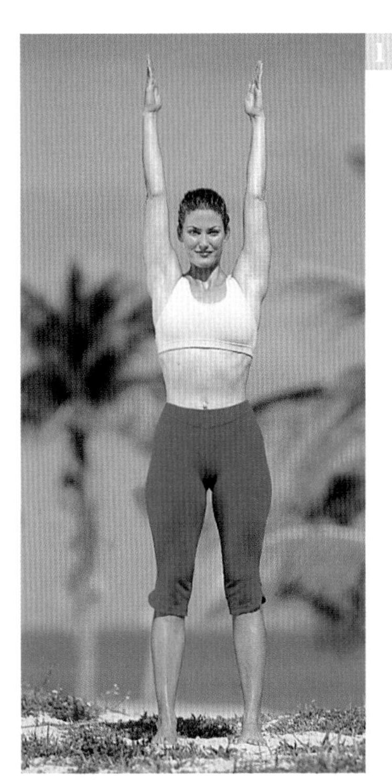

1 Stand straight with the feet shoulder-width apart, weight evenly distributed on all parts of the feet. Extend your arms straight up overhead so that the arms are close to your ears.

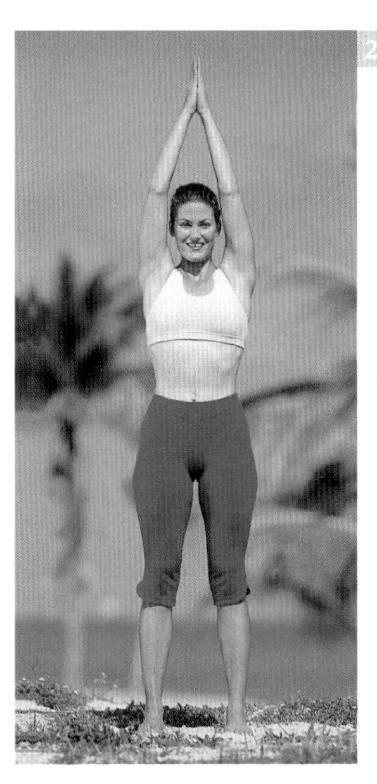

2 Firmly clap the entire surface of the palms together 8 times, chanting *Har* each time.

2 STRIKE THE GROUND

Forward bending relaxes and stretches the spine and invigorates the mind and nervous system. Clapping the ground stimulates meridian points in the hands that connect to the brain and improve your mental clarity.

Following the Overhead Clap immediately bend forwards, keeping the arms close to the ears. Strike the ground with your palms 8 times, chanting *Har*. Make sure that your knees are not locked. If you cannot reach the ground, bend your knees slightly.

AUBERGINE CURRY

The womanly shaped aubergine energizes and benefits hormonal and reproductive health.

1 medium–large aubergine, oven-baked at 350° for 15 minutes, or microwaved
2 medium onions, cut into thin slivers
4cm (1½in) peeled ginger, finely chopped
2 medium tomatoes, peeled and chopped
1–2 mildly hot peppers
½tsp garam masala

Brown onions. Then add ginger, tomatoes, peppers, garam masala, and salt to taste. Cook covered for 5–10 minutes. Take skin off aubergine. Mash flesh, add to pan, and simmer for 5 minutes. Add fresh parsley and serve with basmati rice.

3 ARM FLAPS

In this exercise the lymphatic areas are stimulated, promoting good breast health. Keeping the arms straight activates reflex points associated with the colon, stomach, spleen and liver, and tension is released from the shoulders.

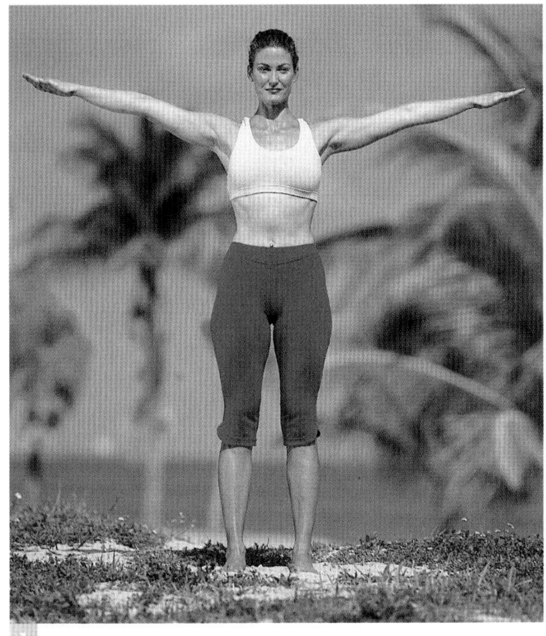

1 After Strike the Ground, straighten the spine and come back into a standing position. Bring your arms out to the sides of your body at shoulder level, parallel to the ground. Your fingers are straight with the palms facing downwards.

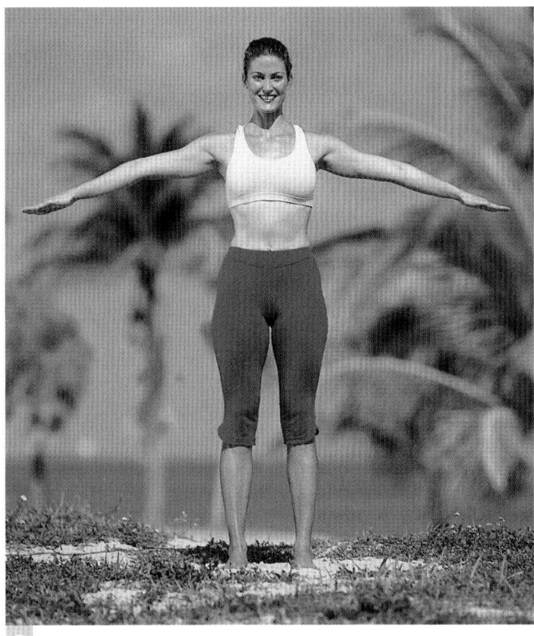

2 Begin flapping your arms without bending the elbows. Move approximately 15cm (6in) up and down from the horizontal in one smooth motion. Each time your arms move up or down chant *Har* for a total of 8 times.

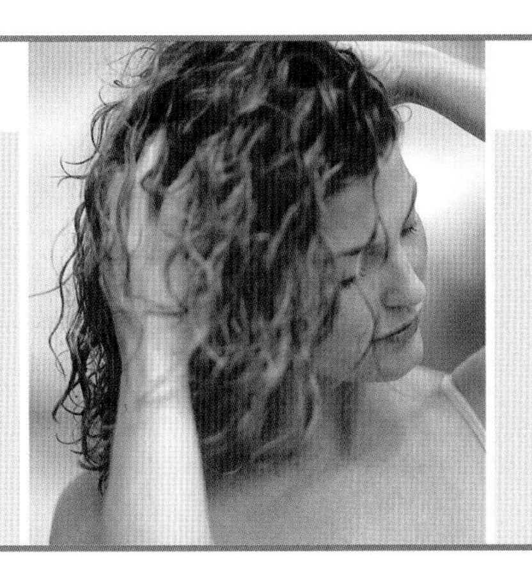

DRYING HAIR IN THE SUN

According to yogic teachings, hair that is dried in the sun absorbs vitamin D, making it directly available to the brain. It is good to massage the scalp as the hair dries, but wait until your hair is fully dry before combing to avoid breaking hair. Women should wash their hair within three days as excess scalp secretions can be subtly irritating to the nervous system. If a woman wants to refresh her outlook, washing her hair and drying it in the sun is a simple place to start!

4 CRISS-CROSS

This is the aerobic section of this yoga set, which strengthens the heart and improves metabolism. If you need to go at a more gentle pace, step the feet into and out of the criss-cross position instead of jumping. Alternate the crossing of opposite arms and legs each time.

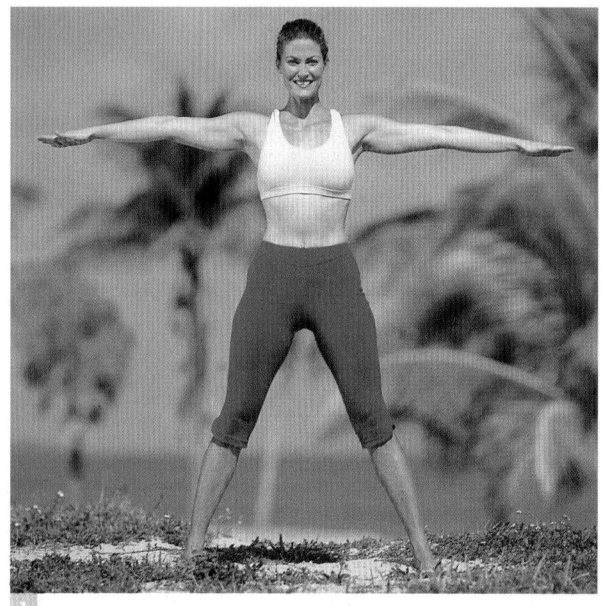

1 Keep your arms extended out to the sides with the palms facing downwards, parallel to the ground. Your feet should be slightly wider than shoulder-width apart.

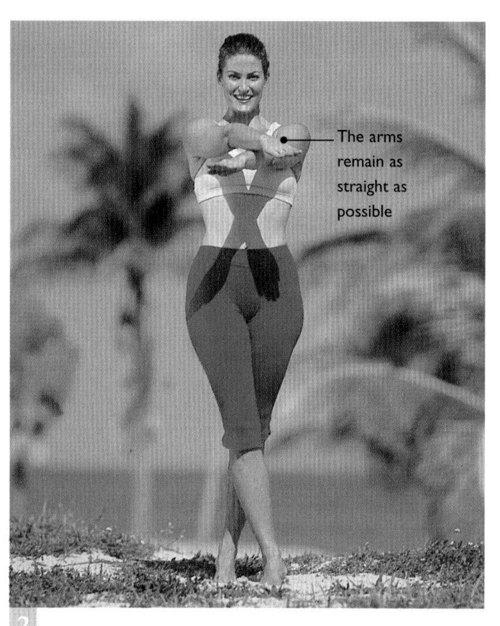

2 Bend your knees slightly as you jump and cross your legs. At the same time, cross your arms in front of your heart centre. Chant *Har* as you cross and uncross the legs and arms 8 times.

JULIE'S STORY (USA)

Several years ago I was working in a government position in biotechnology, a fast-paced, highly stressful job. Hearing that yoga was a way to calm the mind and body, I began classes in Kundalini Yoga. Within the first few months, I could tell that I was gaining a different perspective on my life and reassessing what was important. A year later, I decided that it was necessary for me to leave my job, reduce the stress in my life, and to share yoga with others by becoming a certified teacher. Having previously earned a PhD in Cell and Molecular Biology, I also knew that science needed to be part of my career, though I had no clear idea how it would all fit together. I believe that the practice of Kundalini Yoga and meditation gave me the clarity to make this career change and the confidence to know that I truly was on the right path. Now, seven years later, I teach Kundalini Yoga and have found a way to incorporate the science into a career related to the study of mind-body medicine.

5 ARCHER

This pose helps to maintain the mineral balance of the body, especially that of calcium, magnesium, sodium and potassium. It strengthens the electromagnetic energy field and improves concentration. Archer pose activates and balances all your chakras, and helps you develop courage.

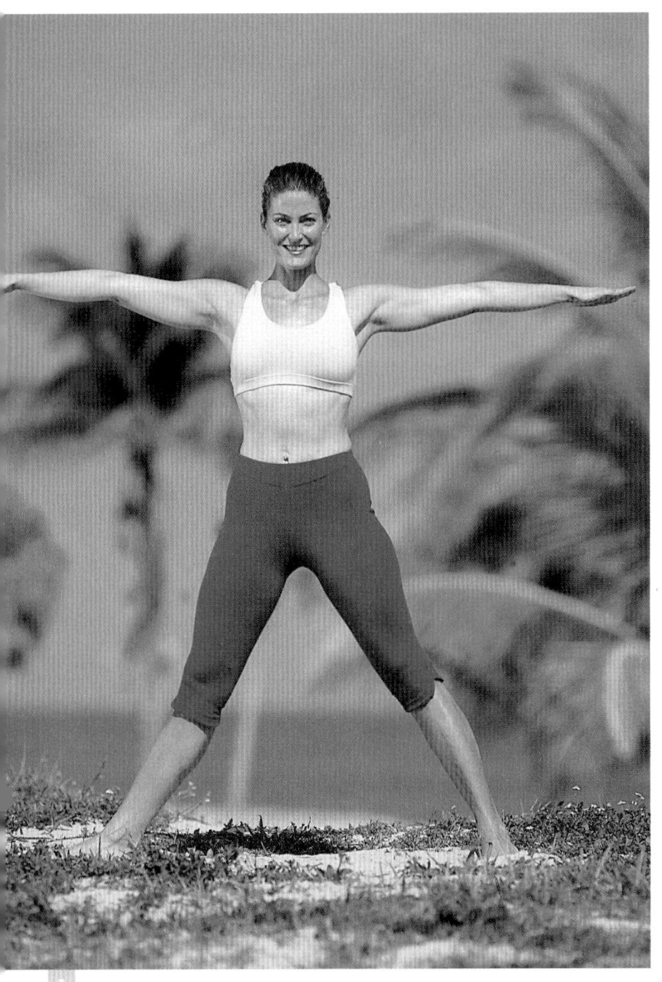

1 Stand with your legs straddled about 75cm (30in) apart, with your right leg forwards and your left leg back at a 45° angle to the front foot. Extend your arms out parallel to the ground.

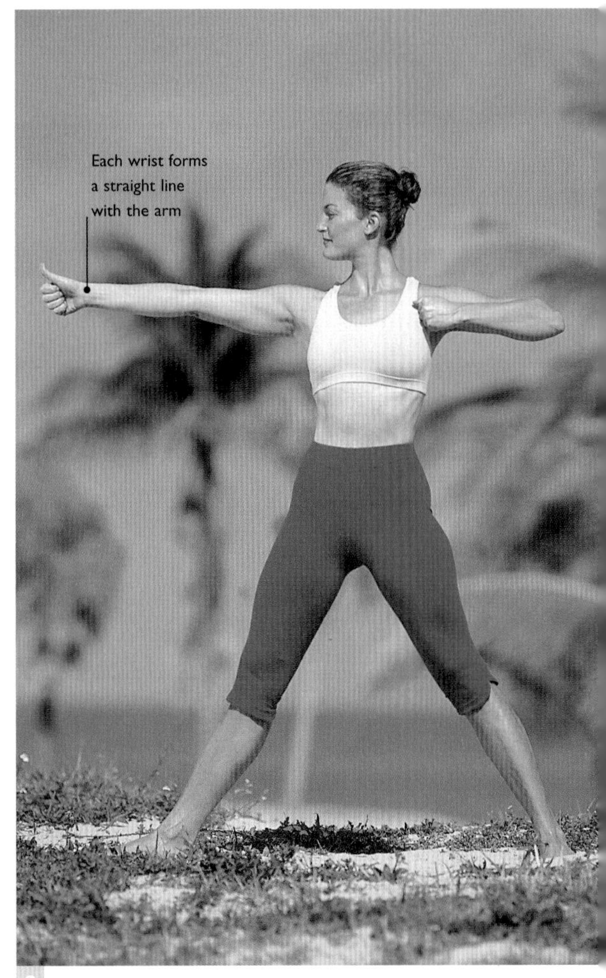

2 Raise your right arm straight in front of you. Make your right hand into a fist, as if grasping a bow, while pressing your thumb forwards. Bring your left arm back as if pulling a bow string back to the shoulder, expanding and lifting the chest. Your left forearm is parallel to the ground, your hand in a fist, again with the thumb pressed forwards.

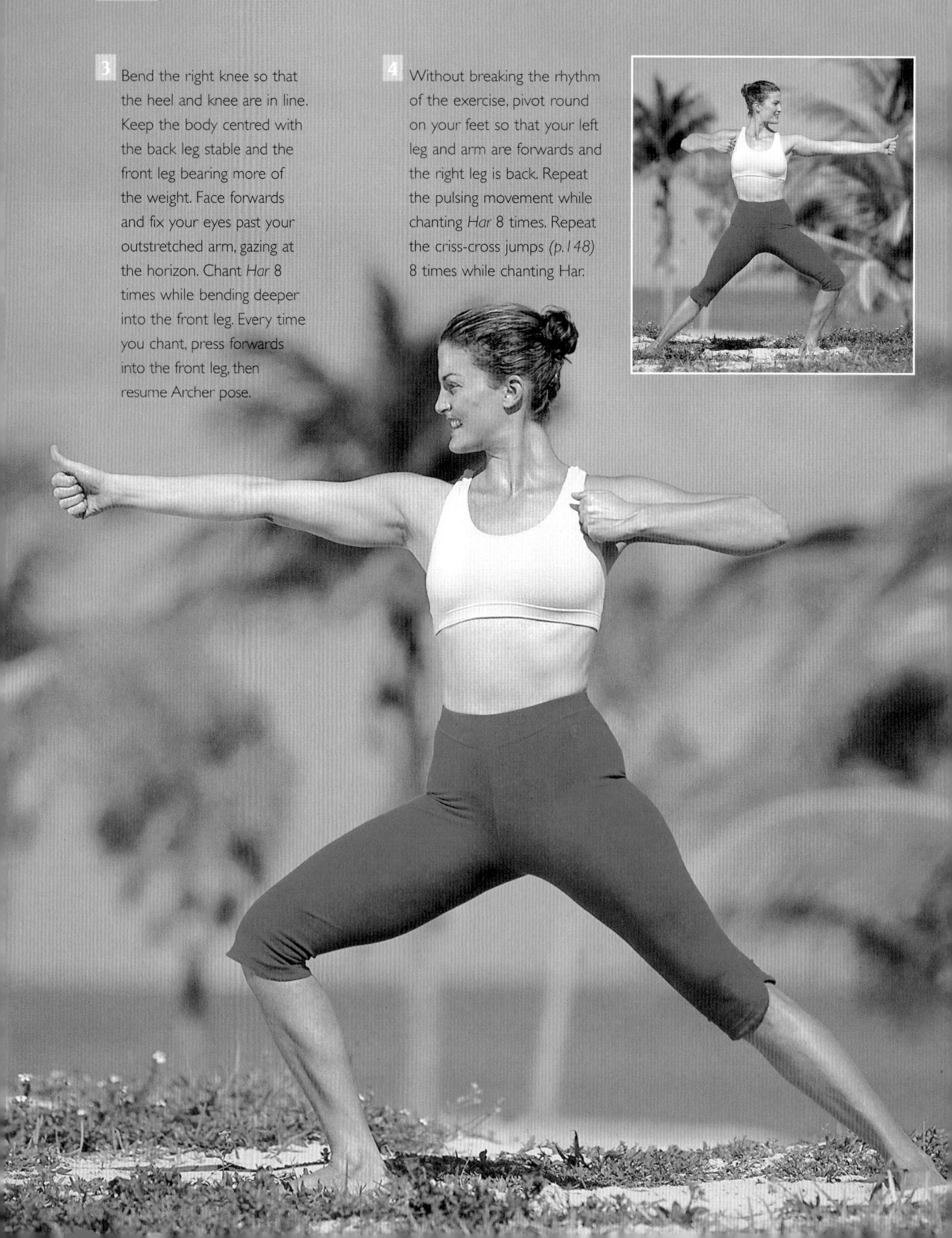

3 Bend the right knee so that the heel and knee are in line. Keep the body centred with the back leg stable and the front leg bearing more of the weight. Face forwards and fix your eyes past your outstretched arm, gazing at the horizon. Chant *Har* 8 times while bending deeper into the front leg. Every time you chant, press forwards into the front leg, then resume Archer pose.

4 Without breaking the rhythm of the exercise, pivot round on your feet so that your left leg and arm are forwards and the right leg is back. Repeat the pulsing movement while chanting *Har* 8 times. Repeat the criss-cross jumps *(p.148)* 8 times while chanting Har.

6 BACKWARD STRETCH

This stretch invigorates and flexes the whole spine, including the cervical vertebrae. Stretching the arms activates the lymphatic system, promoting good breast health.

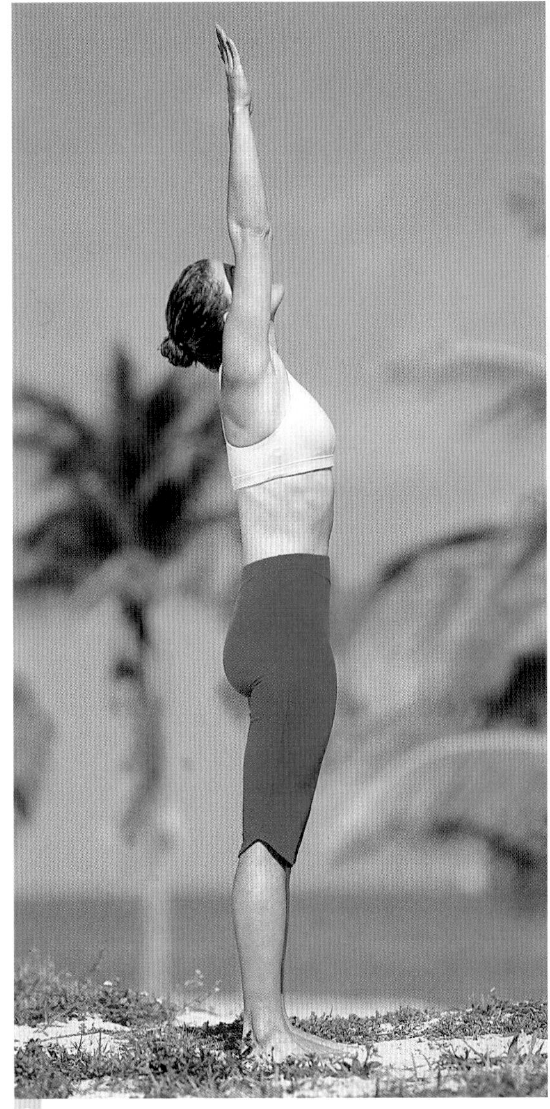

1 With the feet still shoulder-width apart, stretch the arms up overhead and back, arching the spine slightly. Look upwards towards your hands the entire time.

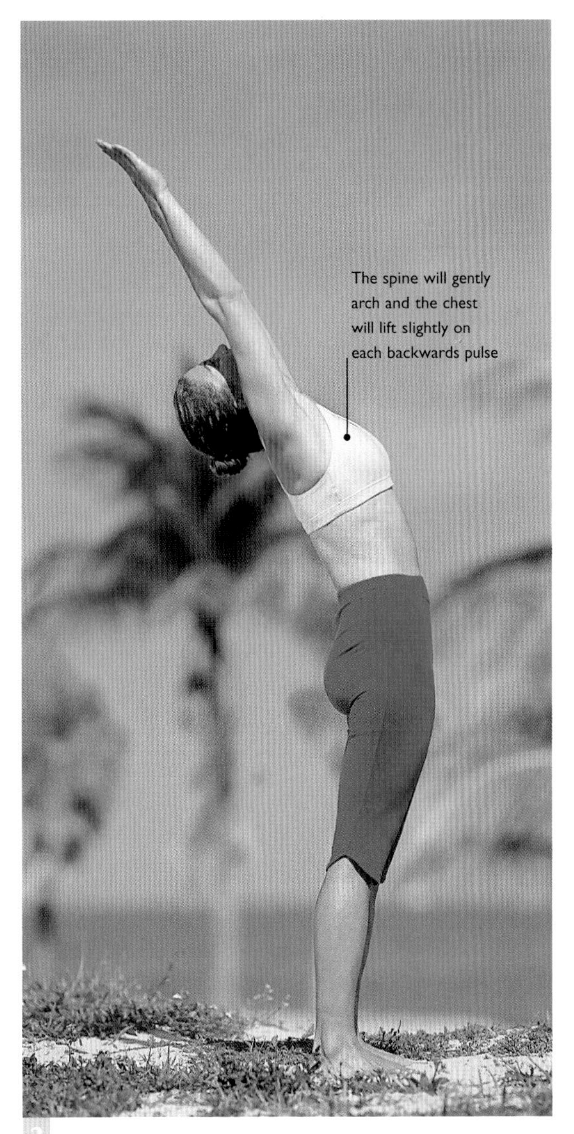

2 Chant *Har* as you pulse the arms back, then release slightly, continuing 8 times. The spine will gently arch and the chest lift slightly on each pulse. Repeat the criss-cross jumps *(p.148)* 8 times while chanting *Har*.

7 SIDE STRETCHES

These lateral stretches improve spinal flexibility, stimulate the lymphatic system, increase muscle tone, and aid digestion. This is the only exercise with a count of four on each side, totalling eight repetitions.

This is the last yoga pose of the set. Begin the set again on page 145 and repeat the entire series 5–25 times.

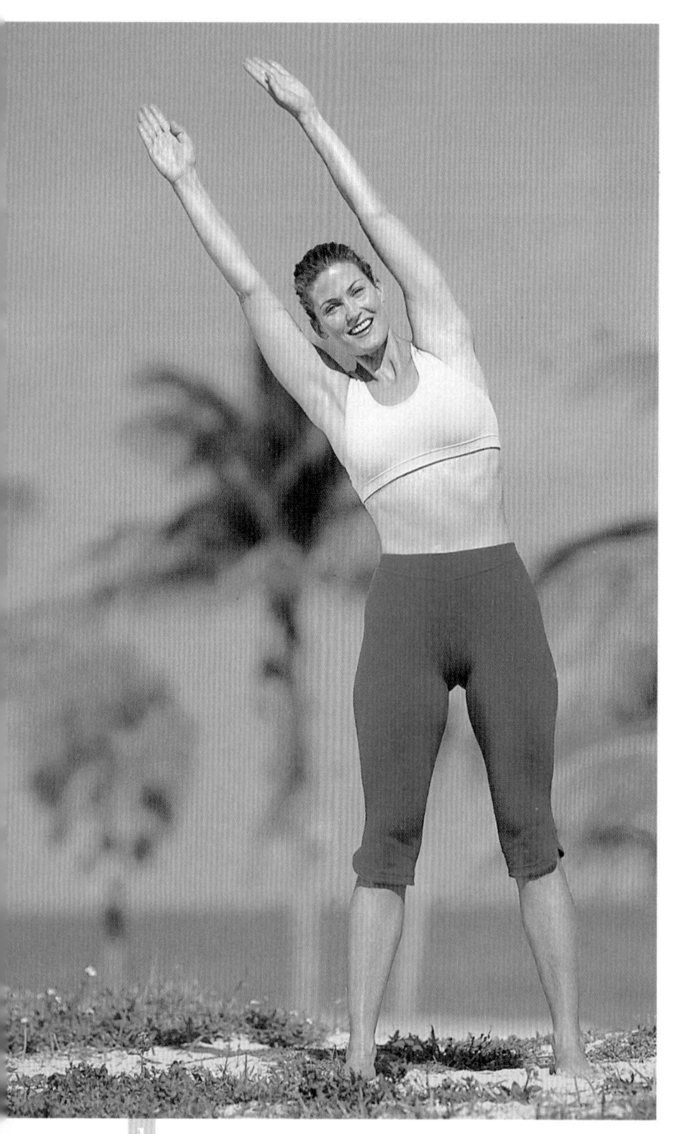

1 Stretch the arms up overhead. Bend directly to the right side so that a lateral stretch is created on the left side of the body. Make sure not to bend forwards or back, but directly to the side.

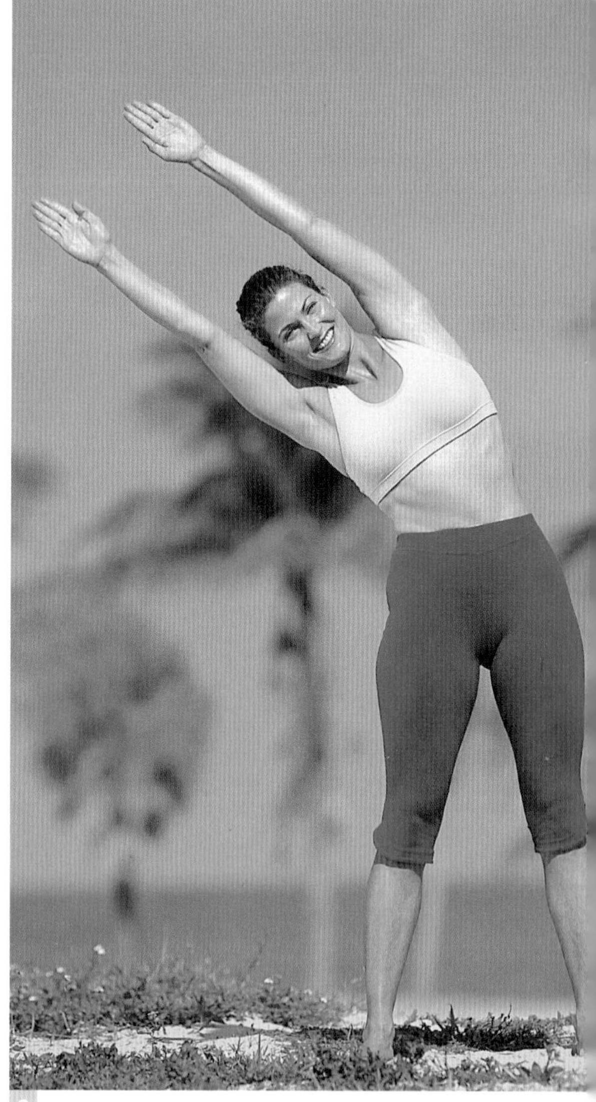

2 Begin to pulse and release slightly for a count of 4, chanting *Har* each time. Without stopping, stretch to the left side for four counts. Repeat the criss-cross jumps *(p.148)* 8 times while chanting *Har*.

8 TO END

After doing this set for an extended period of time it is important to rest. If you practise it on consecutive days, alternate between the following positions for relaxation: on one day rest on your back with the knees pulled into the chest and the arms wrapped around the bent legs. The next day rest in Child's pose *(p.50)*. Relax for at least five minutes, preferably more, and listen to an uplifting piece of music *(see also p.224)*.

ADI SHAKTI MEDITATION

This meditation uses the Kundalini Bhakti mantra, the "female power". It describes four qualities of the feminine aspect of creative power: the power that gave birth to all creation; the power that is forever; the power that cuts through darkness; and the nuturing power of the mother. It can be chanted powerfully from the heart centre in a monotone, or sung (see also Music Resources, p.224).

The mantra has four parts:

1 Adi Shakti, Adi Shakti, Adi Shakti, Namo Namo *("Ah-dee Shah-k tee, Nah-moe") meaning, "To the primal power that creates all things, I bow".*

2 Sarab Shakti, Sarab Shakti, Sarab Shakti, Namo Namo *("Sah-rub Shah-k tee") meaning, "To the total power of Shakti, I bow".*

3 Prithum Bagwati, Prithum Bagwati, Prithum Bagwati, Namo Namo *("Prit-um Bah-g wut-ee") meaning, "To the original Goddess, The Sword of Truth, I bow".*

4 Kundalini, Mata Shakti, Mata Shakti, Namo Namo *("Kun-da-leen-ee, Mah-tah Shah-k tee") meaning, "To the Kundalini, the mother power, I bow".*

Sit in Easy pose, spine straight, chest lifted, chin slightly tucked back towards the neck. Suggested mudras are: hands in the lap; right palm resting inside the left; tips of the thumbs touching; or arms crossed over the heart centre with the left palm underneath; and right overtop of the left. Close your eyes and vibrate the mantra from your heart. Feel the navel pull in slightly with the rhythm. Feel the energy of Shakti within you and all around you as you chant for 5, 11, or 31 minutes.

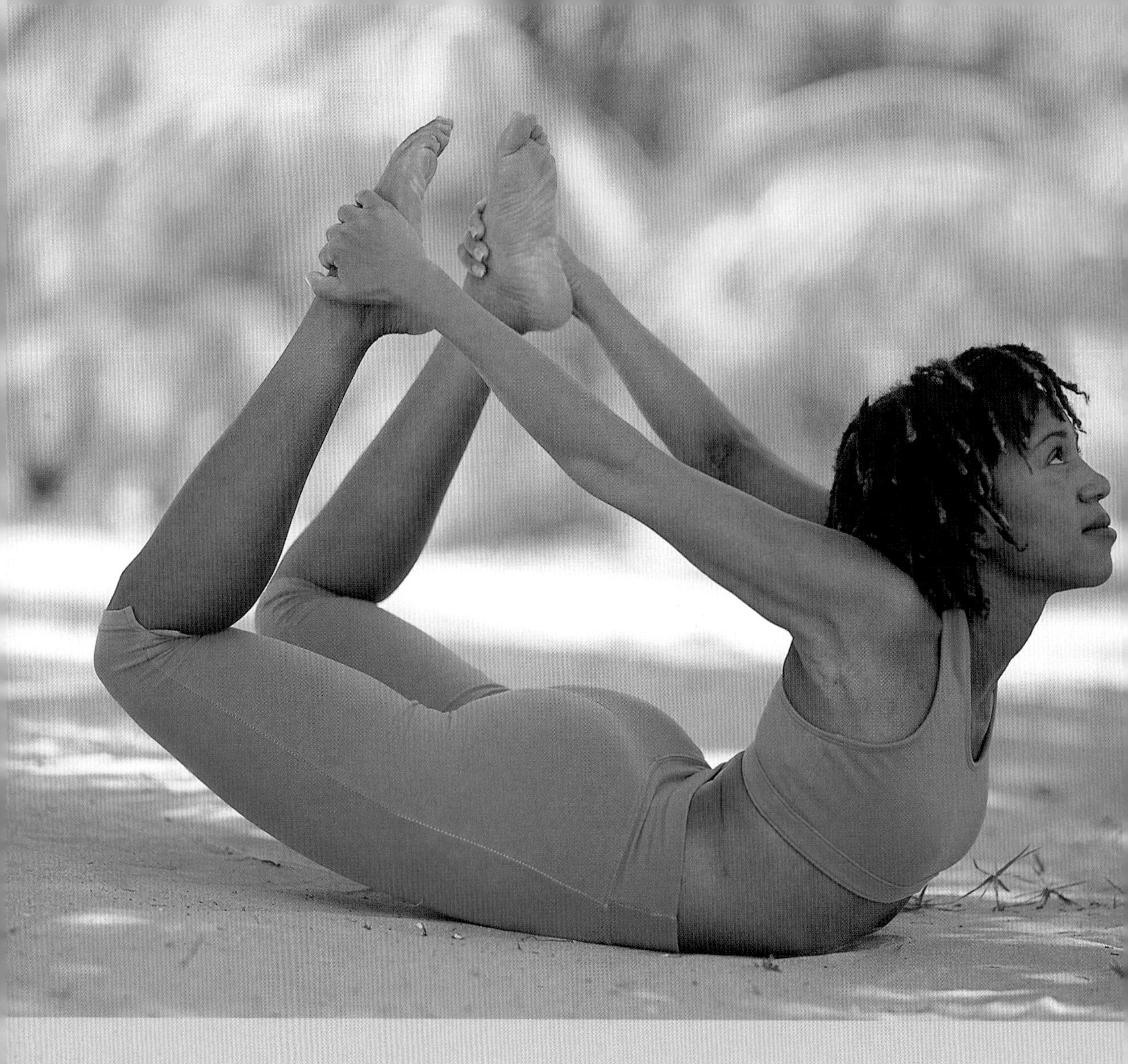

RELEASING FEAR & ANGER

I gratefully count myself among the many women who have found yoga and meditation to work wonders when it comes to strong emotions such as fear and anger. I think of yoga and meditation as partners, my two best friends, who upon finding me in a drama or trauma, roll up their sleeves and get right into the mess with me. They are loyal friends who help me get out all my "stuff", see it for what it is, then efficiently and effectively help me clean it up and send it on its way. My load lightened, I am left with lots of gratitude and a renewed dedication to my yoga practice. The yoga and meditation exercises in this chapter, and this entire book, serve as a means towards that end.

KUNDALINI SALUTATIONS

This set of postures and exercises strengthens and tones the muscles, releases fear and anger, and elevates the consciousness. It is called Kundalini Salutations because it works to awaken the kundalini energy. Once awakened, this energy provides you with the awareness you need to live to your potential.

The yogic numbers 26, 54, and 108 are cycles that have particular effects on your body and mind. Begin with 26 or 54 repetitions and, with practice, move on to 108.

1 UPPER TORSO LIFTS

This pose opens up the meridians of the abdomen, solar plexus, heart centre, and throat, which are associated with the navel chakra (seat of power and passion), heart chakra (home of altruistic love and compassion), and the throat chakra (ability to speak truth).

Lie on your abdomen with your chin on the ground and interlace your hands behind your back. For wrist problems, try grasping your wrists or a short rope or belt instead.

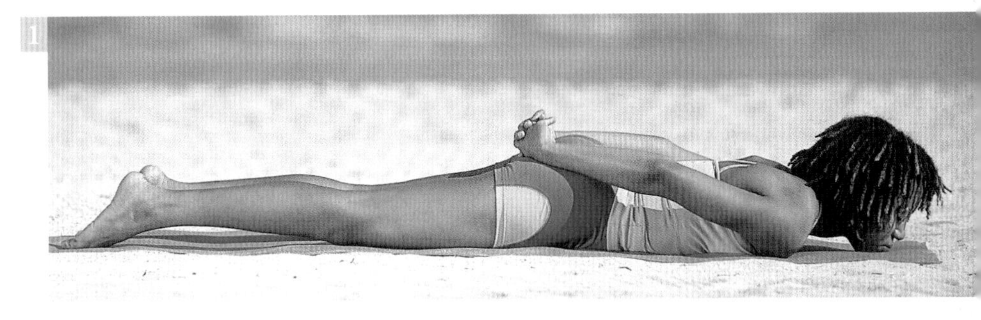

As you inhale, raise your upper torso off the ground as high as possible, using your abdominal, upper chest, and back muscles. Stretch your arms back and up simultaneously, as high as you can without straining. Exhale and relax the body back down with a rolling motion, keeping your hands clasped behind your back.

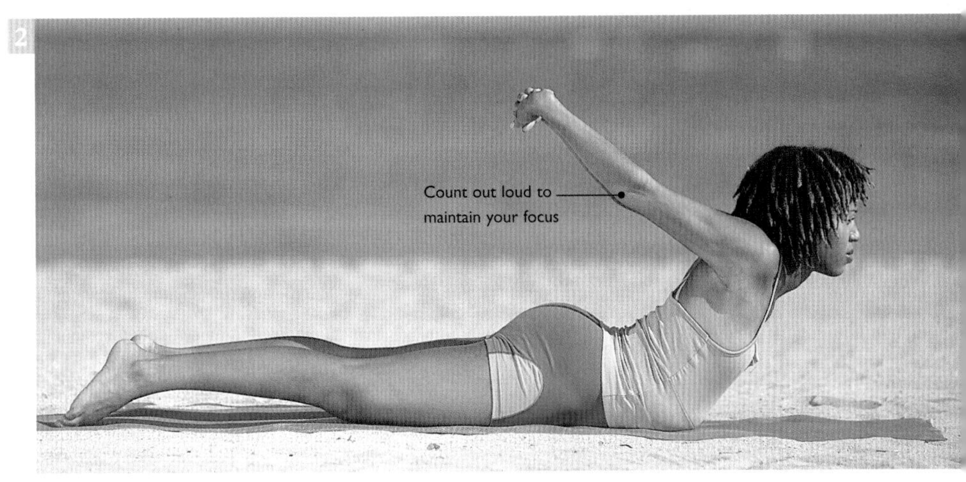

2 ROCKING BOW

This helps regulate a woman's hormones, which play a primary role in her emotional balance. If rocking is difficult, try lifting the body up on the inhale (as in step 4) and relaxing down on the exhale (as in step 5).

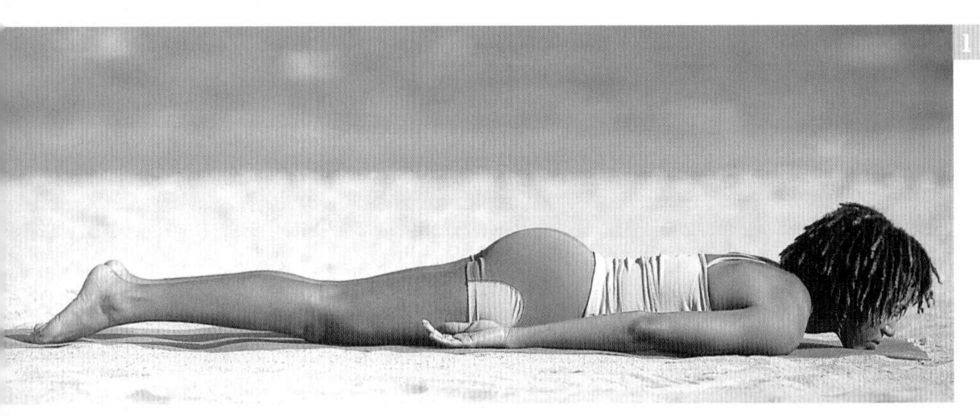

1 Lie on your abdomen with your arms at your sides, palms facing upwards and chin on the ground.

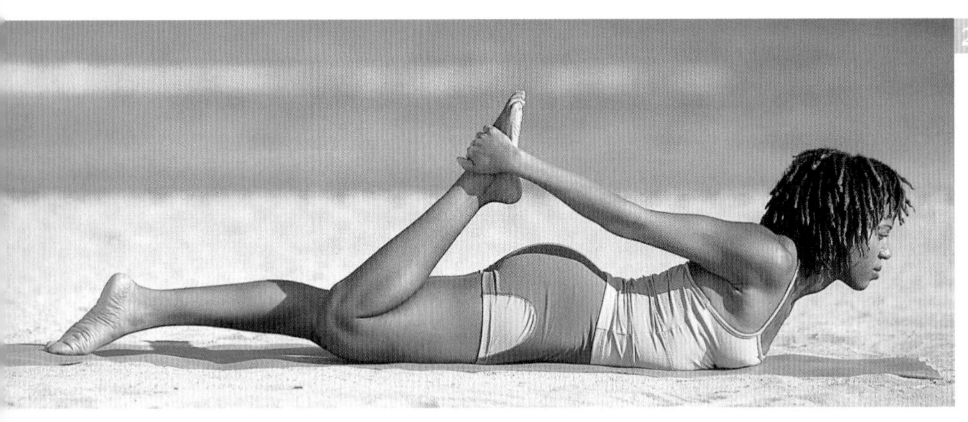

2 Raise your head up off the ground. Bend your right leg at the knee and reach back with your right hand to grasp the ankle.

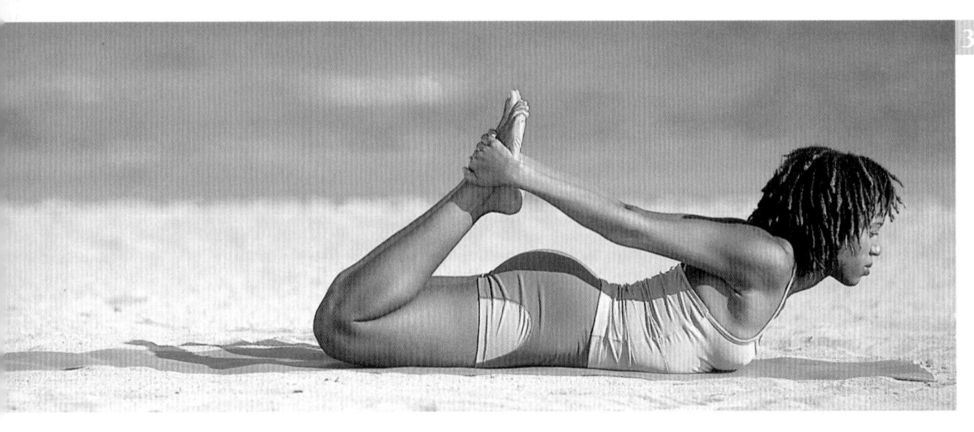

3 Bend your left leg at the knee and grab the ankle with your left hand. Keep the legs as close together as possible. If you cannot reach your ankles, loop a belt around your feet and hold onto the two sides of the belt as close to your feet as possible *(see also p.47)*.

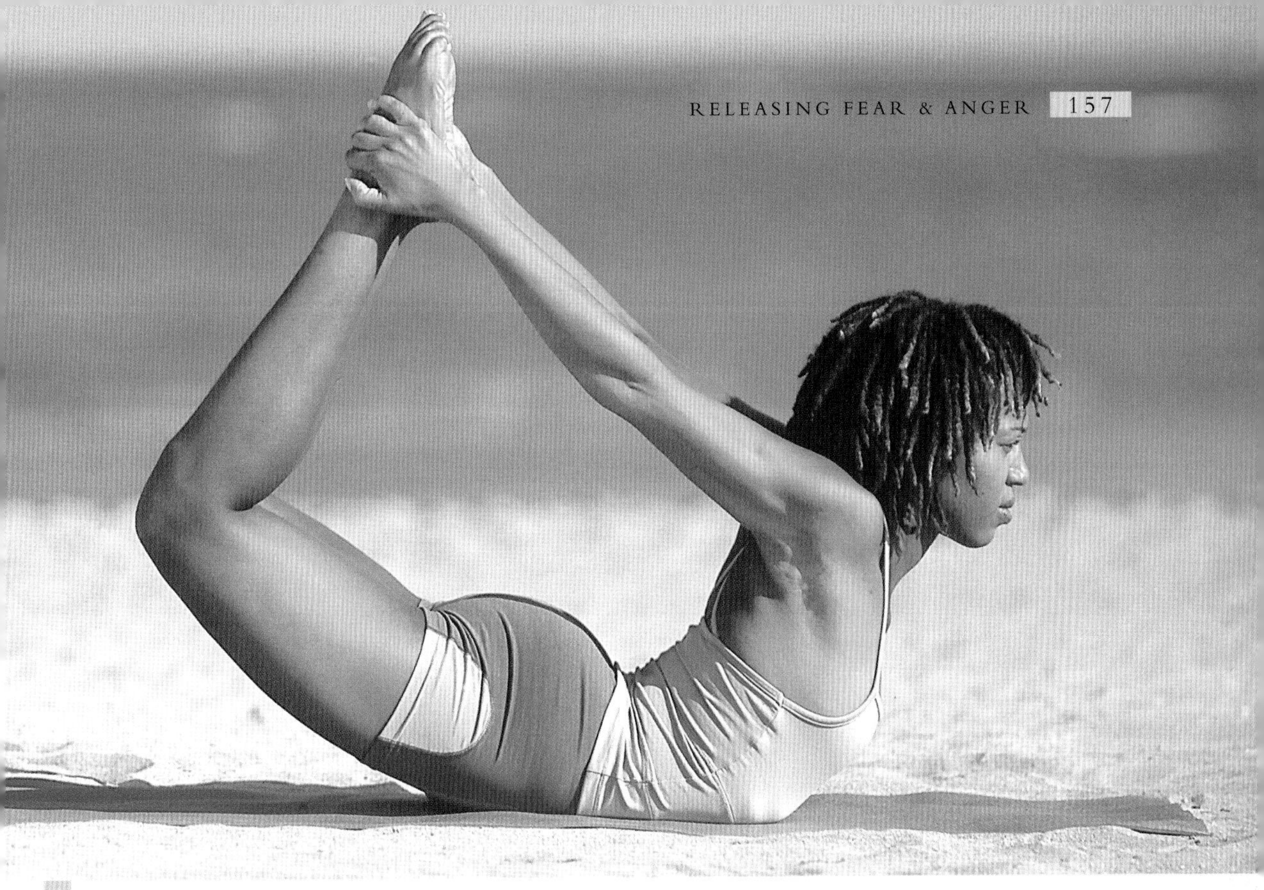

4 Inhale and lift your body upwards, raising your head, chest, and thighs up off the ground. Create a tension between the straight arms and the legs to stretch up higher without straining. Your elbows remain straight. Use your upper body strength to stretch up. Look straight ahead. Prepare yourself to exhale and rock forwards.

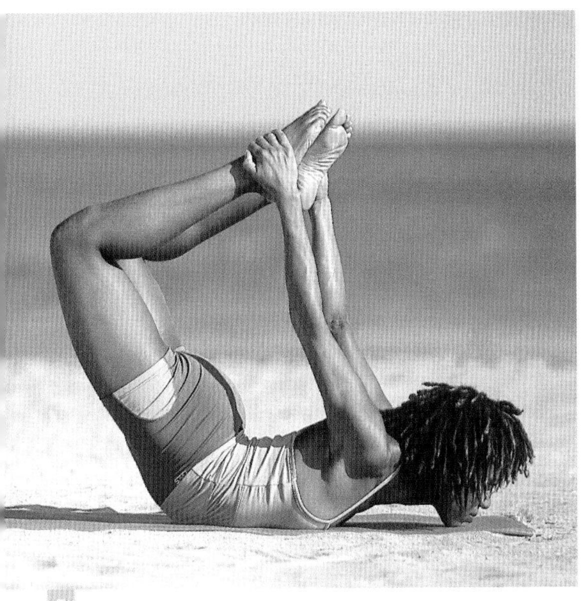

5 As you exhale, rock forwards so that your head comes down and your thighs lift off the ground as much as possible without you straining.

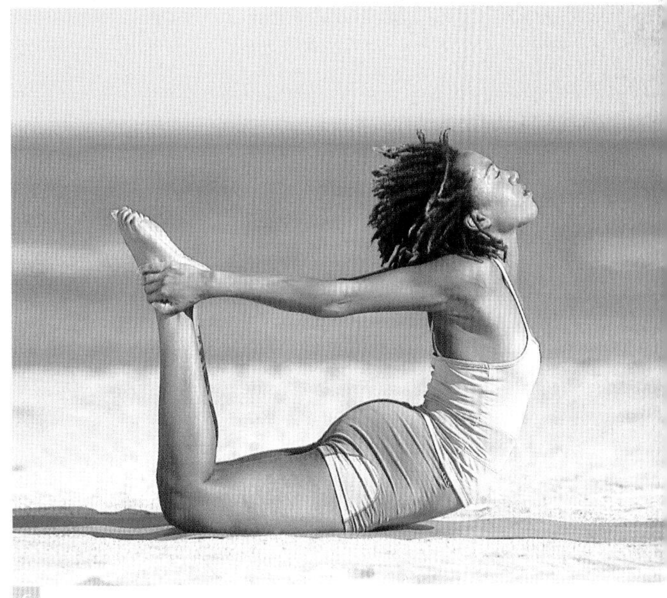

6 Inhale as you rock back and your chest lifts up. Continue Rocking Bow, counting up to 26, 54, or 108 as you rock. Each forwards and backwards movement counts as one.

3 BOWING POSE

This pose generates internal heat or tapas from the base of the spine to the base of the neck. As you bow with arms outstretched, the lymph area under the armpits is stimulated. Be aware of touching your third eye point (located between the eyebrows) to the ground as you bow; this creates a natural focal point for the mind.

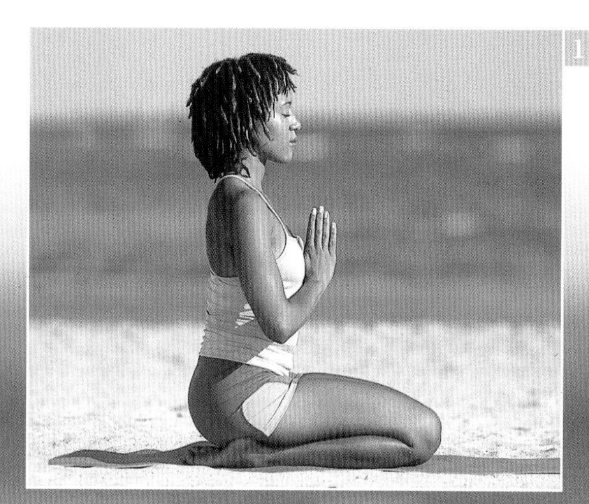

1 Sit on your heels with a straight spine. Press the palms of your hands together in Prayer pose, then bring them to the centre of your chest so that the thumbs are pressing against the breastbone. Inhale deeply in this position.

2 As you exhale, bend forwards, and in one smooth motion bring your torso and your hands down to the ground. As you bow with your hands in Prayer pose, slide the outside edges of your hands forwards until your arms are stretched out straight and your forehead touches the ground. Perform this pose 26, 54, or 108 times.

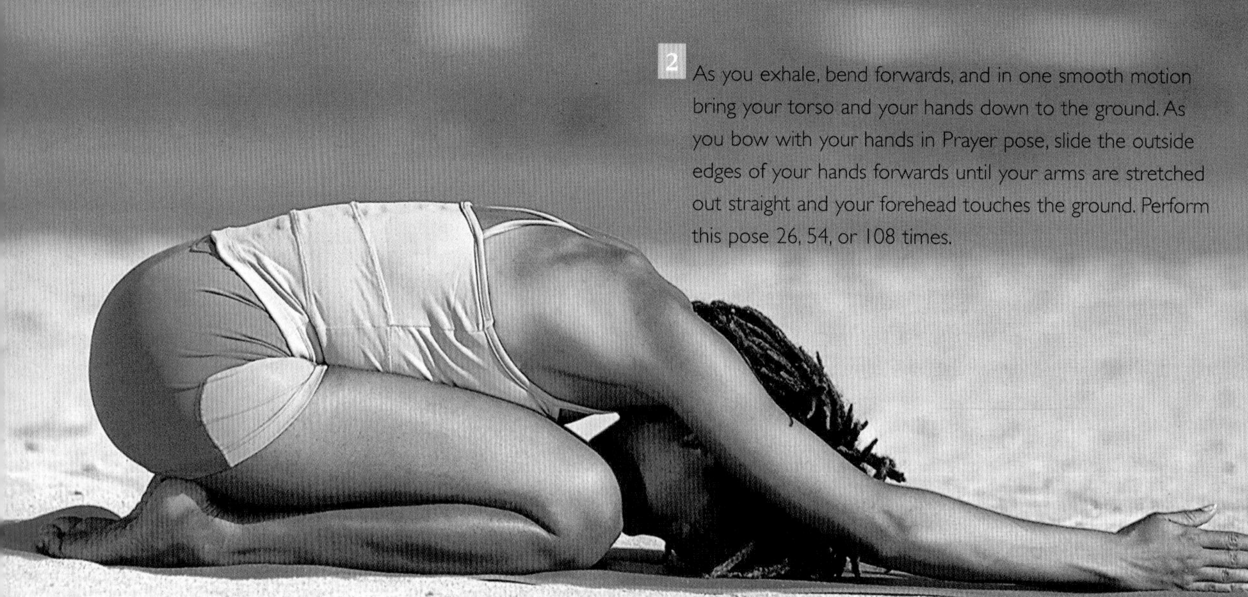

MICHELLE'S STORY (USA)

The first time I went to a yoga class, the strong breathing techniques and poses helped calm my mind for the first time that I could remember. I have always suffered from high anxiety, and unchecked thoughts lead me to worry and self-criticism. Kundalini Yoga hushed my mind to allow for my deeper spiritual purpose to be revealed.

Through my job as an engineer I was working in the Pentagon, Washington DC, on September 11, 2001, when the terrorist plane crashed into it. As I ran away from the building with no purse, keys, or money, I came upon the on-site daycare centre being evacuated.

I was faced with a decision to continue running scared or help the children. Regardless of my own fear, I knew where I should be. So I stayed with the children for the remainder of the day until each child was picked up. During the following week as I neared the Pentagon on my daily train journey into work, I would break out in a sweat, begin to breathe rapidly, and start to cry uncontrollably. Then after that first week, I found myself quickly regaining my mental and emotional balance on the ride to work by using two Kundalini Yoga techniques; long, deep breathing, and Sa Ta Na Ma meditation.

Since the attack in September, I have found that as long as I stay conscious of my breath and meditate, I can keep anxiety to a minimum. Yoga in the wake of disaster has helped me increase my personal practice of yoga and meditation, and has awakened new feelings of gratitude for this precious life.

4 JUMP AROUND

Jumping your body in this way strengthens your nervous system and releases tension and anxiety. Make sure you have a soft surface underneath you before practising this exercise. Then have fun with it!

Lie down on your back with your arms at your sides, palms facing downwards. Begin to freely jump your body all around. Press your legs and arms against the ground to jump your torso. Move your legs and arms. Move your head and neck from side to side, taking care not to jerk or bump your head against the ground. Continue for 1–3 minutes.

5 SITALI COBRA

Sitali breath, the Sanskrit name for Cooling breath (*p. 77*), cools off anger, soothes the nervous system, and calms anxiety and fear. Coupled with the Cobra pose, it stimulates the pranic flow of energy throughout the spine and torso, distributing vital energy to the body and mind.

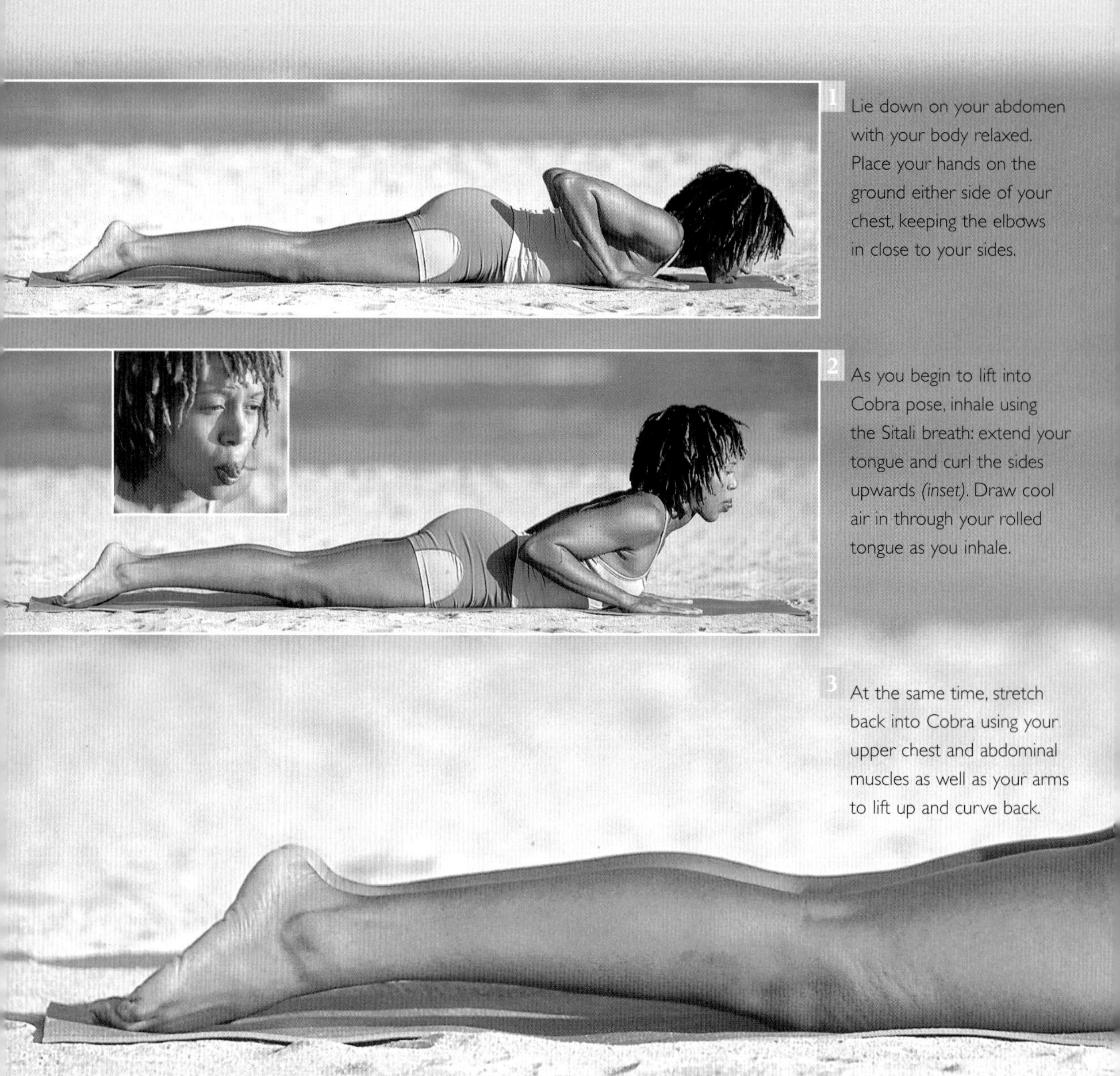

1 Lie down on your abdomen with your body relaxed. Place your hands on the ground either side of your chest, keeping the elbows in close to your sides.

2 As you begin to lift into Cobra pose, inhale using the Sitali breath: extend your tongue and curl the sides upwards *(inset)*. Draw cool air in through your rolled tongue as you inhale.

3 At the same time, stretch back into Cobra using your upper chest and abdominal muscles as well as your arms to lift up and curve back.

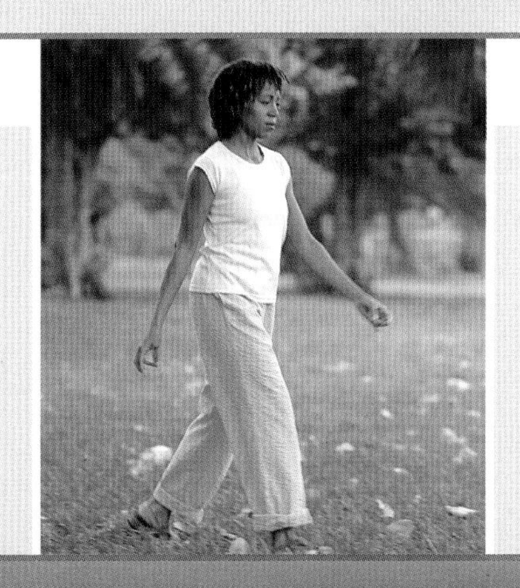

WALKING MEDITATION

A fun and effective form of meditation can be done by walking in rhythm as you breathe, inhaling to the count of two or four steps and exhaling for the same length of time. Or add a mantra: try chanting Sa Ta Na Ma *while pressing your fingers* (p.97)*. You may chant silently or out loud. Keep your eyes gazing out in front of you to maintain your meditative state. The yogic science of walking meditation is called Breathwalk, and has helped many people reduce stress and increase calmness just by the simple act of walking* (see also p.224).

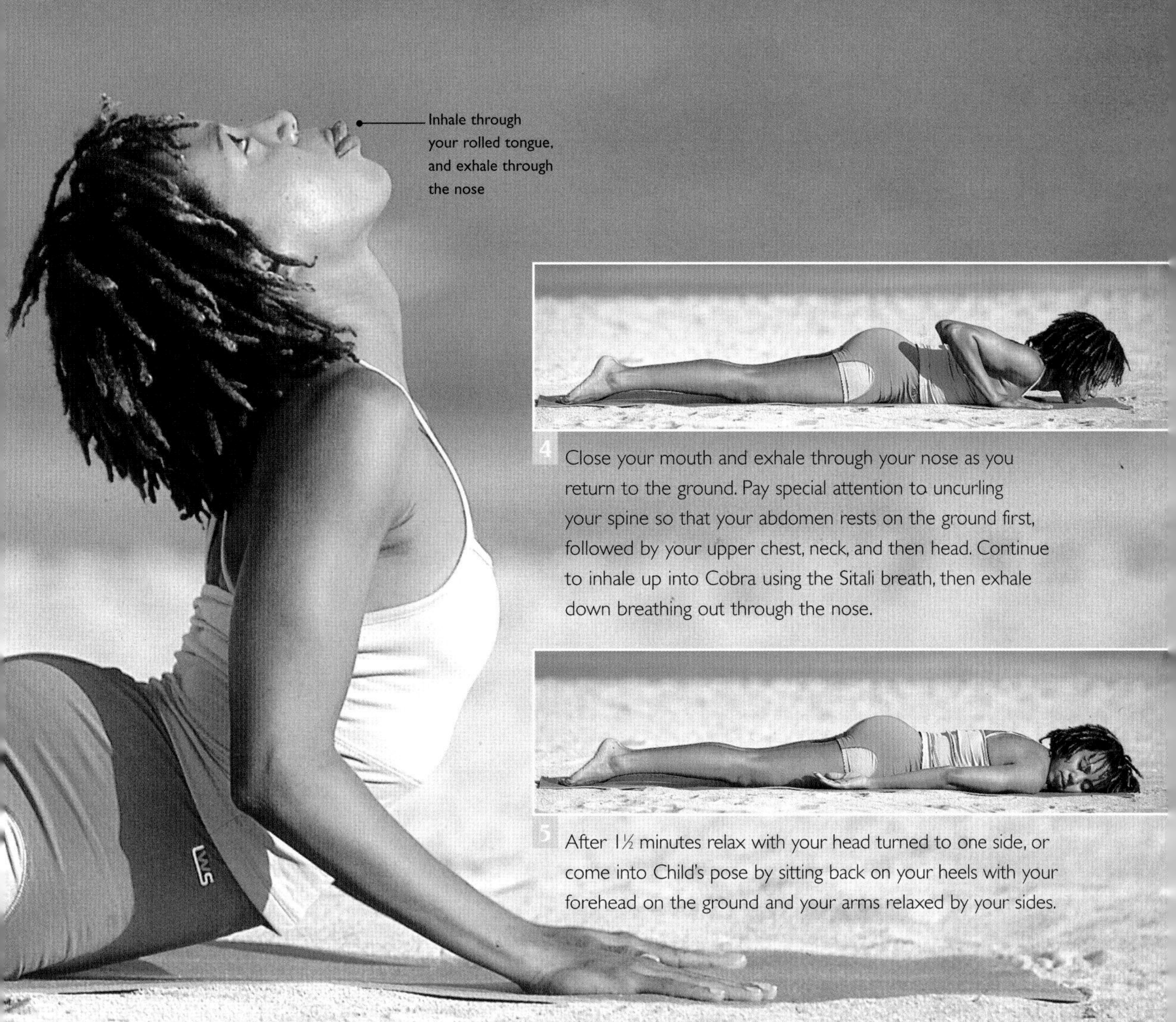

Inhale through your rolled tongue, and exhale through the nose

4 Close your mouth and exhale through your nose as you return to the ground. Pay special attention to uncurling your spine so that your abdomen rests on the ground first, followed by your upper chest, neck, and then head. Continue to inhale up into Cobra using the Sitali breath, then exhale down breathing out through the nose.

5 After 1½ minutes relax with your head turned to one side, or come into Child's pose by sitting back on your heels with your forehead on the ground and your arms relaxed by your sides.

6 MANTRA MEDITATION

In this meditation at the end of the set you learn to direct an internal sound into your chakras using your imagination. The result is that you become more self-aware and in control of your thoughts and actions. Start with one repetition of the mantra on the held inhalation and exhalation. As you become familiar with this process, try to repeat the mantra three times or more on each inhalation and exhalation.

After this, sing along to the music Naad: The Blessing (see Music Resources, p.224) *or sit silently for three minutes, then relax on your back for 10 minutes.*

1 Sit in Easy pose. Straighten the lower vertebrae, lift the chest, and draw the chin slightly in towards the neck to bring the cervical vertebrae in line with the spine. Rest your hands on your knees in passive Gyan Mudra *(p.21)*, first finger and thumb touching and the other fingers extended but relaxed. Close your eyes.

2 Inhale deeply and hold your breath. Mentally chant the mantra *Har Har Wahe Guru*: pull your navel slightly towards your spine and upwards as you mentally sound *Har* (rhymes with "car") at your navel point, then sound *Har* at your heart centre. Mentally project the sound *Wa* ("la") at your throat centre, then *He* ("hey") at your brow point, or intuitive centre. Finally, imagine the sound *Guru* ("gu-roo") at the top of your head.

3 Repeat the mantra mentally as many times as you can on the held inhalation, then exhale and hold the breath out, repeating the same process. Continue for 11 minutes.

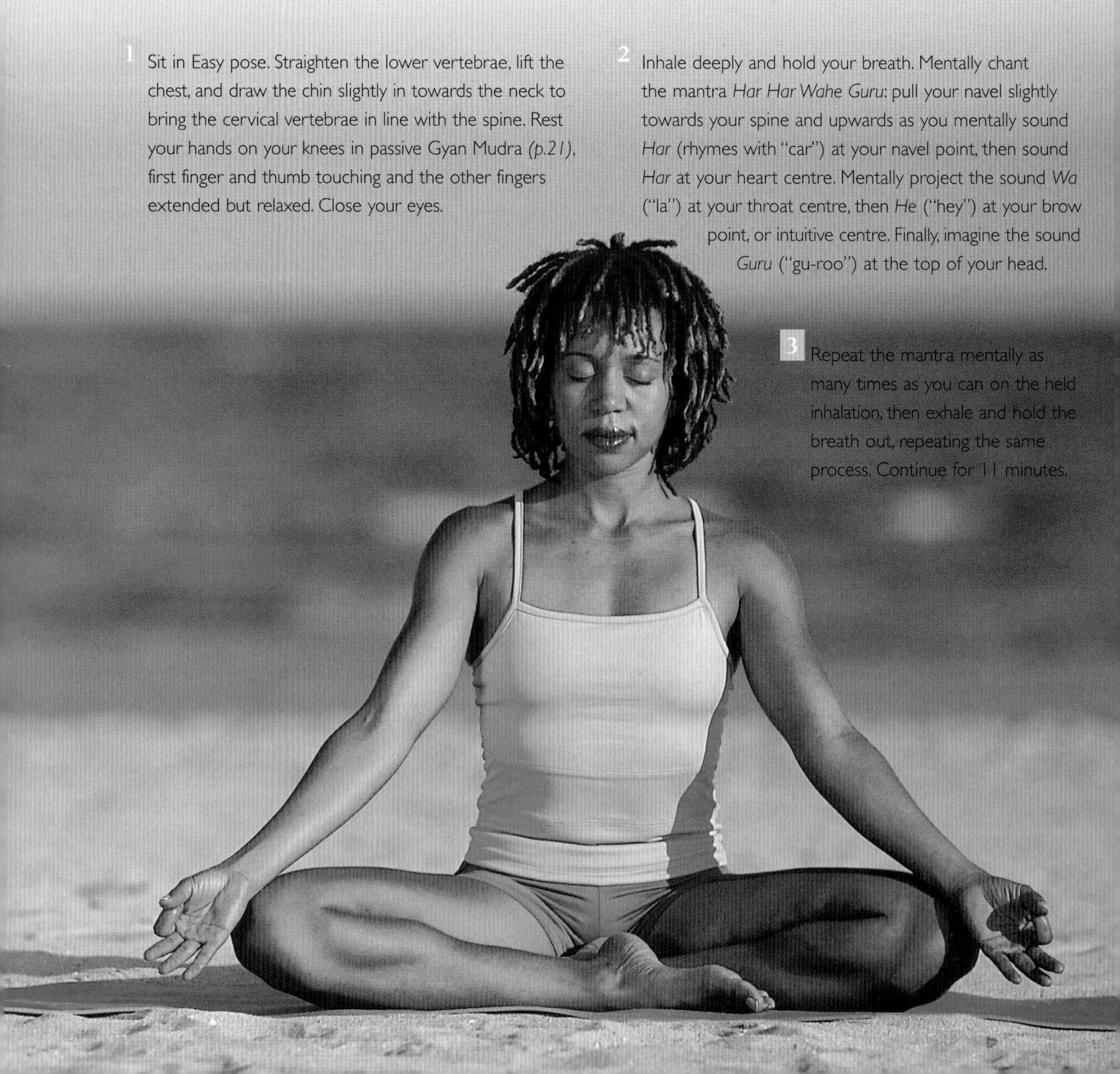

PRANAYAMA TO EXPEL NEGATIVITY AND DISEASE

This pranayama, or breathing exercise, uses the circle breath, which cleanses out whatever is the root of the problem within you. It has a purgative effect, ridding your body of disease and your mind of anger, sorrow, and fear. On the four-part inhalation, your lungs will fill in one continuous motion as follows:

On the initial part of the inhalation, the lowest part of the lungs are filled and the abdomen expands outwards.

On the second part, the lower rib cage expands.

On the third, the chest begins to expand.

On the last part of the inhalation, the top of the chest is filled with the breath and the throat and shoulders feel an expansion.

1 *Sit up straight in Easy pose. Bend your right arm up at the elbow and bring it close to the side of your body with your open palm facing forwards, as though you are taking an oath. Then raise your left arm with the elbow bent, and bring the forearm round in front of the chest, parallel to the ground, with the fingers straight and the palm facing down. Keep your eyes closed. Form an "o" shape with your mouth and begin to inhale powerfully and deeply in four distinct parts* (see above). *Then exhale with one long breath. Continue for 11–22 minutes.*

2 *To end the pranayama, inhale as deeply as you can, relaxing your diaphragm and opening up the chest cavity. Hold your breath and stretch your arms up straight and as high possible, with your fingers spread wide and as tight as steel. Stretch your entire spine upwards. Exhale strongly through the mouth like a firing cannon. Repeat two more times, then relax.*

"People who do breathing exercises will have the capacity for very long breaths. They will have extra prana.... If prana is less in you, then you are less in you."

Yogi Bhajan

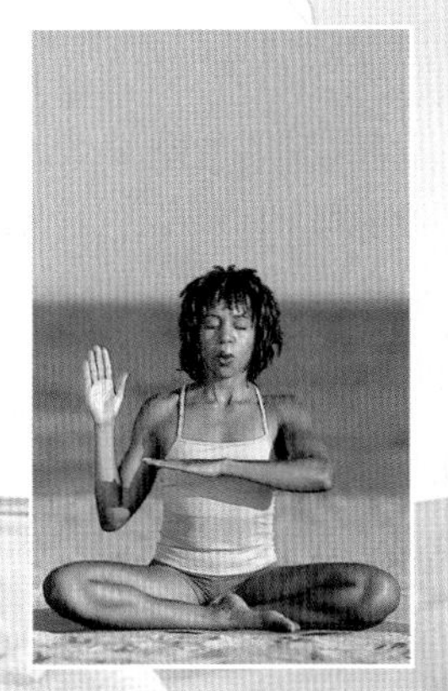

Step 1

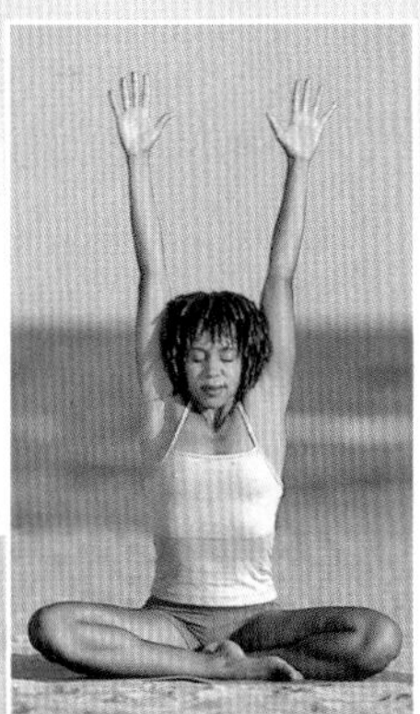

Step 2

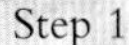

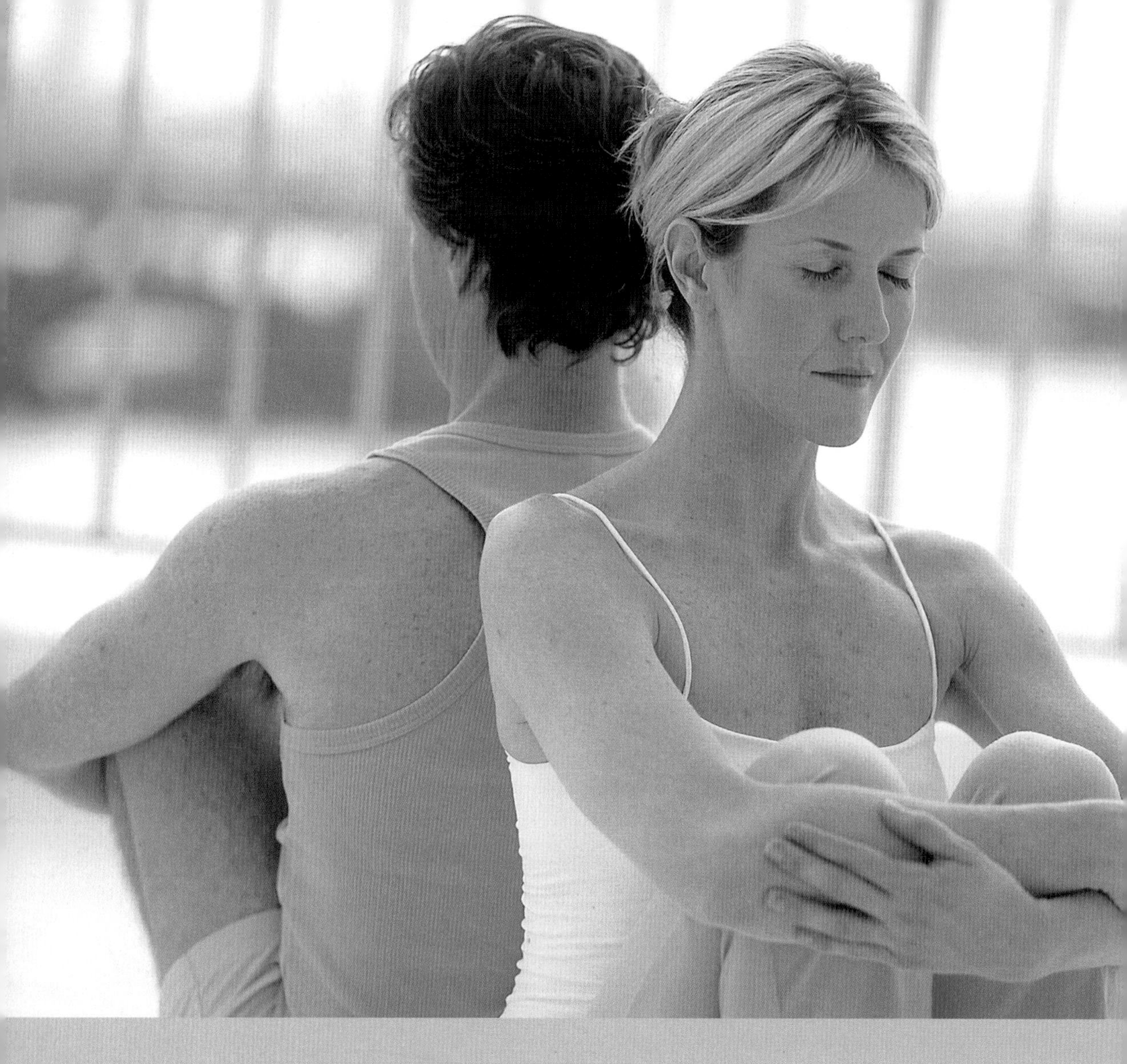

RELATIONSHIPS

Every challenge, every conflict, every dream, every prayer that you have comes from you and resolves with you. It all comes back to you. Nowhere is this more apparent than in relationships with your partner. Other chapters in this book will help you to become a woman who is solidly prepared for enlightened relationships. This chapter will help you blend your male and female sides, and strengthen your inner resolve. Partner yoga and meditations allow your energies to blend and your hearts to open to each other. This is also the place to turn to when you are not getting along in your relationships, or when there may be discord, dissatisfaction, or disappointment.

VENUS KRIYAS

Venus (meaning love) Kriyas are exercises that are shared between partners. The internal energy is drawn and directed positively towards subconscious cleansing and the raising of energy through the chakras to higher consciousness. Each of the kriyas is complete in itself; choose just one or two to do and practise each for no longer than three minutes. Begin by tuning in (p.22).

If your partner is willing to join you, be grateful. If not, be grateful anyway. You'll feel happy and happiness is contagious. Your partner may be curious about what's making you feel so good.

GETTING RID OF GRUDGES

When you and your partner have felt discord between you, whether spoken or not, this exercise helps you both to clear the air and start over afresh. All it takes is a willingness to practise.

Sit back to back with your partner, with the length of your spines touching. Put your feet flat on the ground in front of you, bring your knees up and wrap your arms around them. Close your eyes and breathe.

Meditate on your heart – hear it and feel it. Meditate on the sun, bringing it into your heart. Burn out all the bitterness and grudges that you may have been carrying. Continue for 3 minutes.

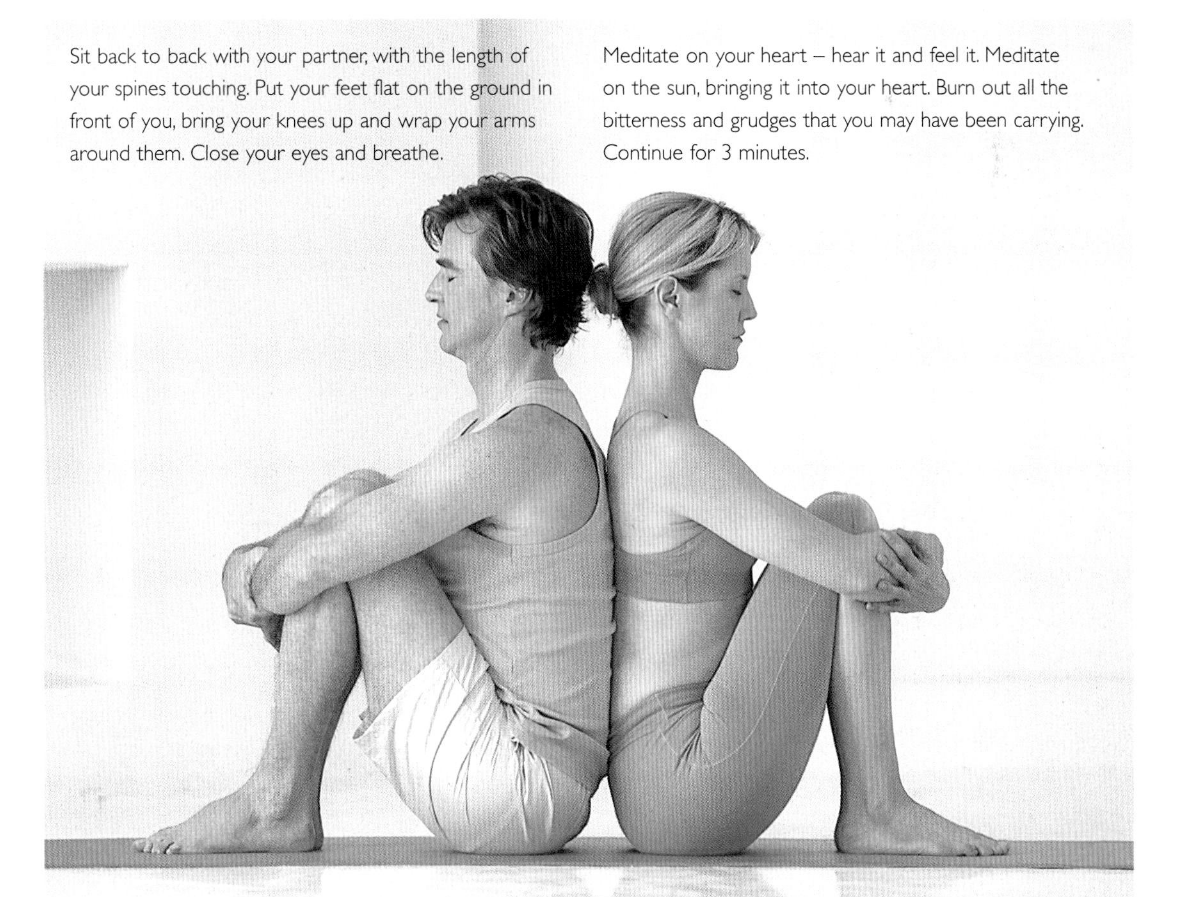

SENDING PRANA

In this exercise you use your hands and eyes to energize each other and build a healing energy between you. Keeping the arms straight increases nerve strength in the arms and pranic energy in the hands.

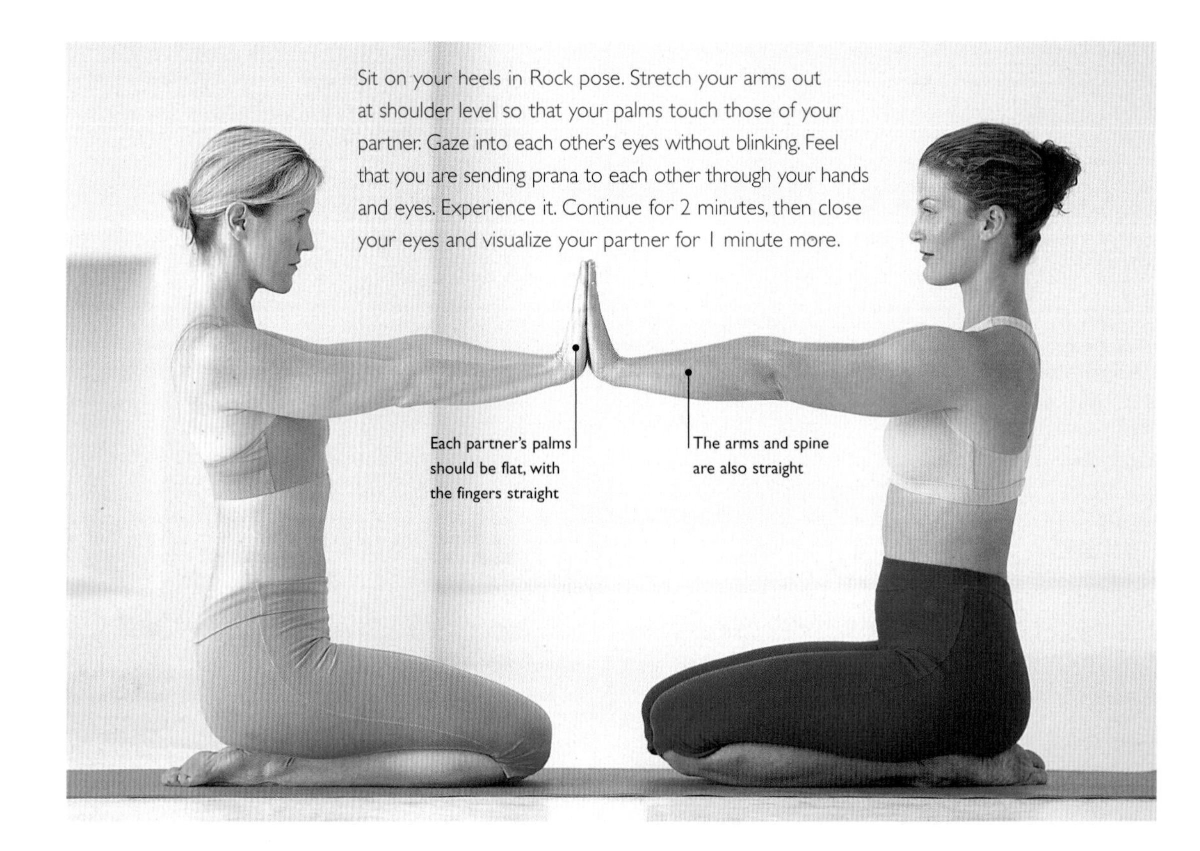

Sit on your heels in Rock pose. Stretch your arms out at shoulder level so that your palms touch those of your partner. Gaze into each other's eyes without blinking. Feel that you are sending prana to each other through your hands and eyes. Experience it. Continue for 2 minutes, then close your eyes and visualize your partner for 1 minute more.

Each partner's palms should be flat, with the fingers straight

The arms and spine are also straight

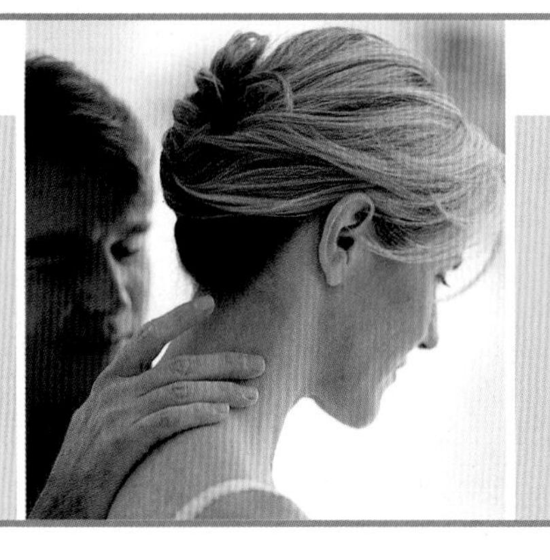

MOON CENTRES

According to yogic teachings, a woman has eight moon centres, extra-sensitive areas that, when kissed and caressed, arouse her sexual desire. They are the hair on her head, her lips, ears, and the back of the neck, her breasts, the navel, the lower back, and her inner thighs. Though it may feel natural to begin at the top moon centre and move downwards, keep in mind that when it comes to intimacy, there are no set rules to follow.

CROW SQUATS

Crow squats benefit your hips, lower spine, and leg muscles by opening, stretching, and toning them. Energy in the lower chakras is stimulated and circulated to the upper chakras. This exercise can be aerobic and heart-strengthening.

1 Stand facing your partner with your feet shoulder-width apart. You may have to adjust your feet in order to maintain balance while squatting. Join hands and look into each other's eyes with love. Verbally greet each other, then continue talking to each other throughout the exercise.

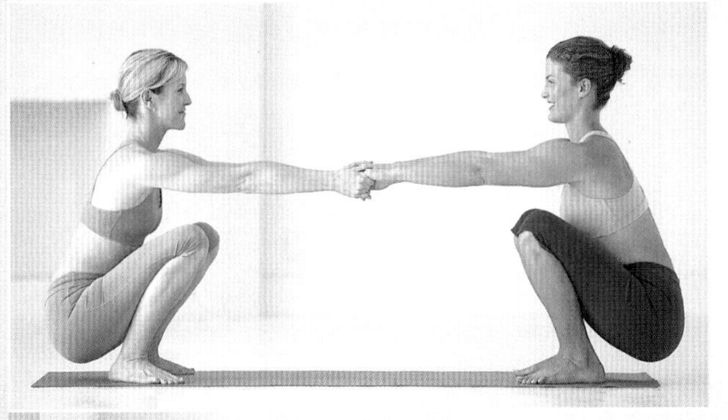

2 Bend your knees and squat down together so that your buttocks are close to the ground. Ideally your feet will be flat on the ground. Your body will naturally lean forwards a bit, but keep the spine as straight as possible. Return to standing and continue for 3 minutes. If possible, each complete up and down cycle should take 4 seconds. If you have a medical condition you should exert caution and move slowly, or try half-knee bends if you have a knee problem.

HEART LOTUS

This kriya slows you down from your busy daily lives and brings an awareness of the shared heart. Adjust your height using a pillow if you cannot comfortably see into each other's eyes.

The place where opposites meet is called Tantra. Venus Kriyas are similar to the meditative exercises of White Tantric Yoga (see p.224.)

These are the only fingers that touch, creating a heart lotus

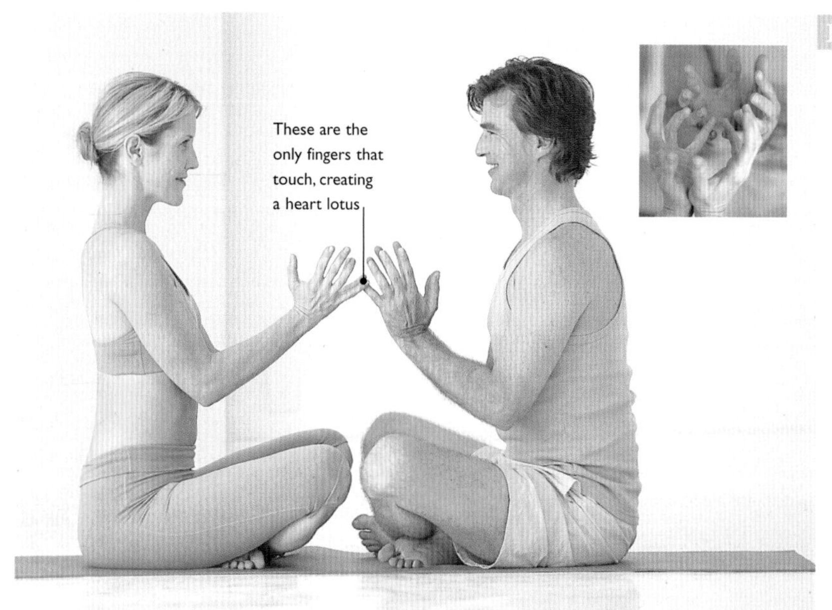

1 Sit in Easy pose with your knees almost touching. Put the base of your hands and wrists together and spread the hands to form a lotus flower *(inset)*. The man positions his little fingers under those of the woman. Look into the soul of your partner through their eyes for 1–1½ minutes.

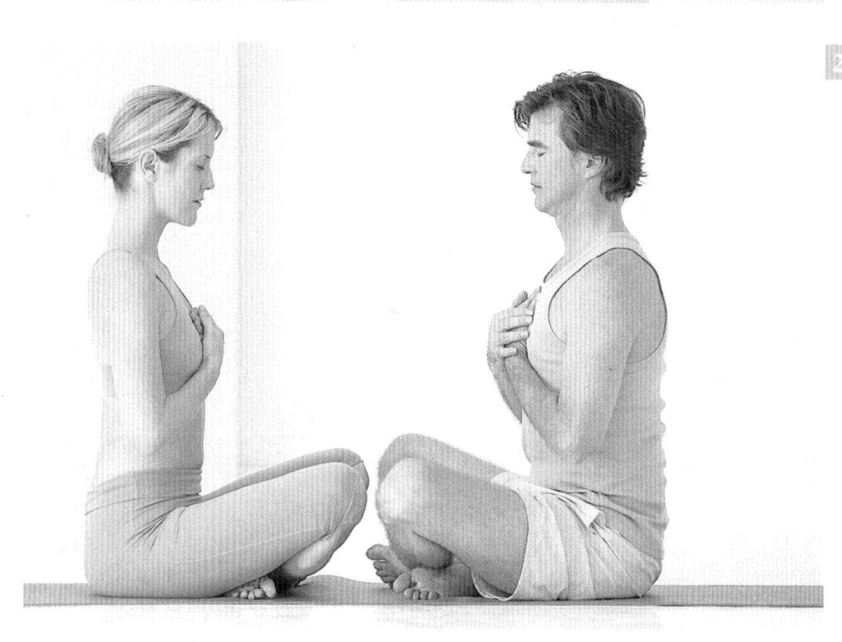

2 Then place one hand over the other at your heart centre. Close your eyes and meditate on your heart. Go deep within to the centre of your being. Continue for 1–1½ minutes. Then inhale and exhale deeply 3 times, relax the posture, and thank your partner.

COUPLES' KUNDALINI LOTUS

This exercise helps channel sexual energy and maintain potency, and brings depth and lightness to your relationship. It requires flexibility, so warm up with Spine Flex *(p.31–32)* and Spread Stretch *(p.36–37)* first.

1. Sit fairly close across from each other and hold hands. With the legs positioned outside the arms, bend the knees and place the soles of your feet together with those of your partner. Lean back slightly, straightening the arms.

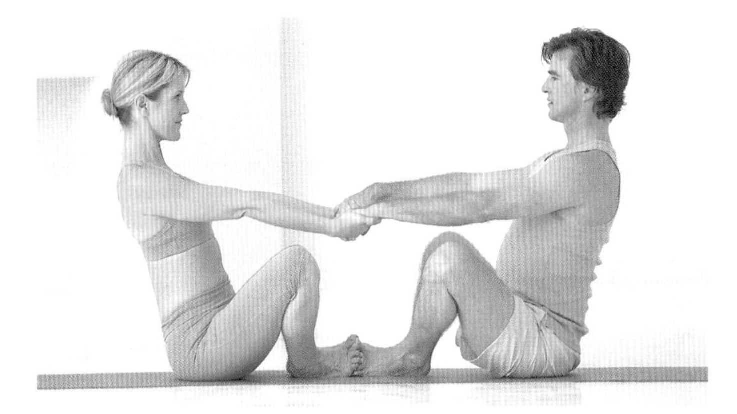

2. Slowly stretch the legs up straight to a 60° angle from the ground, with the soles of the feet touching. Look into each other's eyes with love and joy. See yourself in the other person. Lift your partner's energy with your love, and realize that you two are one. Continue for 3 minutes with either Breath of Fire or long, deep breathing. (Decide before you start which type of breathing you do; both partners should do the same.) Then relax.

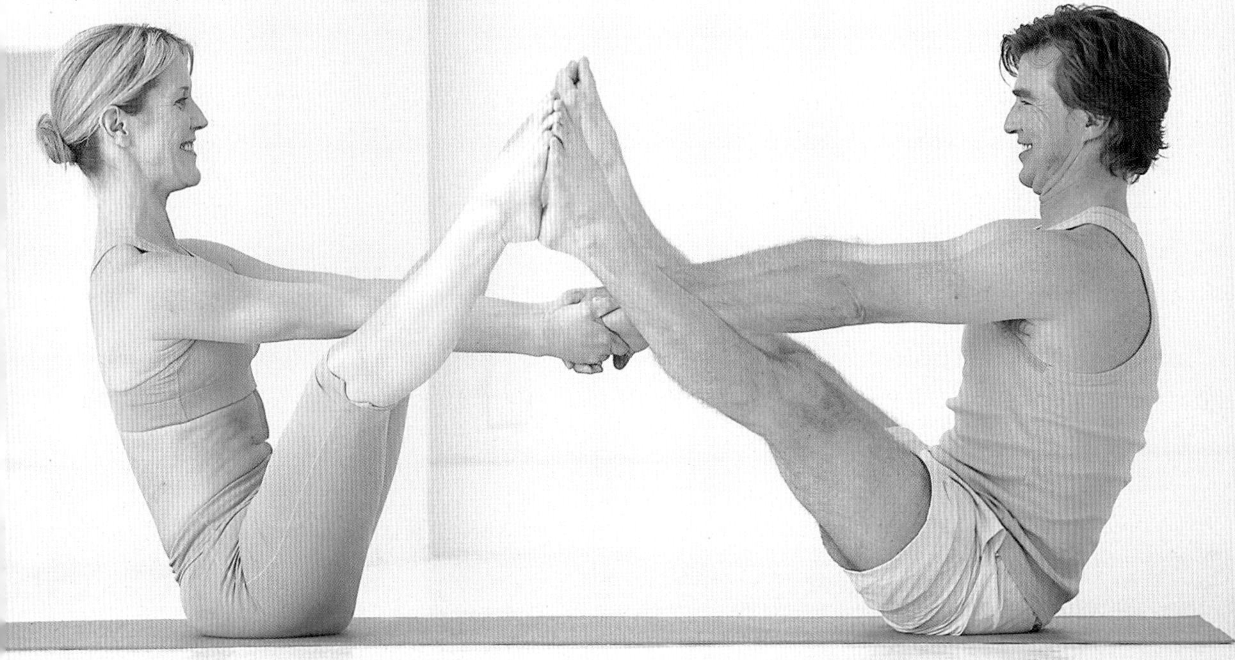

FOR INTERNAL STRENGTH

These individual exercises and poses have been chosen for their ability to build balance, endurance, and positive energy, which are essential for a woman whether she is single or in a relationship.

WARRIOR

A regular practice of Warrior pose develops an intensity of focus, mental strength, and endurance. It relieves cramps in the calves and thighs, brings elasticity to the leg and back muscles and makes the legs strong, and tones the abdominal organs. To prevent your bent knee from over-working, keep it directly over the ankle to distribute the weight evenly.

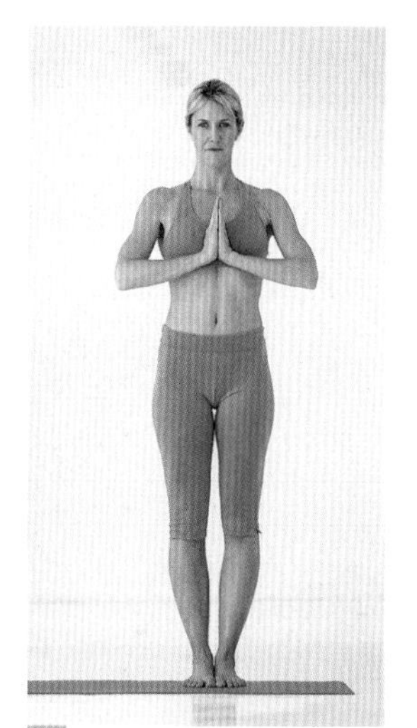

1 Stand straight with your feet together. Bring your hands together in Prayer pose at the centre of your chest and inhale.

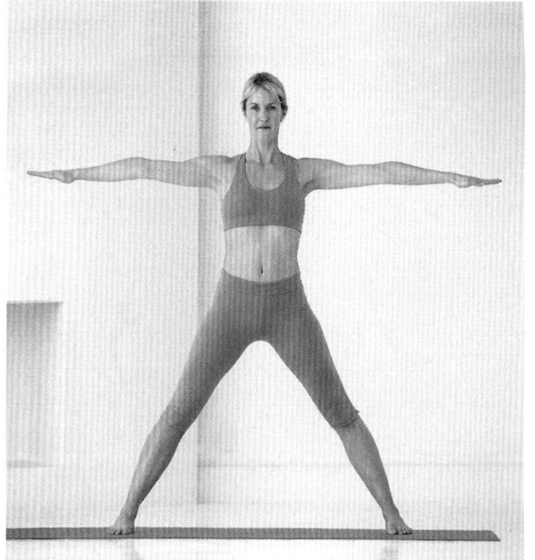

2 Exhale as you spread your legs apart sideways 1.2m (4–4½ft), with your feet parallel and facing forwards. Raise your arms sideways in line with your shoulders, palms facing down and shoulders relaxed.

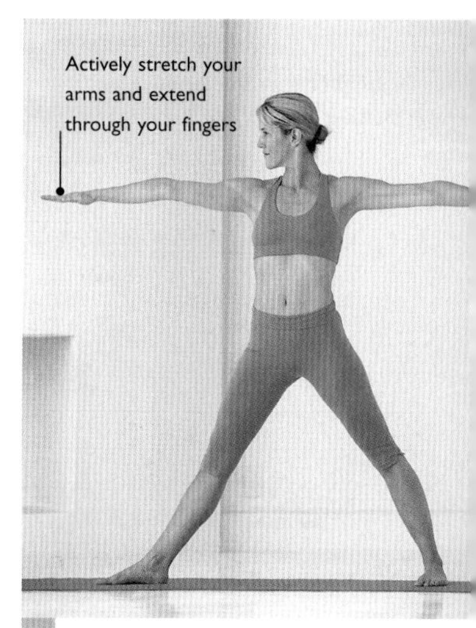

3 Inhale and turn your right foot 90° to the right and your left foot slightly to the right. Keep your hips and chest facing forwards while turning your head to the right. Slightly tighten the muscles around your left knee.

MICHELLE'S STORY (CANADA)

One of my first experiences with Kundalini Yoga was at the organization's summer camp for women. I saw a flyer for the camp and decided it was for me, even though I didn't know anyone else who was going and it was out of character for me to try something I knew little about.

Attending the camp, waking up before dawn and practising yoga and meditation, learning about men and women, was an amazing transformational experience. But the single thing that affected me most was the space created in the company of women. Looking back, I realized that this was the first time in my life that I had been surrounded by women only. I had grown up interpreting the message "women can do anything that men can do" to mean that women and men are the same. That summer I realized that we have a different energy and attunement from men.

In the past, I often felt that I was competing with the man in my life. Now I see that my energy is complementary to his. This understanding has helped me to value what I bring to the relationship. I honour and value my feminine energy and what I can bring to a situation as a woman.

Stretch out your hands sideways as though you are being pulled from opposite ends
Your knee is directly over your ankle, but not extended beyond it

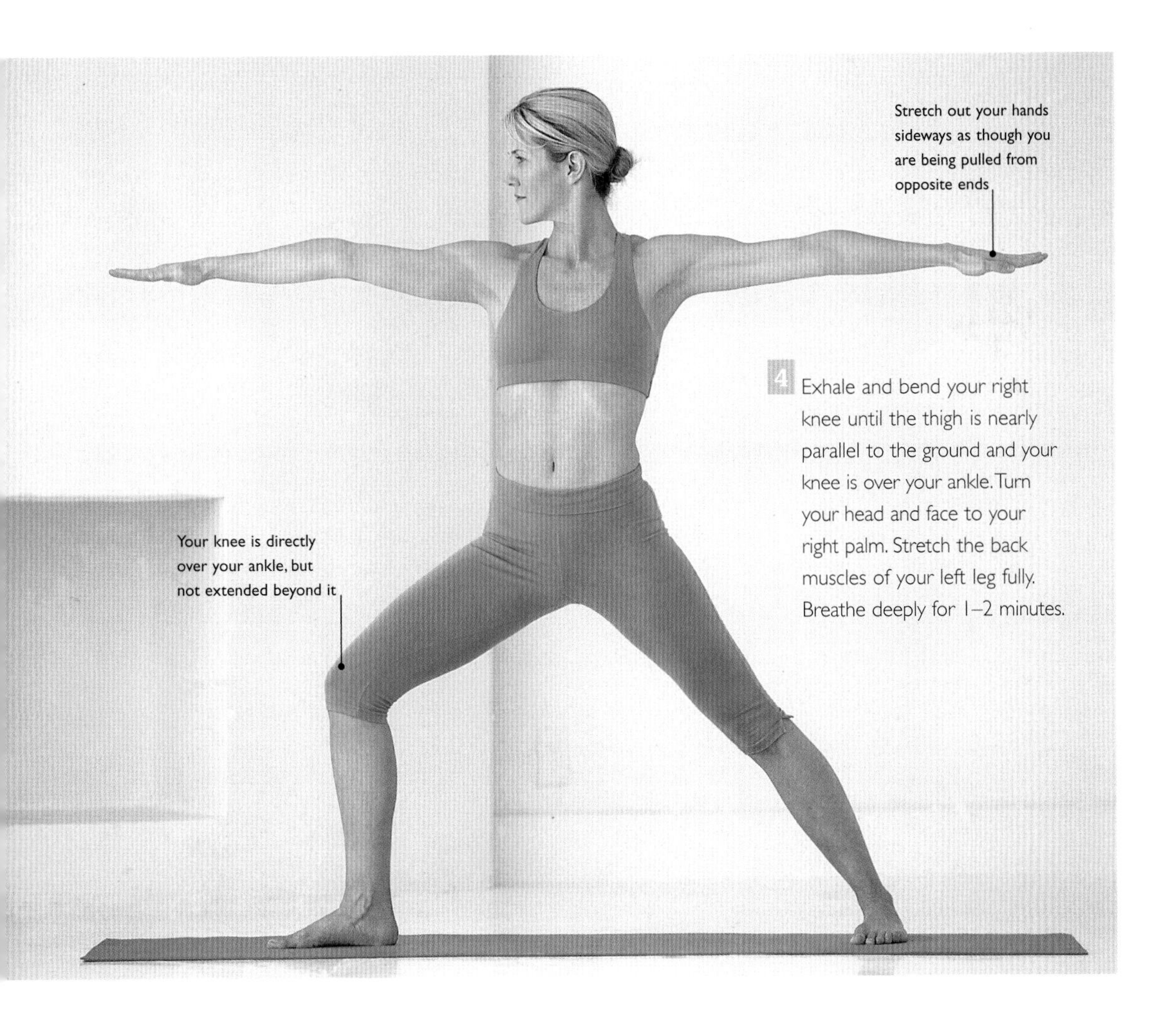

4 Exhale and bend your right knee until the thigh is nearly parallel to the ground and your knee is over your ankle. Turn your head and face to your right palm. Stretch the back muscles of your left leg fully. Breathe deeply for 1–2 minutes.

VARUYAS KRIYA

This kriya can cause a cleansing sweat. The amount of time spent practising Varuyas Kriya can be slowly increased up to 7½ minutes on each side. There is a strong tendency to shake while practising this pose as it adjusts and strengthens your nervous system. The practice and perfection of this kriya is said to improve the functioning of the pituitary gland, regulate excessive sexual energy, and increase general immunity to disease.

Similar in action and effect to Sat Kriya (p.56–57), *Varuyas ("Var-uh-yas") Kriya is a powerful, somewhat strenuous pose. Stand on a thin, non-slip mat beside a wall in case you feel unsteady.*

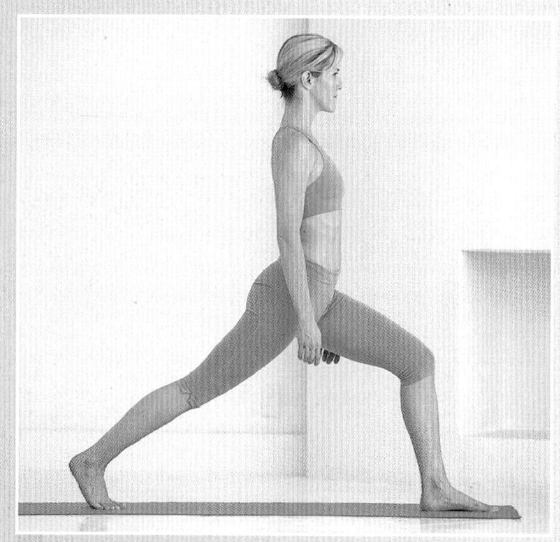

1 Stand straight with your arms at your sides. Place the right leg as far back as you can while maintaining your balance. Bend your front leg so that your knee is bent directly over the foot, but not extended beyond that point.

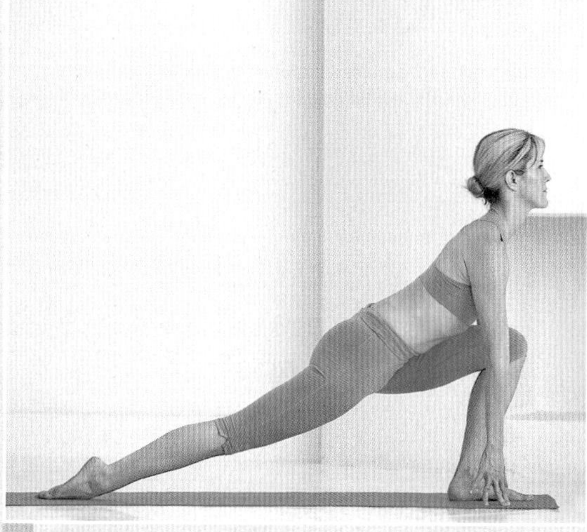

2 Bring your hands to the ground by your front foot for balance. Place the top of your right foot on the ground so that the leg and foot extend out behind you in a straight line. Take a deep breath in.

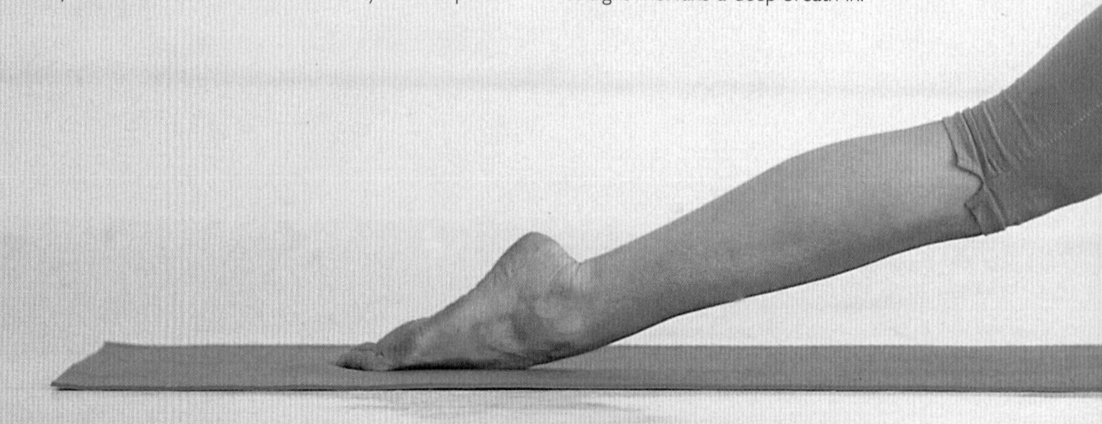

The arms and hands form a straight line with the palms together, fingers pointing straight ahead, and thumbs side by side
Pull the navel in and pull up slightly on the perineum

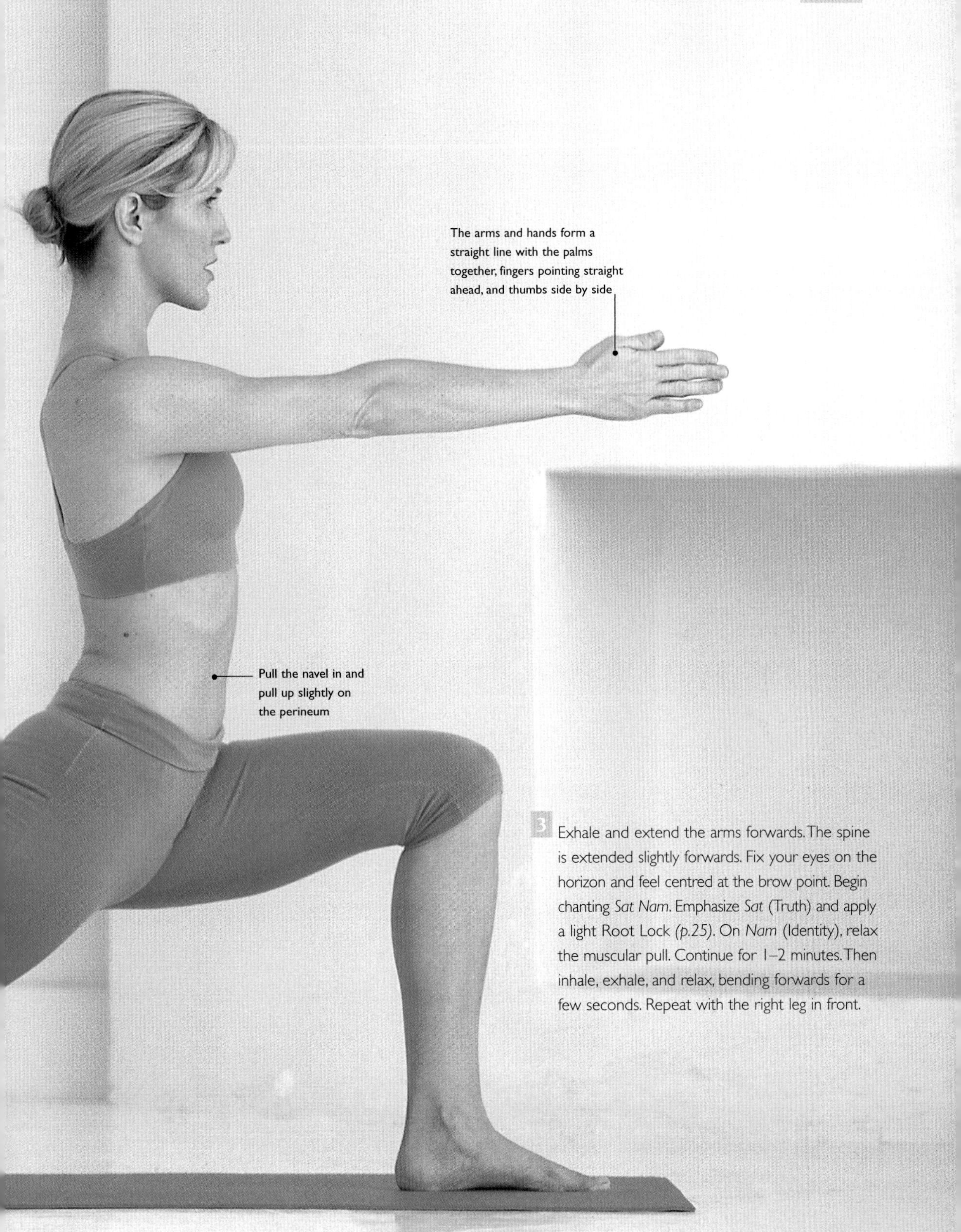

3 Exhale and extend the arms forwards. The spine is extended slightly forwards. Fix your eyes on the horizon and feel centred at the brow point. Begin chanting *Sat Nam*. Emphasize *Sat* (Truth) and apply a light Root Lock *(p.25)*. On *Nam* (Identity), relax the muscular pull. Continue for 1–2 minutes. Then inhale, exhale, and relax, bending forwards for a few seconds. Repeat with the right leg in front.

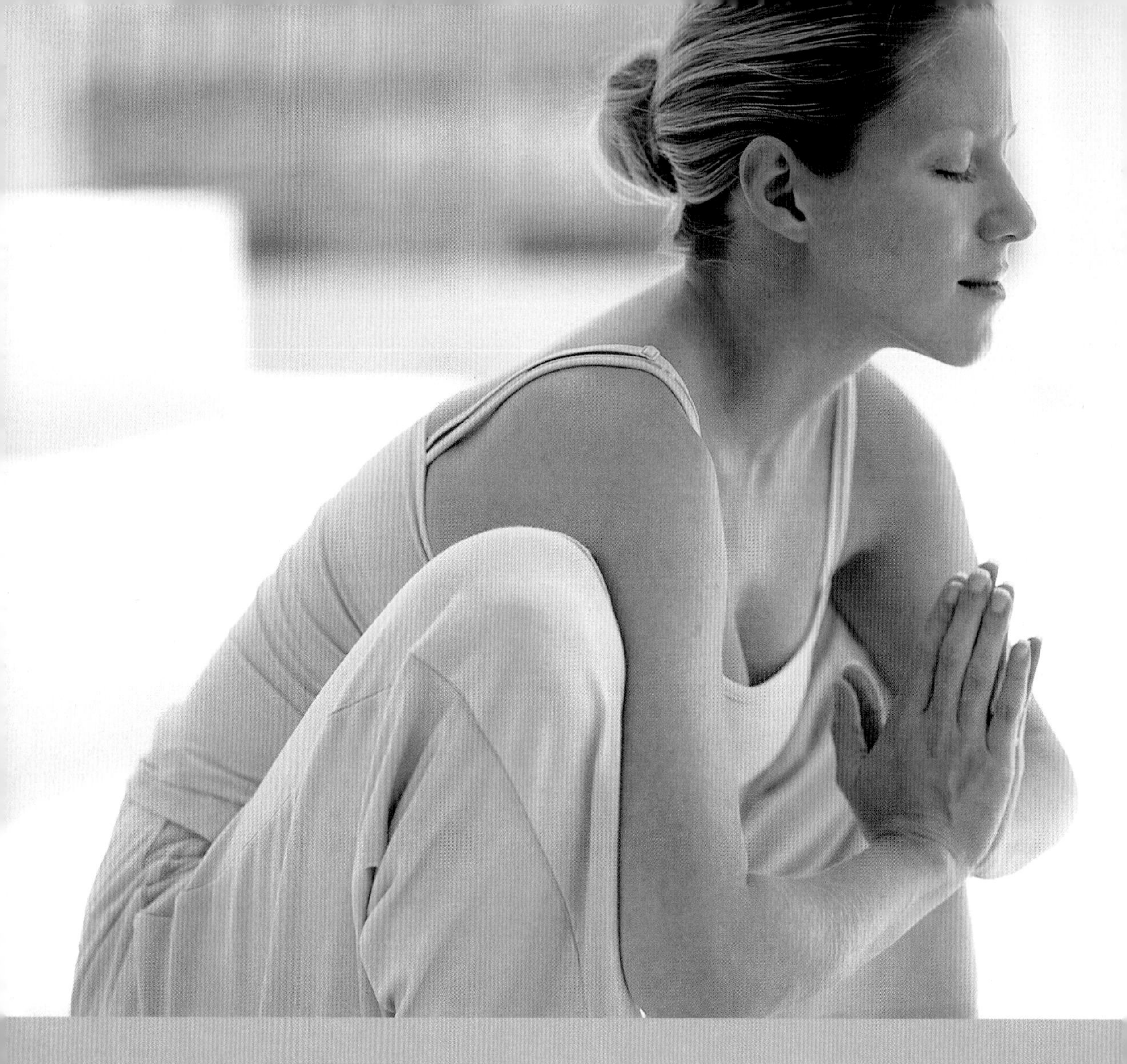

PREPARING FOR BIRTH

Pregnancy is a most extraordinary time of a woman's life: dramatic hormonal and bodily changes week by week and even day by day can make her life pretty topsy-turvy. Yoga provides a calm sanctuary where she can experience a peaceful, loving union with her baby, discover her inner resolve, and delve into the practice of breath awareness. Yoga's primary gifts of increasing flexibility and decreasing tension are perfectly compatible with the needs of a pregnant woman. Here are postures that open and relax the pelvic area, strengthen muscle tone, and release back tension, together with deep breathing and a meditative focus to enhance your experience of the life growing within you.

ACTIVE STANDING POSE

When you are pregnant, most of the extra weight you carry is all in one place. Since your abdominal muscles (which normally hold your lower torso in place) are missing in action, so to speak, you may develop a swayed back or exaggerated spinal curve. This can cause lower back pain and sciatica. As often as possible, practise this pose to lengthen your spine downwards.

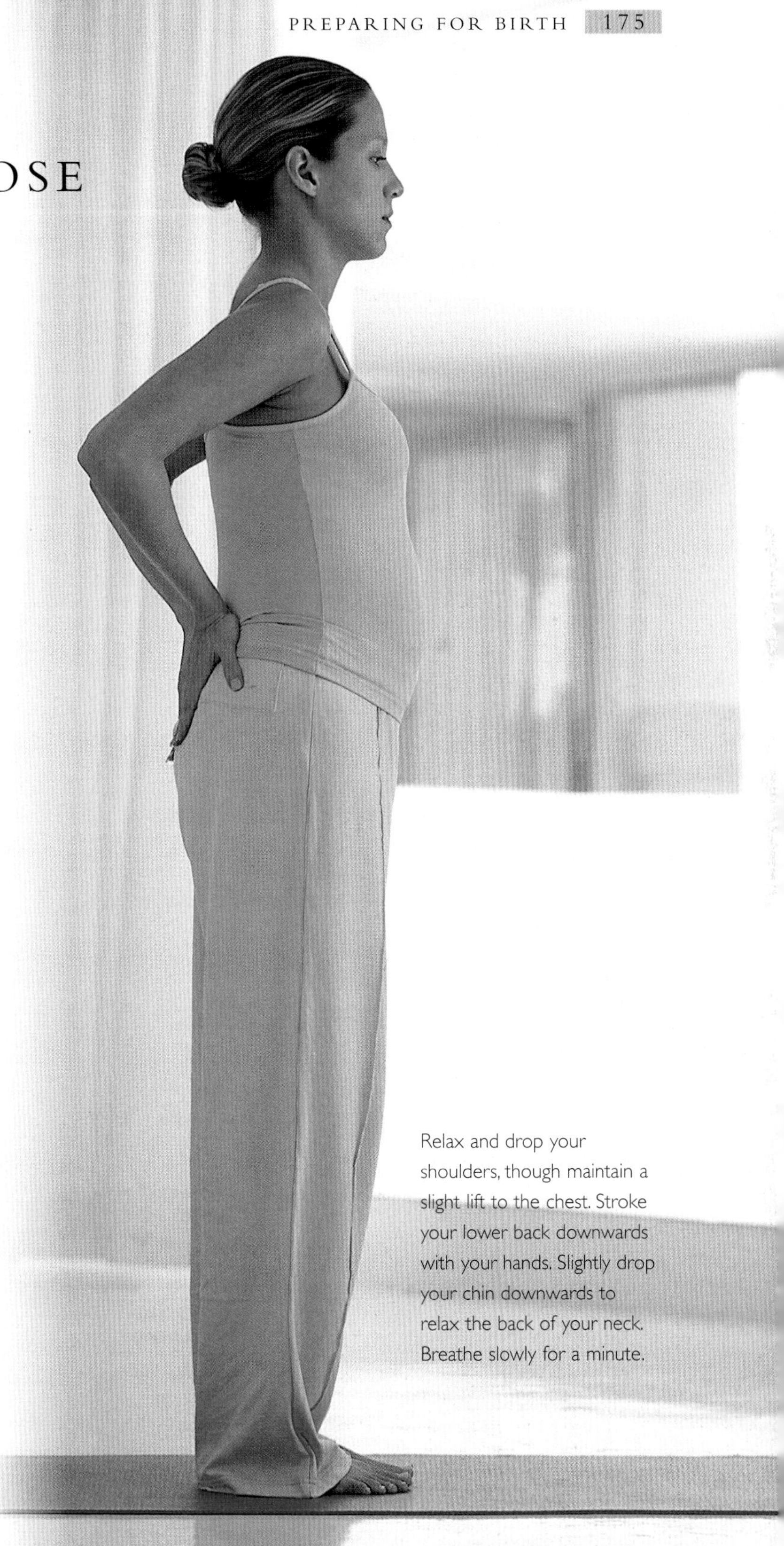

Relax and drop your shoulders, though maintain a slight lift to the chest. Stroke your lower back downwards with your hands. Slightly drop your chin downwards to relax the back of your neck. Breathe slowly for a minute.

Be aware of any personal limitations when practising pregnancy yoga. Consult your GP if necessary. Stop exercises that cause discomfort. After the first trimester avoid retaining the inhalation, abdominal exercises, poses done lying on your front, inverted poses (like Downward Dog, Plough, Shoulder-stand), and knee to chest positions. Light Breath of Fire may be practised, but check with a GP first.

PRENATAL POSES

The following poses are helpful during pregnancy. For example, poses done while kneeling on all fours will help to relieve tension in the back and strengthen back muscles, which aids labour. Because your pelvic floor supports the weight of your baby during pregnancy, squeezing the pelvic floor muscles (rectal and vaginal) to strengthen them should be done as often as possible, both on and off the mat.

"I'm pregnant!" These few words herald a magical journey in a woman's life that is like no other. It is a moment held forever in her heart, a passage of time during which her precious child takes shape in her body and becomes, from then on, inexorably linked to her heart and soul.

CAT POSE

This exercise brings great flexibility to the spine – including the cervical vertebrae, circulates the spinal fluid, and serves as a great warm-up exercise. For added benefit, at the end of the exhalation gently squeeze your buttock muscles for 1–2 seconds and then release as you inhale.

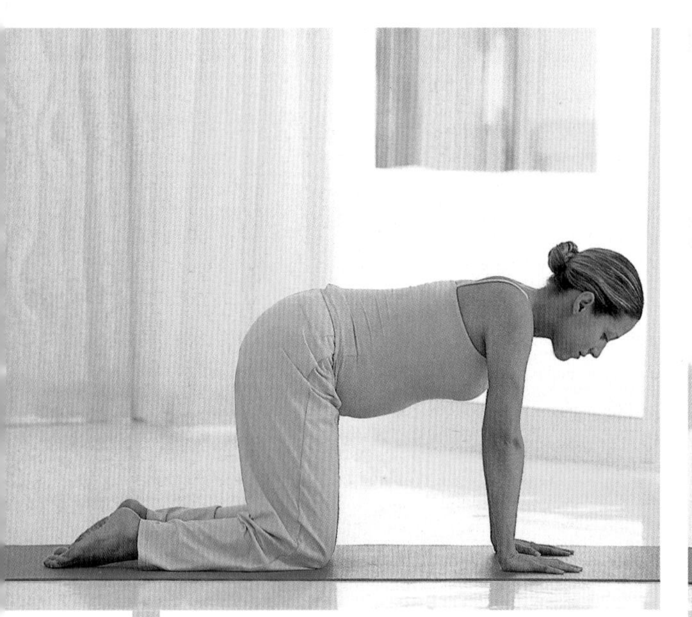

1 Begin on your hands and knees with your knees directly under your hips and your hands under your shoulders. The hands, feet, and knees are in line with each other. Relax your neck and inhale, keeping your spine in a horizontal position. Do not let your spine sag since this can put pressure on the lower back during pregnancy.

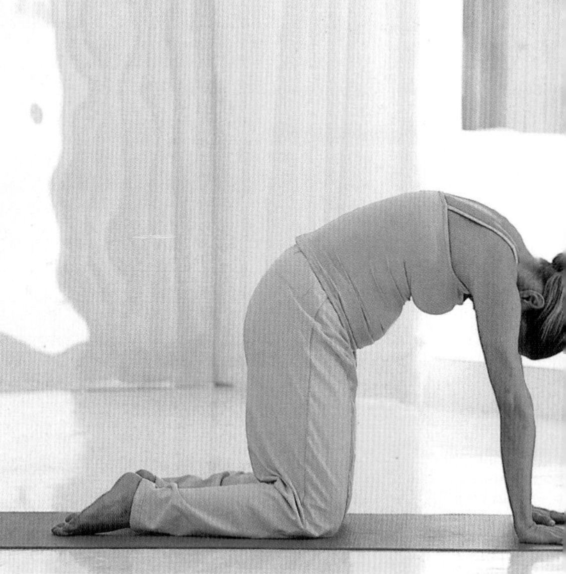

2 As you exhale, lengthen the base of your spine gently downwards and tuck your pelvis under so that your back is rounded like that of a cat. Inhale and return to the original position. If you experience pain in the wrists in this position, use your knuckles to support you so that your wrists remain straight.

BALANCING CAT

This posture is challenging and requires concentration. It develops balance and focus, both important areas for pregnancy and childbirth. For a good diagonal stretch, practise slowly with deep breaths.

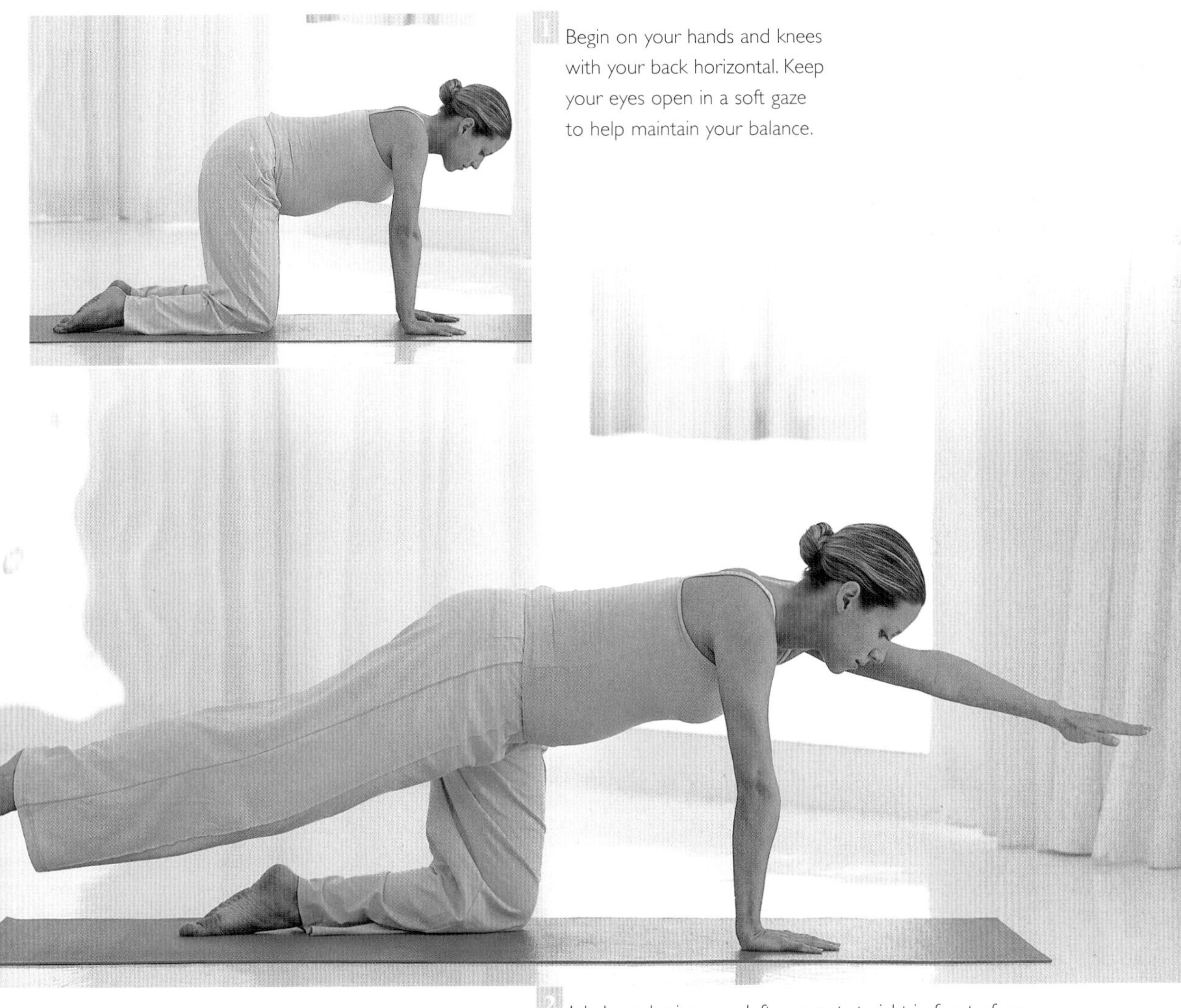

1 Begin on your hands and knees with your back horizontal. Keep your eyes open in a soft gaze to help maintain your balance.

2 Inhale and raise your left arm out straight in front of you. At the same time raise your right leg straight out behind you. Lift only as high as you can without bending your spine. Exhale and return your hand and leg to the ground. Inhale and raise the opposite arm and leg. Exhale and return to the original position. Continue for 1–2 minutes.

SUPPORTED BUTTERFLY

This pose helps to open the pelvis and hips and release tension from the area. This natural widening of the pelvis will help make it easier for your baby's head to engage in late pregnancy. Leaning back allows your lower back to relax and encourages the sacral vertebrae to self-adjust.

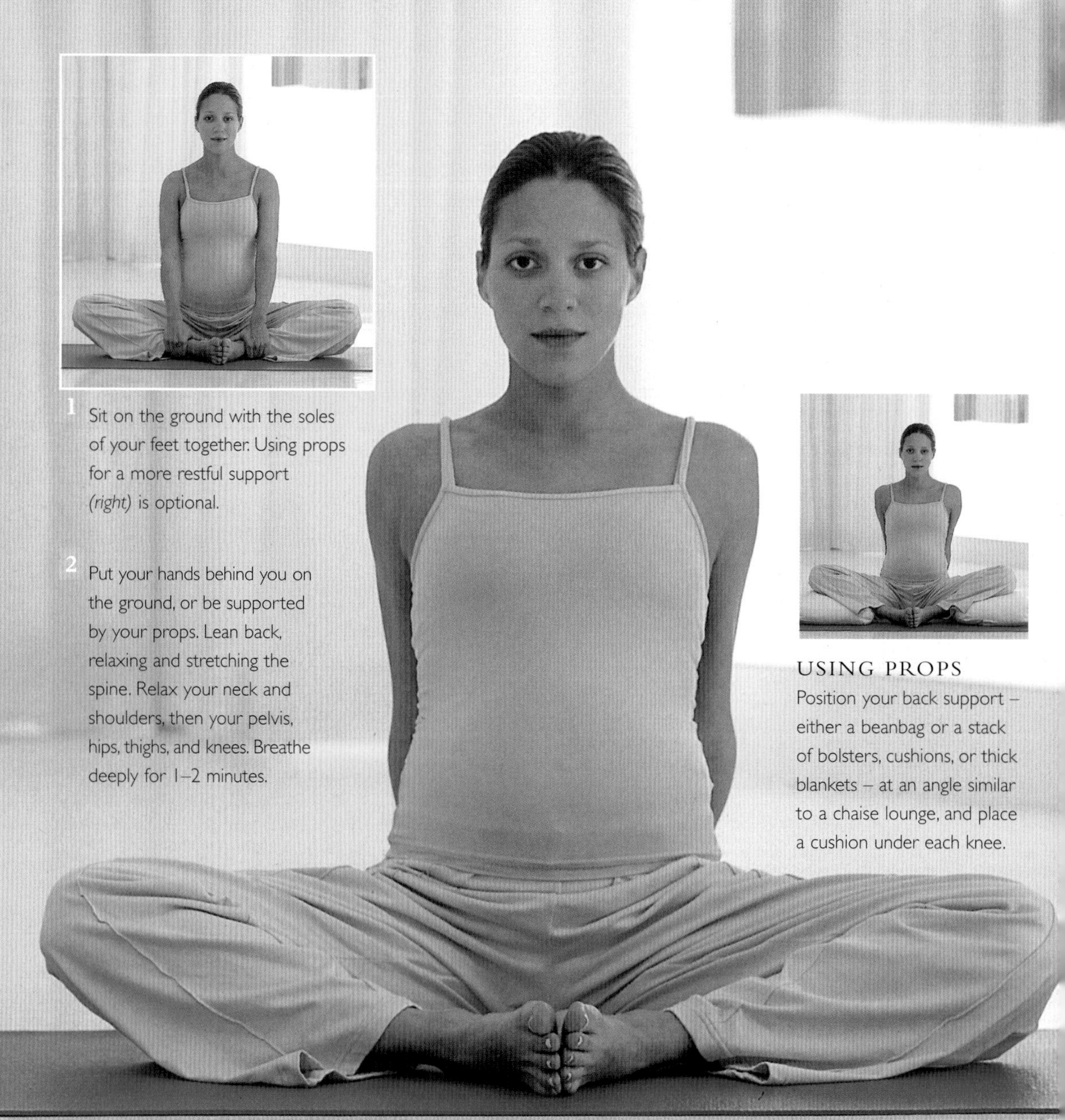

1 Sit on the ground with the soles of your feet together. Using props for a more restful support *(right)* is optional.

2 Put your hands behind you on the ground, or be supported by your props. Lean back, relaxing and stretching the spine. Relax your neck and shoulders, then your pelvis, hips, thighs, and knees. Breathe deeply for 1–2 minutes.

USING PROPS

Position your back support – either a beanbag or a stack of bolsters, cushions, or thick blankets – at an angle similar to a chaise lounge, and place a cushion under each knee.

SQUATTING WITH A PARTNER

Squatting in childbirth is instinctive for a woman because it naturally allows the pelvis to open and the baby's head to engage. In the last six weeks of pregnancy it is better to squat on a bolster to reduce pressure on the cervix and pelvic floor. Avoid squats if you have haemorrhoids, and check with your GP first if you have a high-risk pregnancy.

Use a rolled towel under your heels if they do not reach the ground, or a bolster for your bottom to rest on as you squat.

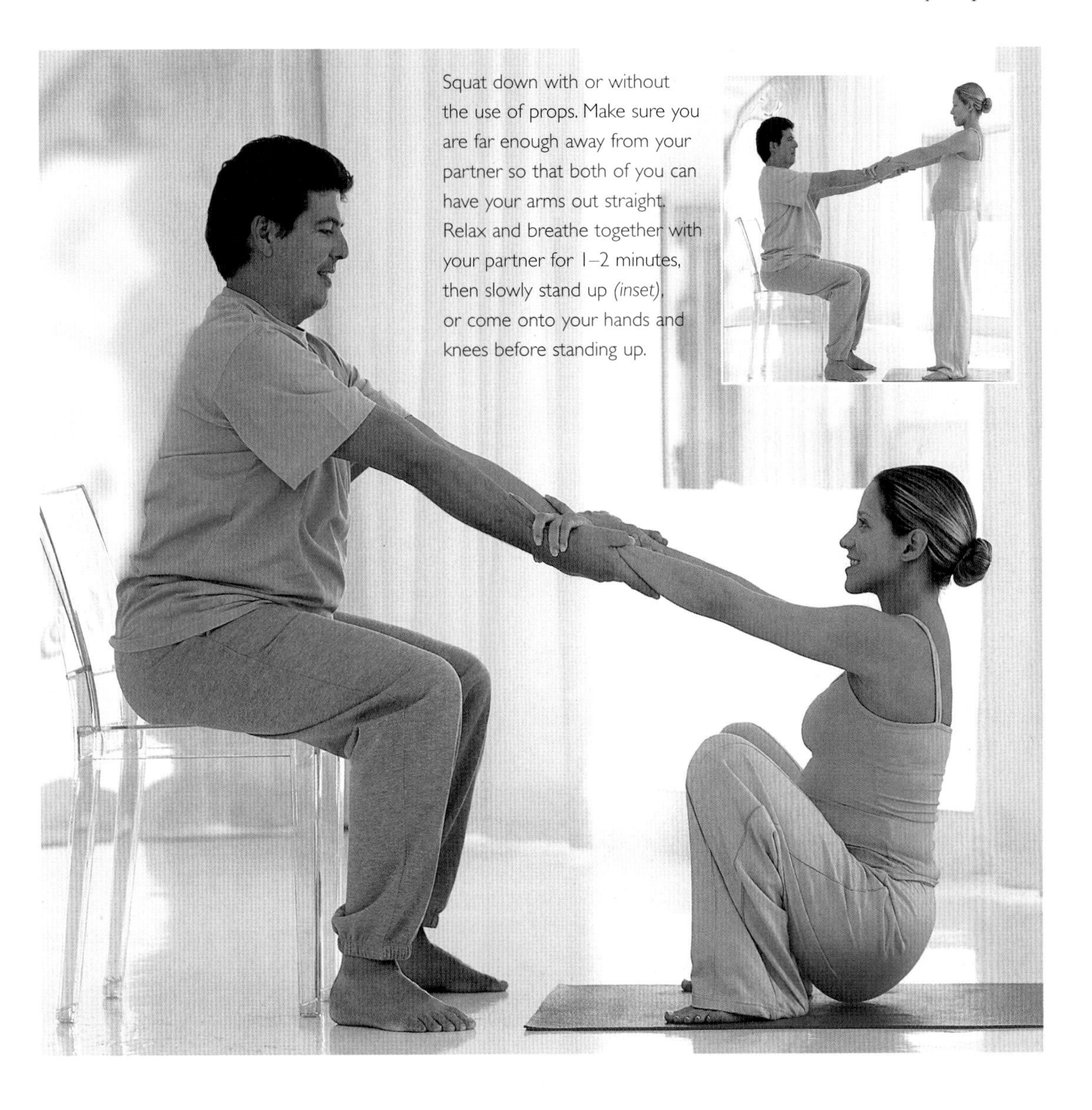

Squat down with or without the use of props. Make sure you are far enough away from your partner so that both of you can have your arms out straight. Relax and breathe together with your partner for 1–2 minutes, then slowly stand up *(inset)*, or come onto your hands and knees before standing up.

SQUAT WITH PRAYER POSE

This pose helps to increase your hip and pelvic flexibility by applying moderate pressure against the knees. As you squat down, feel a gentle expansion in the hips. See also cautions regarding Squats on page 179.

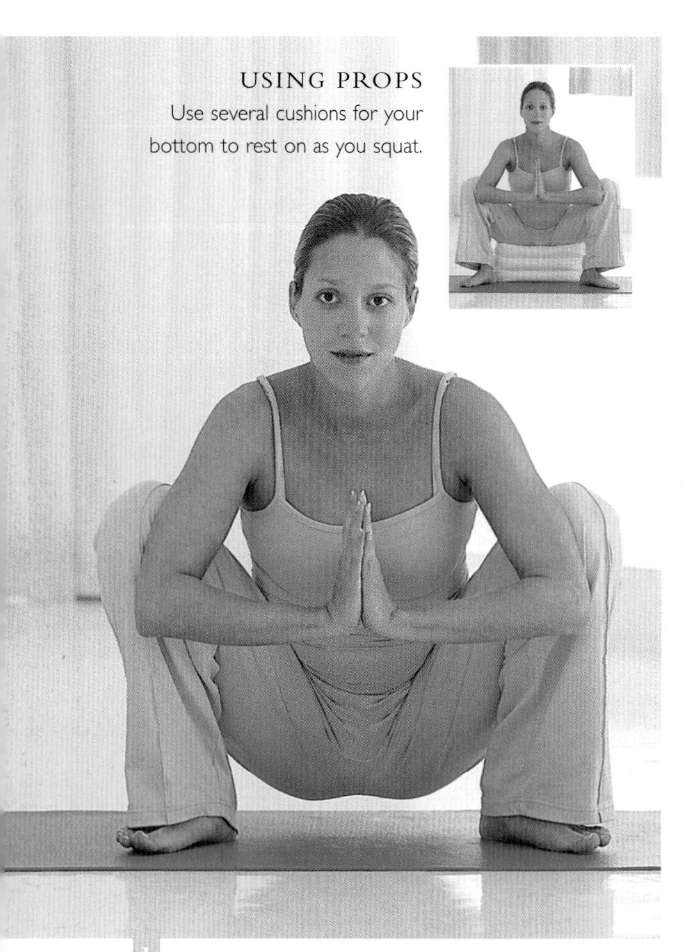

USING PROPS
Use several cushions for your bottom to rest on as you squat.

1 Using props if needed *(inset)*, squat down so that your buttocks are close to the ground. Bring your palms together in Prayer pose and rest the thumbs at the heart centre in the middle of your chest. Your elbows will be out to the sides and touching the inside area of your knees. Inhale, then exhale and with the elbows exert a moderate pressure against the knees. Do this 5–10 times.

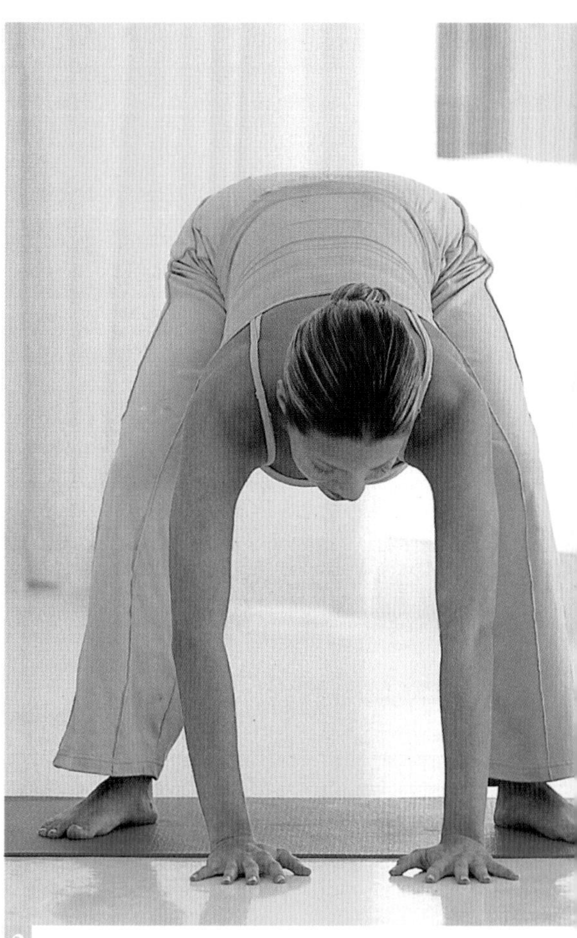

2 Inhale deeply and exhale. Place your hands on the ground, straighten your legs and slowly stand up. Alternatively, you can come onto your hands and knees as in step 1 of Cat pose *(p.176)* before standing up.

FORWARD BENDS

Practise these Forward Bends daily to release tension in the back, stretch the muscles and nerves of the legs and arms, and to relax your shoulders. Do not practise if you feel dizzy or light-headed.

Keep the spine straight, not arched

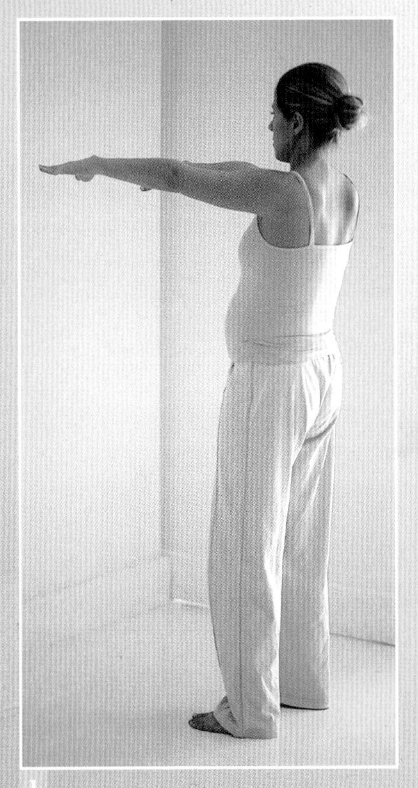

1 Stand up straight with your legs about shoulder-length apart, arms stretched out in front, and facing a wall or table.

2 Slowly exhale, lean forwards, and put your hands on the wall – or hands and forearms on a table. Allow the weight of your lower back to sink downwards through your heels and into the ground. Lengthen your spine without arching towards the ground. Let your neck relax. Feel a strong stretch in the arms and legs. Breathe deeply for 1–2 minutes. Let your head relax forwards and feel a strong stretch in the arms and armpits. Breathe deeply for 1–2 minutes.

EAR TO KNEE POSE

Besides being a great lateral stretch, this pose opens up much-needed breathing room in the lungs. Be aware that you want to stretch directly to either side of the body – avoid forward stretching after the first trimester since it puts pressure on the abdomen and womb.

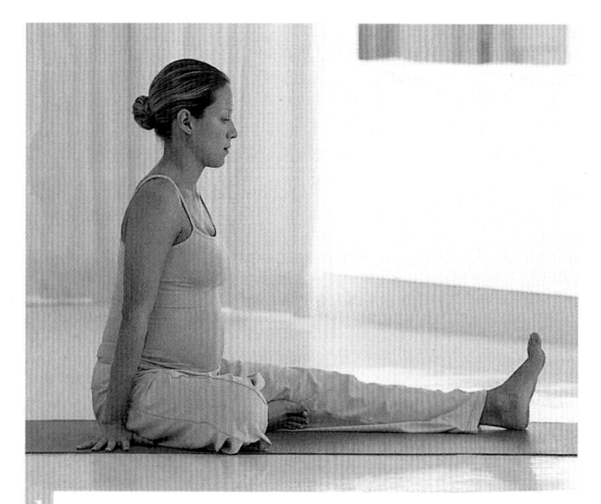

1 Sit with the legs extended and the spine straight. Place your hands on the ground with fingers slightly spread. Then bend your right knee and tuck it in so that the foot is close to or against the inner thigh of the left leg.

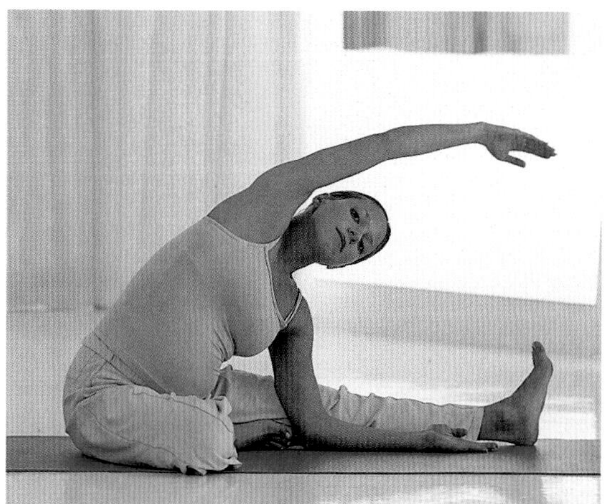

2 Stretch your arms overhead. Exhale, keep your body facing forwards, and stretch to the left, bringing your left ear towards your left knee as far as is comfortable. Rest your left arm on the ground inside your left leg. Breathe deeply and stretch for 3–5 breaths. Repeat on the right side. Continue for 1–2 minutes.

CLARE'S STORY (UK)

Practising yoga during my pregnancy not only opened my eyes to a whole new form of exercise and way of life, but also gave me and my baby more benefits than I could have imagined. Yoga kept me fit, supple, and relaxed through my pregnancy, and prepared my mind and body for a very positive birth. I was able to keep much more active in my last few months of pregnancy than I had expected, and even up until the day before I went into labour I was practising yoga. Except for my "bump", my body had never been in better shape!

Also because of my yoga practice, I believe I have been much better able to cope with postnatal recovery and look after my new baby.

I truly believe that yoga has provided me with a calm frame of mind all through my pregnancy and blessed me with a very happy and contented little baby. As well as the benefits of doing the poses, the music, the mantras, and the general positive energy surrounding yoga continue to help me and my baby to relax and stay happy and healthy postnatally.

RESTING POSES

Relax in Side or Front Lying pose as many times a day as possible, especially during the last few weeks of pregnancy when you are fatigued from carrying extra weight or your sleep is often disturbed. Lying on your left side during the last six weeks will help to encourage your baby's spine towards the left side of your abdomen, which is the best position for labour. You may wish to vary this sometimes by lying on the right. Many women find the Side Lying position helpful for labour.

You will need several cushions, pillows or folded blankets for these resting poses. Create enough height with the pillows so that the shoulder you lie on does not feel crushed.

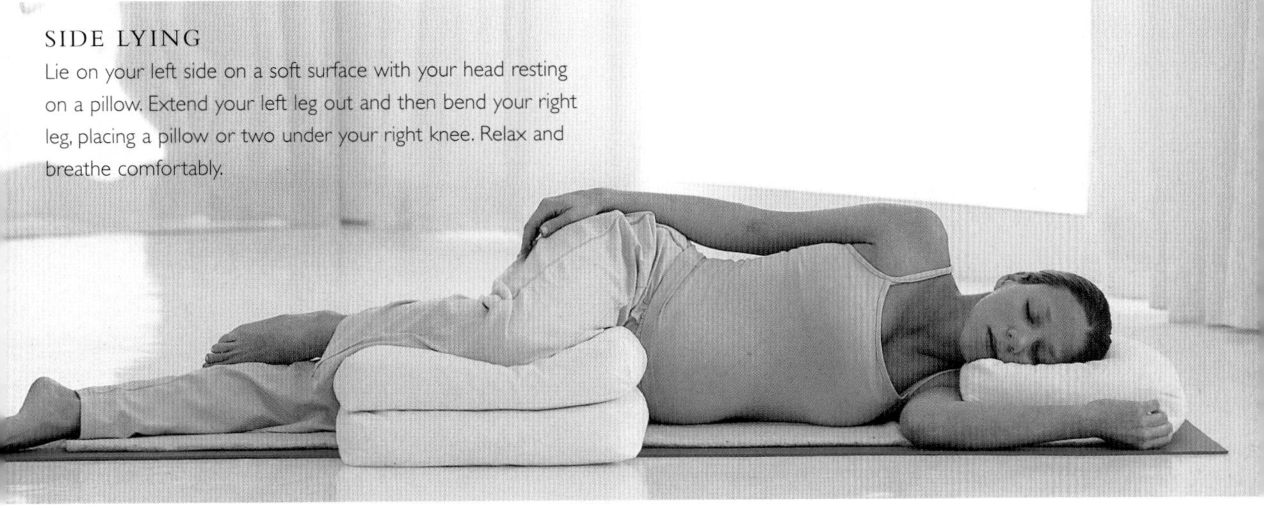

SIDE LYING

Lie on your left side on a soft surface with your head resting on a pillow. Extend your left leg out and then bend your right leg, placing a pillow or two under your right knee. Relax and breathe comfortably.

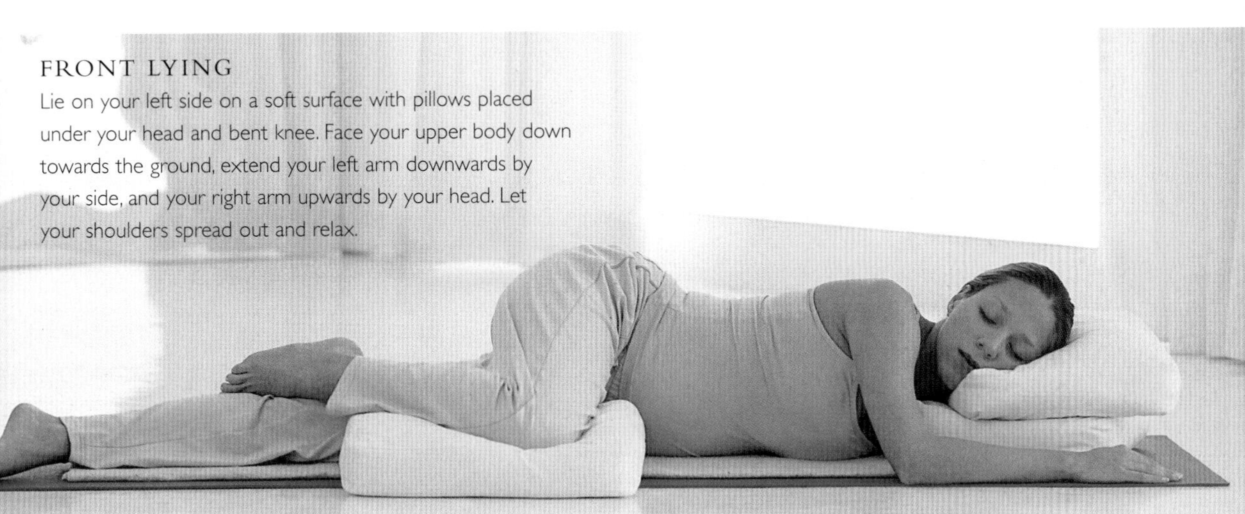

FRONT LYING

Lie on your left side on a soft surface with pillows placed under your head and bent knee. Face your upper body down towards the ground, extend your left arm downwards by your side, and your right arm upwards by your head. Let your shoulders spread out and relax.

A THREE-WAY CONNECTION

Practise this with your partner for a cozy feeling of togetherness. Share the space of love with your unborn child through voice, touch, massage, and meditation for as long as you wish.

Have your partner sit against a wall with his legs apart and slightly out to the sides. Use pillows for support if desired. Sit inside your partner's arms with your back supported by his chest. Your partner's hands may rest on your abdomen and your hands may rest on his. Cross your legs or leave them outstretched, whichever is comfortable. Focus on breathing together in a deep and relaxed manner. Let go of tension or tightness. Focus on the presence of your baby. Suggestions for a three-way connection are: stroking, feeling the energy of your hands surround and bless your child, or talking out loud or internally to your child.

RESPONDING TO FAMILIAR SOUNDS

A couple about to have a baby played a musical box before they fell asleep every night. When the baby was born, she cried through her mother's attempts to nurse her and her father trying to rock and walk her to sleep. Finally her father wound up the musical box. Within minutes, the baby's cries subsided and she fell peacefully asleep on her father's chest.

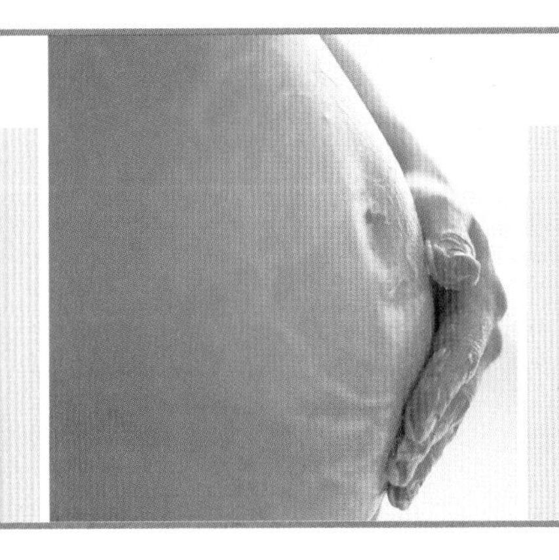

SKIN CARE DURING PREGNANCY

Massage yogurt, lemon, and honey on the breasts, abdomen, and thighs once a week to prevent stretch marks, or take a yogurt bath (p.65). Oil your body regularly with a quality oil such as almond or sesame oil. Do not use soap on the nipples as it dries the skin. If skin becomes dry or cracked, use the homeopathic salve Calendula. In preparation for breastfeeding, "toughen" up the nipples by squeezing and pinching them regularly, and rub well with a towel after bathing.

COMMUNING WITH YOUR UNBORN BABY

Make a special time in your day to sit with your baby, sending love and feeling the love your baby has for you. Your intuition, which is extra-strong during pregnancy, will lead you naturally to your favourite ways of communion with your baby. Perhaps this special connection happens during a sitting meditation early in the morning, as you sit in the rocking chair that you bought especially for nursing your baby, or as you float in a swimming pool while imagining your baby floating inside of you – whatever speaks to you as the most true way for you and your baby to connect.

Sit in Easy pose. Place your hands gently on your lower belly and cradle your baby. Close your eyes and let your head relax forwards naturally. Focus on the rhythm of your breath and imagine how your baby experiences your heartbeat, your breath, and the sensation of floating in the warm fluid of your womb. Be aware of the deep connection between you. Realize that you chose each other, that you are the best mother for the soul that is taking birth through you. Talk out loud or internally to your child and speak from your deepest heart and soul. Bless your child, yourself, your partner, your family. Thank him or her for coming to be with you. Allow the communion to continue as long as is natural, 10 minutes or more.

When you are ready, slowly return your focus to your breath and the room and open your eyes. Know that you remain connected even in your busiest moments.

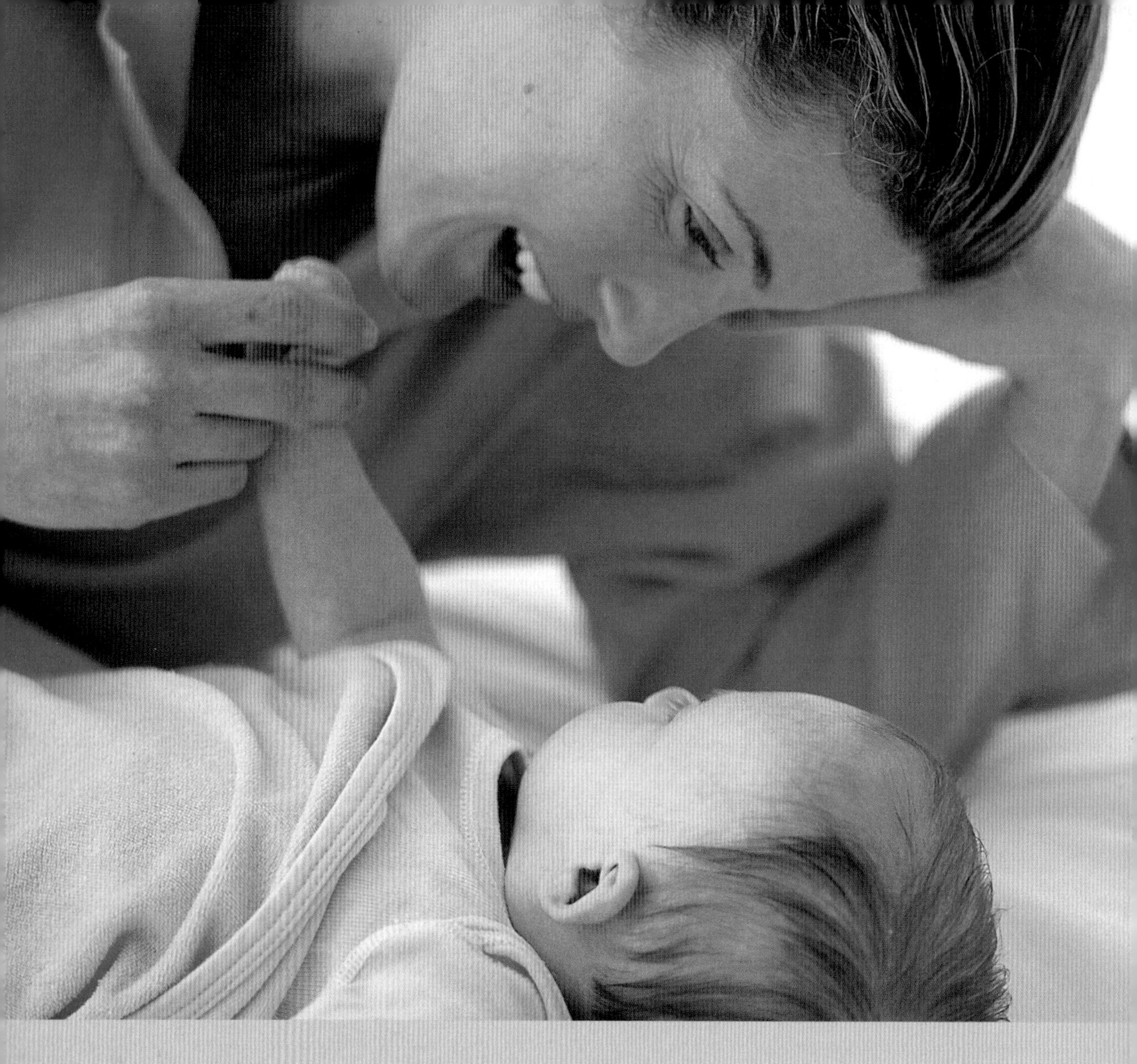

NEW MOTHER & BABY

It is truly remarkable how adaptable a woman's body is, and how much it changes in one brief year of pregnancy, birth, and lactation. I distinctly recall the day I arrived home with my three-day-old son, looked in the mirror, and laughed in the delightful realization of what an amazing and wondrous thing a woman's body is. Common sense tells a woman that she has to take it slow and easy when it comes to exercise after her baby is born. She may wish to look and feel as she did before her pregnancy, but the reality is that it took nine months to make the baby and it will probably take at least that long for her body to return to a pre-pregnancy state of health and fitness.

Barring complications, most women may begin pelvic floor exercises *(p.25)* and gentle exercise within a few days or weeks of birth. Women's concerns about exercise in the post-partum phase usually have to do with three basic practicalities: having time for exercise; having the energy; and knowing which exercises will be safe and effective.

Having energy can be a real challenge for a new mother. There is so much to adjust to that it can easily become overwhelming. Suddenly there is a small being who is completely dependent on you. That alone would be enough, but huge hormonal changes are going on in your body that can wreak havoc on your emotional state of mind. You may alternate between feelings of blissful contentment and frenzied anxiety, and everything in between. Just remember, you are handling a lot of change; go easy on yourself and ground yourself in your meditative mind as often as possible.

As for finding time to exercise, find a few minutes here and there for stretching, maybe while waiting for the kettle to boil with your baby in a carrier on the kitchen table. Hold onto the table and stretch your lower back *(see* Preparing For Birth, *p.181)*. In fact, most of those exercises are great to do after the birth, with one important difference: the emphasis during pregnancy is on poses and exercises that open the pelvis, like Squats and Butterfly pose; the focus in postnatal yoga is on healing and strengthening the pelvic area and pulling it back together. The postnatal phase is a recovery period. Be gentle with yourself and have patience and appreciation for your body.

BREASTFEEDING

Hopefully you are breastfeeding your baby; there is nothing like breastfeeding to bond mother and baby. Mother's milk naturally has everything that the baby needs – and the milk is always available! To stay healthy while breastfeeding, remember these two very simple but important points:

* ***Eat well.*** *Fruit, vegetables, whole grains, and foods high in protein. Organic milk products, soy products, beans, legumes, nuts, and seeds are your healthiest choices for protein.*
* ***Rest well.*** *Rest whenever your baby does, at least for the first few months. Relaxing time is important, too. Let Dad have his special time with the baby while you take a break and have a warm bath, read, visit a friend, and have a little time to yourself in whatever way you most enjoy.*

SPECIAL NURSING DRINK

180ml (6fl oz) organic milk (dairy or non-dairy)
6–8 blanched almonds (soaked and peeled)
2tsp ghee (clarified butter)
1–2tsp honey
Blend well and drink to help produce rich, nourishing milk for your baby. Makes 1 cup.

POSTNATAL YOGA

If your labour and delivery were uncomplicated, you may be able to begin to exercise within the first few weeks of delivery. Every woman's body and every birthing story is different, so check first with your GP. Go slowly and stay aware of your body as you practise. Stay in a pose for 3–4 breaths to begin with, and work up slowly to 15 breaths.

The Kegal exercise is a short, upward vaginal squeeze and release technique. Try to do 100 a day – anytime, anywhere – to regain essential muscle tone after pregnancy.

HAND GRASP

This adjusts the vertebrae of the middle and upper spine, opens the chest and shoulder areas, and counteracts any tendency to slump while breast-feeding or carrying your baby. It may be helpful to use a prop *(inset)*.

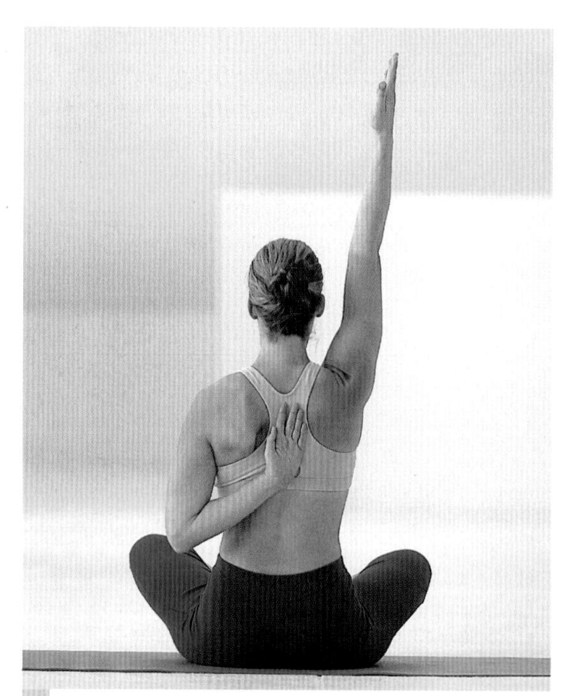

1 Sit on a chair, or on the ground, or stand. Keep your spine straight and chest lifted the entire time to perform this pose. Bend your left elbow and reach your left arm behind your back. Draw the upper part of your arm close to the side of your body. Raise your right arm up.

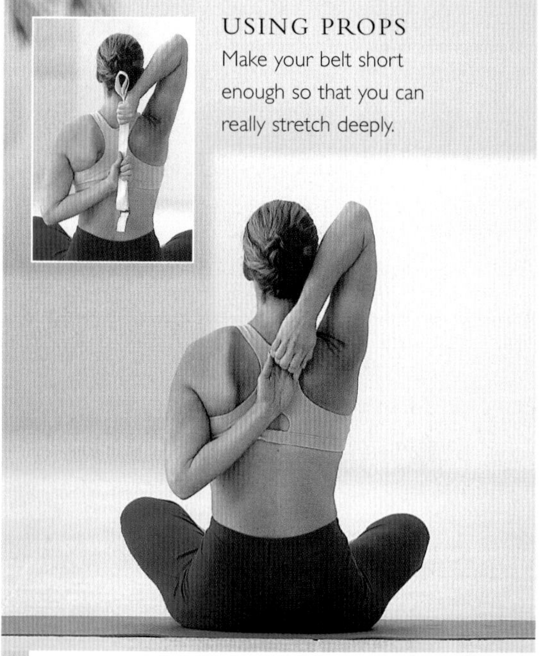

USING PROPS
Make your belt short enough so that you can really stretch deeply.

2 Bend your right arm at the elbow so that your right hand reaches towards your shoulder blade and faces your back. Interlock your fingers. If they do not reach, touch your fingers together, or use a belt or rope. Breathe deeply with your eyes closed for 5–8 breaths, then reverse the hands.

LOCUST LIFTS

Recovering muscle tone after pregnancy is key, especially in the core muscles that support the pelvis and torso. Locust Lifts are particularly beneficial for strengthening and toning the abdominal and back muscles. To build strength and to prepare for holding this pose, try inhaling up into the pose and exhaling down several times beforehand.

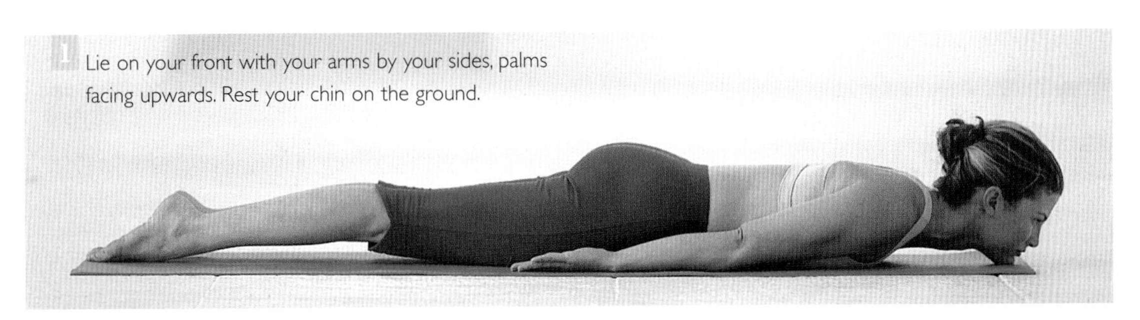

1 Lie on your front with your arms by your sides, palms facing upwards. Rest your chin on the ground.

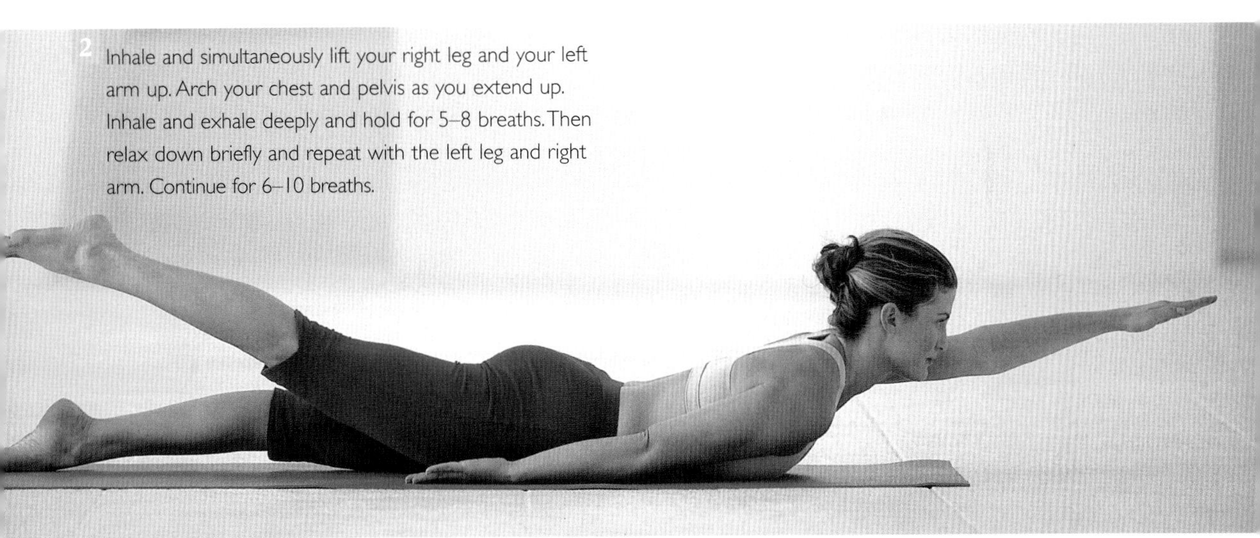

2 Inhale and simultaneously lift your right leg and your left arm up. Arch your chest and pelvis as you extend up. Inhale and exhale deeply and hold for 5–8 breaths. Then relax down briefly and repeat with the left leg and right arm. Continue for 6–10 breaths.

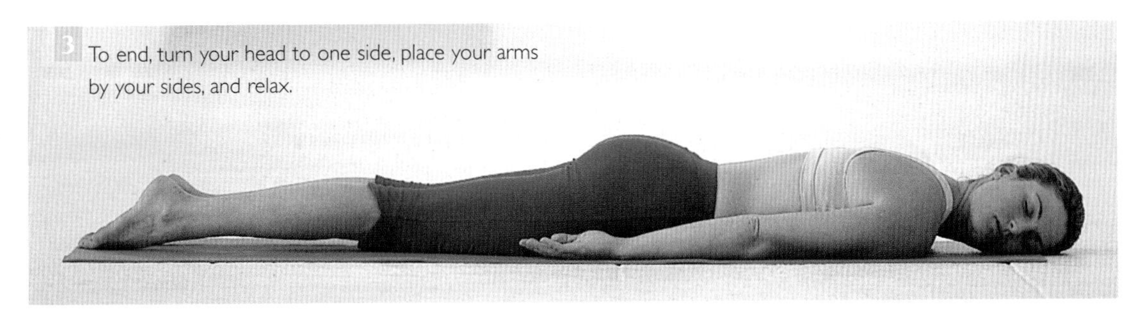

3 To end, turn your head to one side, place your arms by your sides, and relax.

SPINAL TWIST

This gives a lateral stretch to the vertebrae, back muscles, and hips, keeps the spine elastic, and helps to retain side-to-side mobility. It also massages the abdominal muscles, aids digestion, and induces calm nerves.

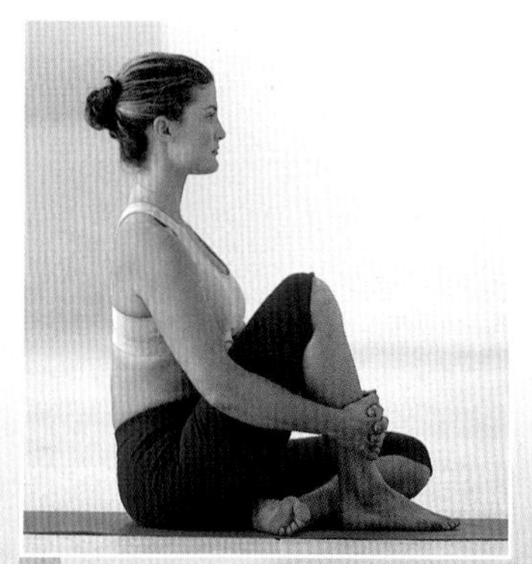

1 Sit in Easy pose with your spine straight. Raise the right knee. Place the right foot flat on the ground.

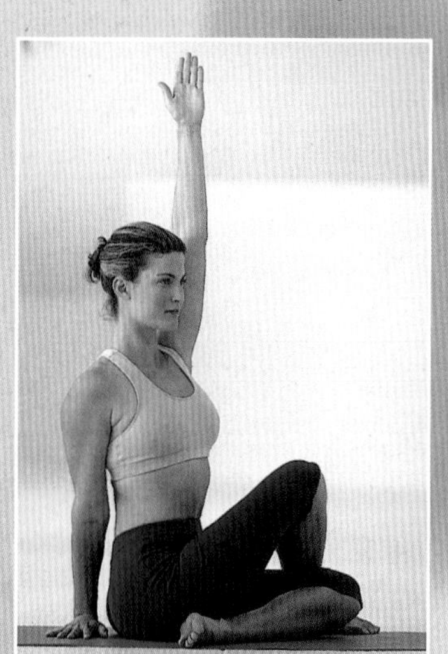

2 Place the right foot on the ground outside your left thigh, your right knee bent over your left leg. Place the right hand on the ground just behind your back. It should bear no weight. Raise the left arm up.

3 Bring your left arm over to your right knee, and reach round to catch hold of the right ankle if possible. Your left arm will push against your right knee. Your head is erect and turned to look over your right shoulder. Your chest is lifted and the shoulders are parallel to the ground. Hold for 5–10 deep breaths. Release and repeat on the other side.

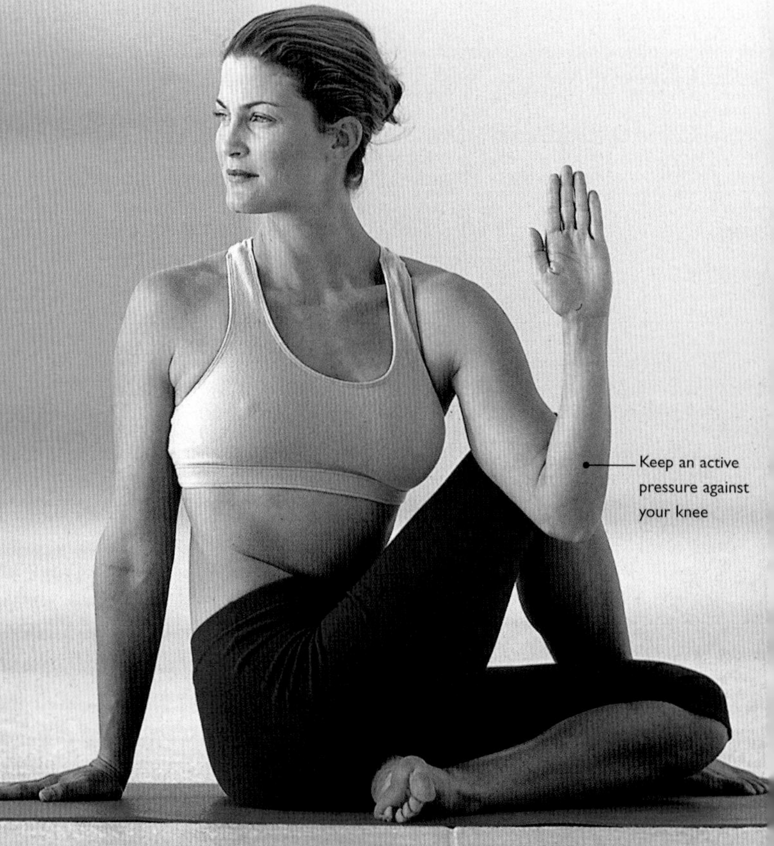

Keep an active pressure against your knee

DATE MILK

Soothing and delicious, this helps wean babies off breastfeeding. It gives energy, provides nourishment, helps ward off colds, and is a healthy, youth-maintaining drink for people of all ages.

Heat together:
250ml (8fl oz) organic milk (dairy or non-dairy)
6 dates, sliced in half.
Simmer on a low heat for 20 minutes. Add a little water if needed. Strain. Makes 1 cup.

BUTTERFLY-COCOON

This gentle movement strengthens your navel chakra and abdominal muscles. If your abdominals need more gradual strengthening, straighten your legs to a 90° angle instead, then bring them back into your chest.

Keep the toes pointed
Use the abdominal muscles to control the gradual extension of the legs

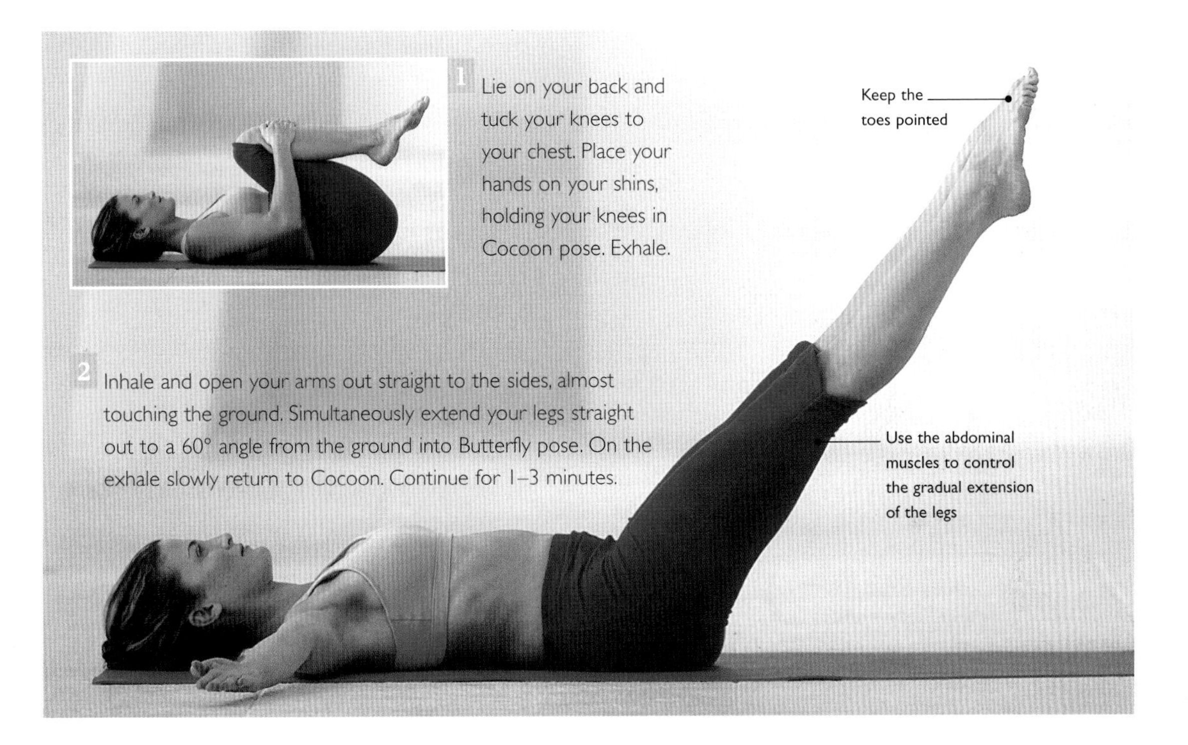

1 Lie on your back and tuck your knees to your chest. Place your hands on your shins, holding your knees in Cocoon pose. Exhale.

2 Inhale and open your arms out straight to the sides, almost touching the ground. Simultaneously extend your legs straight out to a 60° angle from the ground into Butterfly pose. On the exhale slowly return to Cocoon. Continue for 1–3 minutes.

ATMA'S STORY (USA)

I am a Kundalini Yoga teacher and teacher trainer of 24 years, so it was only natural that I should practise yoga during pregnancy. I was so grateful for my practice of yoga all throughout pregnancy, as it made for such a happy, relaxed time. Labour flowed so smoothly, allowing me to squat comfortably and release much tension in my hips. Meditating with deep breathing during and between contractions helped me to maintain a calm, steady awareness, and to reduce pain considerably. Just a couple of weeks after my son was born, I was sitting on the bed beside him, watching him, and feeling how cozy he was laying there all dreamy. So yoga just flowed into my mind. Since it was so soon after the birth, I felt like something very simple and gentle was appropriate – a little bit of spine flexing. I was astonished! Energy flooded my body. One of the basic principles of Kundalini Yoga, and one that I myself have said many times to my students, came to mind at that moment. This time I truly understood: you don't have to be a gymnast to experience great results with yoga.

BABY YOGA

You will have your baby by your side most of the time, so why not enjoy your time together in a way that benefits both of you? When assisting your baby to move her body, never move her with force. Don't be discouraged if she resists: she is adjusting to the wide open spaces of a new life, so help her relax and uncurl and learn about her environment in a natural, flowing way with gentle touch, eye contact, your voice and your love.

Through the years of mothering and teaching children, these words of wisdom have given me guidance: think of children as super-sensitive, fully-fledged people, with high potency antennae that record every single vibration within their vicinity.

HEART CROSSES

Crossing the centre of the body strengthens crossover connections between the right and left brains. This exercise stretches and strengthens your baby's arms and upper back.

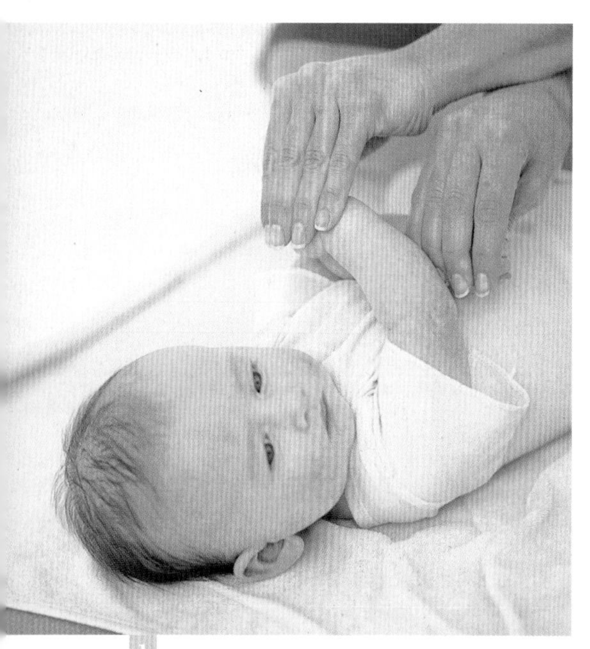

1 Lay your baby on a blanket facing you, and sit or kneel in front of her. Hold her hands and cross her arms over her chest.

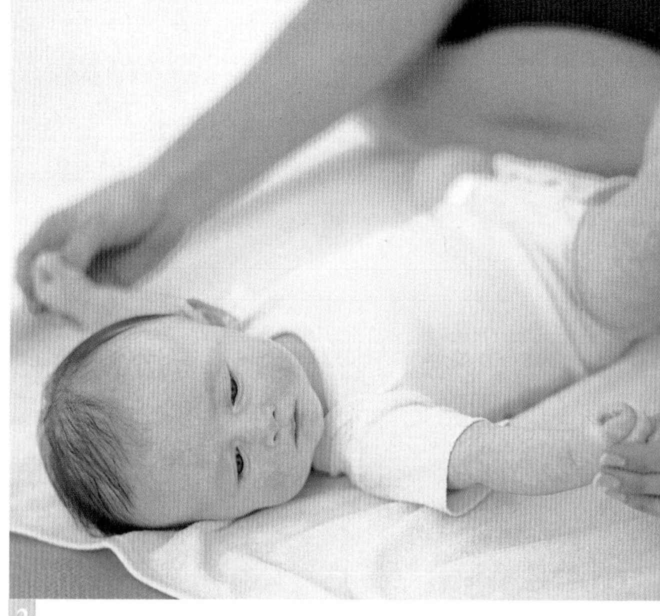

2 Bring her arms out to the sides. Chant a mantra such as *Sat Nam* in rhythm with the movement. Repeat the sequence of steps 1 and 2 for as long as you both like.

BICYCLES

Moving your baby's legs in a bicycling motion and rocking her knees up to her chest helps to relieve and trapped gas. It also helps your baby to strengthen her leg and abdominal muscles.

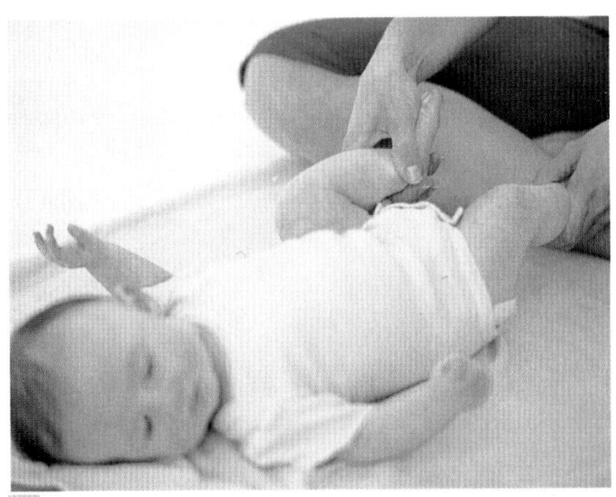

1 Lay your baby on a soft blanket. Smile and look in her eyes. Talk to her about what you are going to do. Gently rotate her legs alternately in a bicycling motion. Sing or chant in rhythm with the motion.

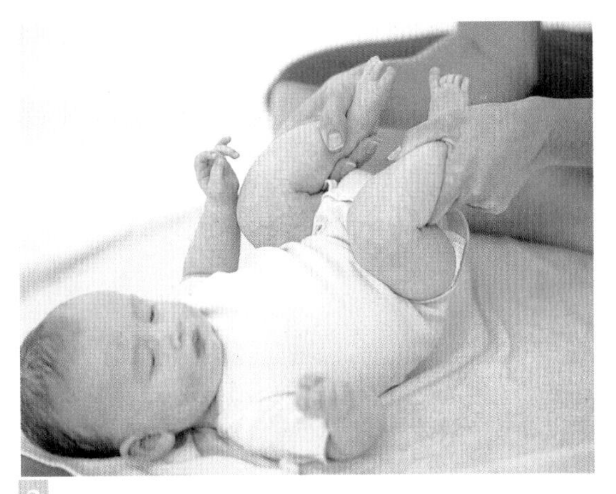

2 To end, bring both of her knees up towards her chest and rock her slightly back, so her bottom comes off the floor. Do this a few times, then let her legs relax down.

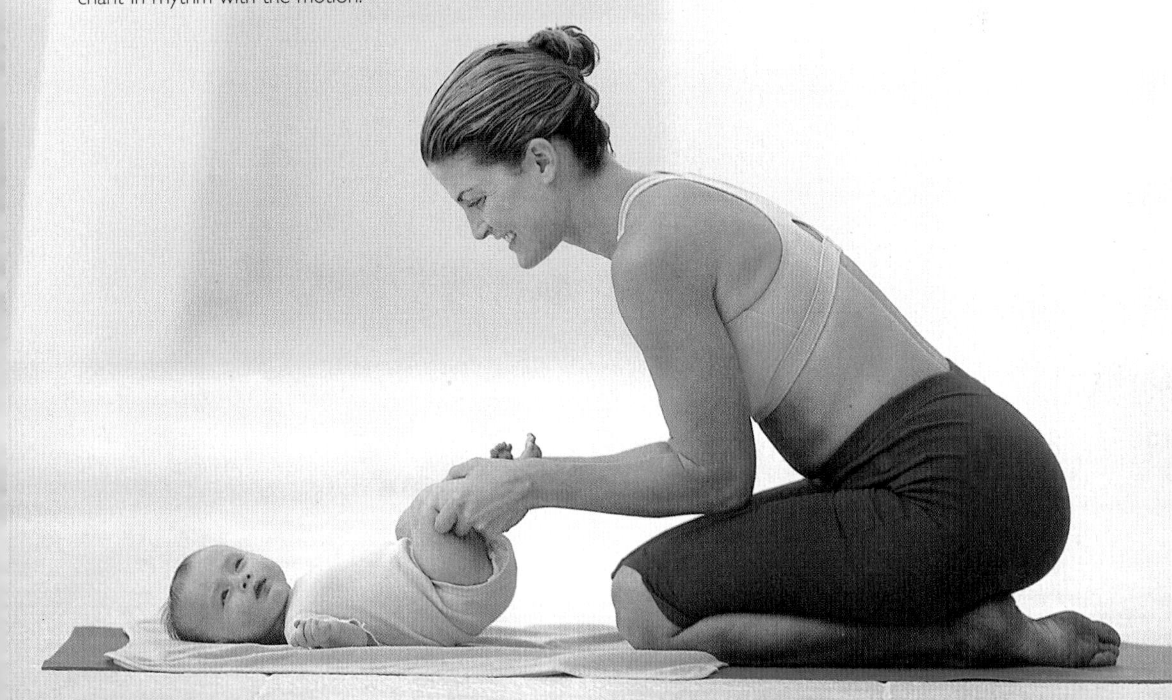

BABY AND ME PELVIC LIFTS

Pelvic Tilts enhance the flexibility in your spine and tone your abdominal and leg muscles. After giving birth, practise Pelvic Tilts against the wall before trying them with your baby.

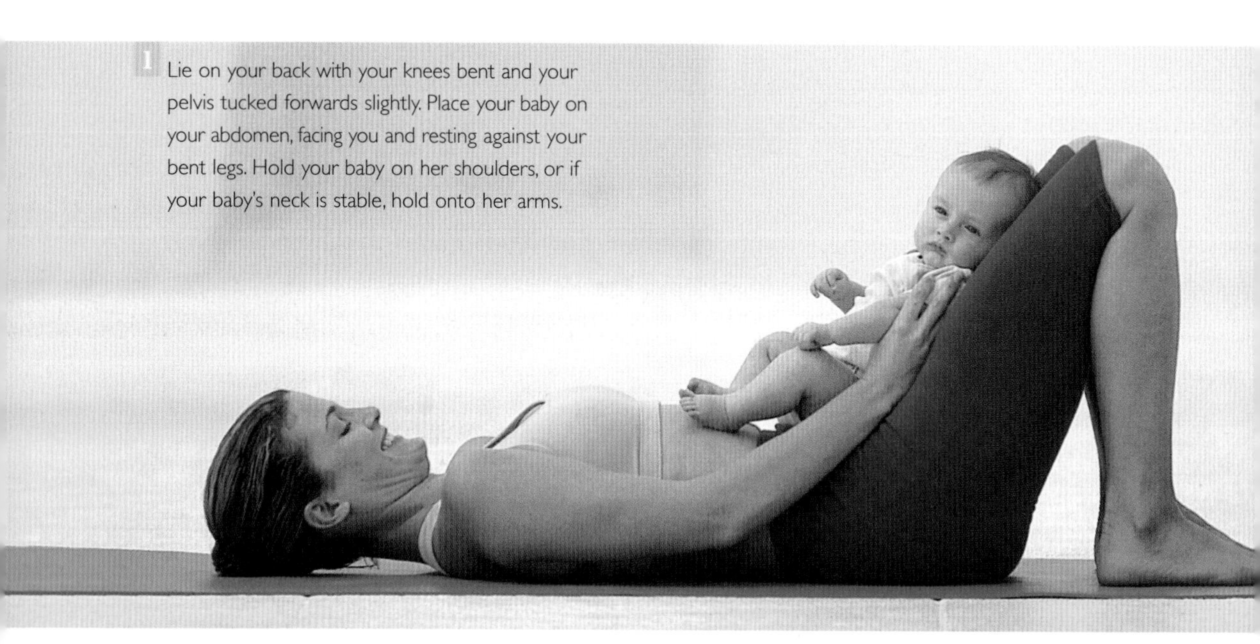

1 Lie on your back with your knees bent and your pelvis tucked forwards slightly. Place your baby on your abdomen, facing you and resting against your bent legs. Hold your baby on her shoulders, or if your baby's neck is stable, hold onto her arms.

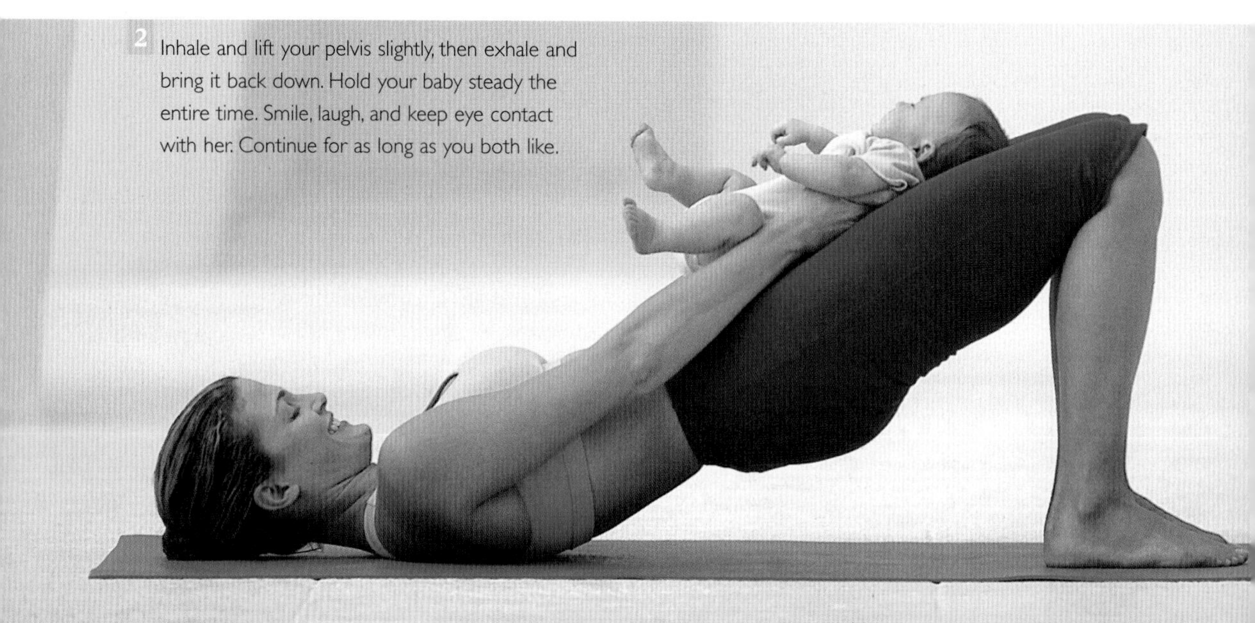

2 Inhale and lift your pelvis slightly, then exhale and bring it back down. Hold your baby steady the entire time. Smile, laugh, and keep eye contact with her. Continue for as long as you both like.

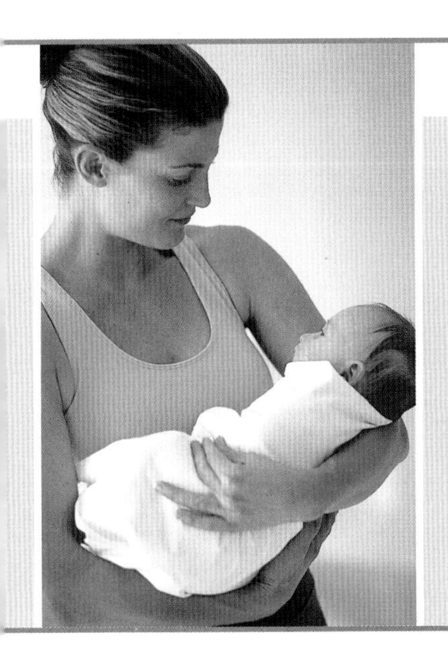

BUNDLE WRAP

In many indigenous cultures mothers wrap their babies in cloth, with their arms and legs straight down at their sides. This is also a yogic technique that provides cozy security for a baby from one or two months onwards. Cut a piece of lightweight cloth (sheeting works well) in a rectangle long enough to wrap around a few times from shoulder to foot. Lay your baby near one edge with enough cloth to bring across the front side and tuck it between his arm and side. Then roll him up. For a peaceful sleep, hold your baby at your chest, heart to heart, and pat him as you sing or hum. Any resistance he gives to the wrap is beneficial as it builds muscle and nerve strength. A wrap may be used before a night-time sleep, but your baby should be unwrapped after an hour or so.

THE GRACE OF GOD MEDITATION

This is perfect for a busy, new mum. It is quick and potent, and you can do it lying down. It helps to positively channel your emotions. There are two parts, and although it is recommended to do them together, they can be done separately or whenever you have a spare five minutes. It uses the mantra "I am Grace of God". The optimum times for this meditation are at sunrise and sunset, preferably practised twice a day.

1 *Lie on your back with your arms at your sides. Relax your face and body. Take a few deep breaths. Inhale, hold the breath in, and repeat silently to yourself "I am Grace of God". Exhale and repeat the affirmation silently 10 times. Continue for five breaths. This will make a total 100 times that the mantra/affirmation is repeated.*

2 *After the cycle is completed, or at a different time during the day, sit in Easy pose. Bring your right hand into Gyan Mudra (p.21). Hold the left hand up by the left shoulder, palm flat and facing forwards, as though taking an oath. The chest is lifted and the spine is straight. Your breath is relaxed and normal. Beginning with the index finger of the left hand, tense the finger and repeat out loud, "I am Grace of God" five times. Then proceed to do the same with each of the other fingers, including the thumb. Inhale to end and feel the reality of the affirmation you have just repeated. Exhale and relax.*

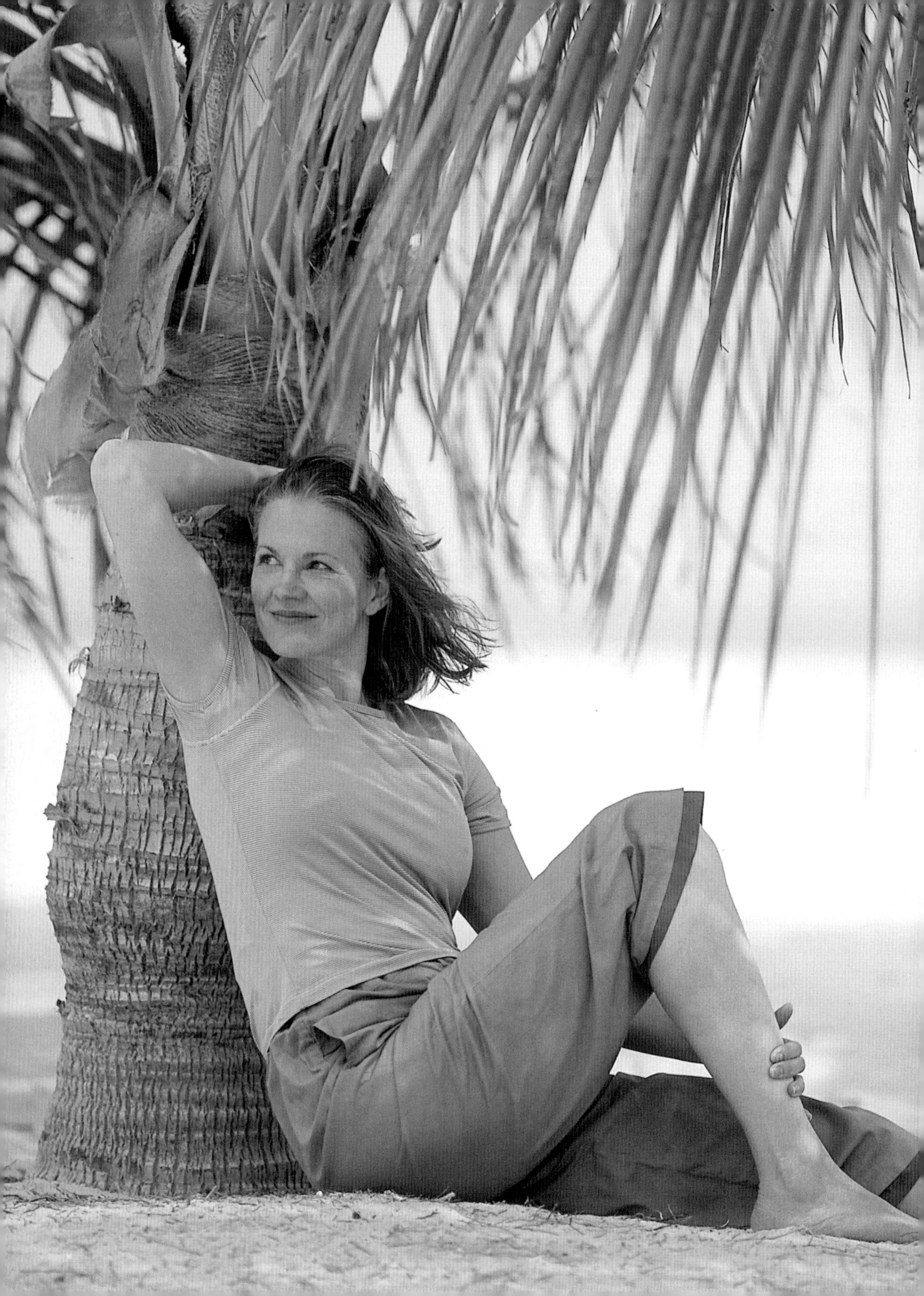

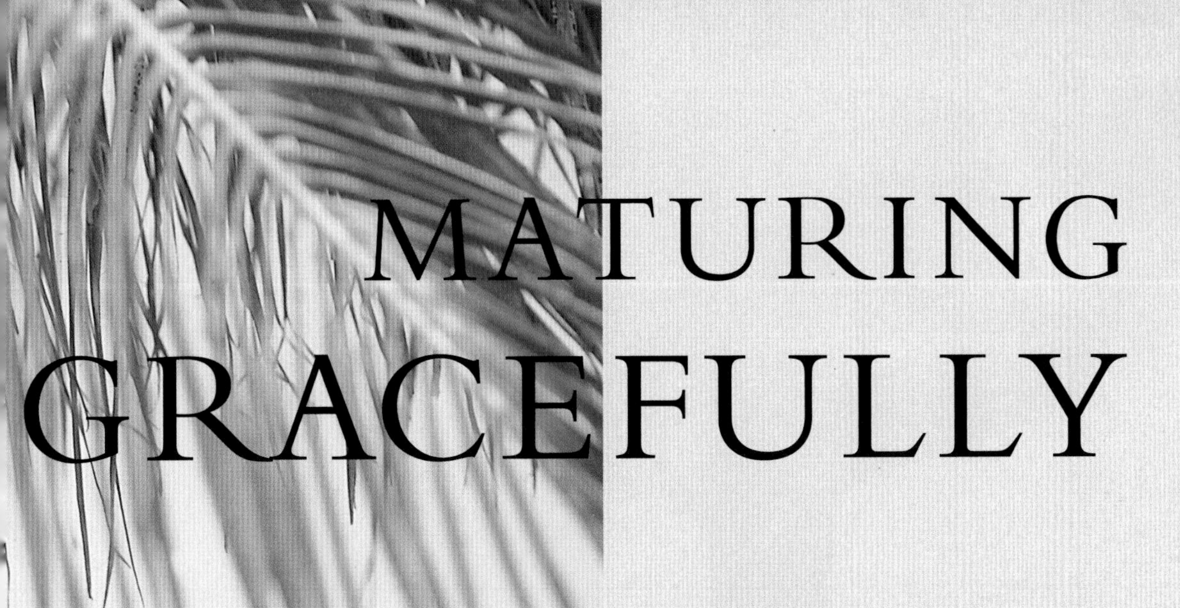

MATURING GRACEFULLY

Many women say that as they grow older, life takes on a richness previously undreamed of, that the second half of life really can be better than the first. Major changes in responsibilities such as children, home, and work open the door to new opportunities for women at this stage. How well a woman can appreciate and enjoy the second half of life depends very much on the quality of her health and wellbeing. This is where yoga plays a part in maturing with grace. In this last section you can practise yoga that helps you maintain strong physical health, glowing inner and outer beauty, and a mind that's clear, calm, and able to live in a timeless state of consciousness.

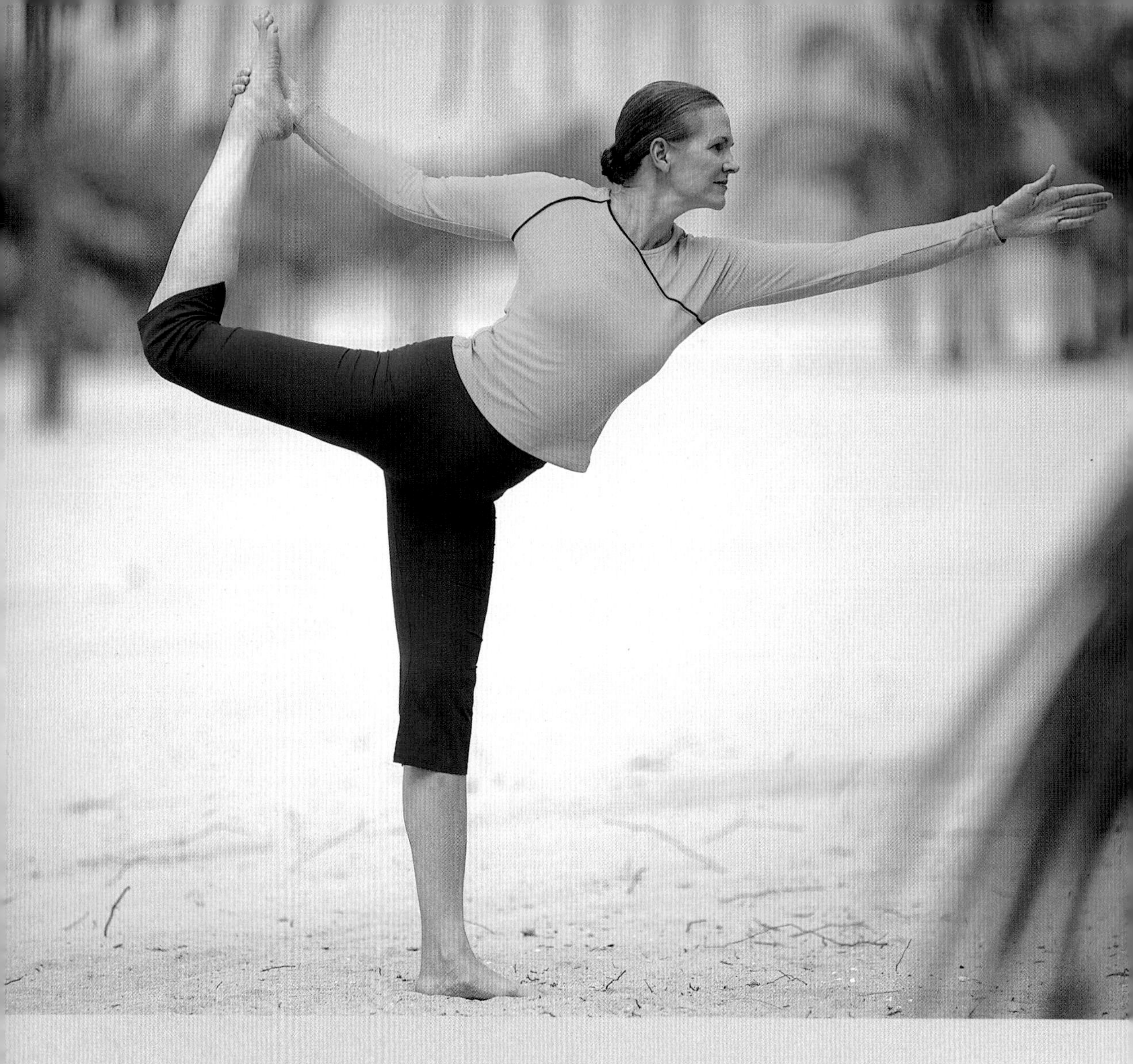

AGELESS BEAUTY

Staying young for a long time is a wonderful, blessed way to live. As women, we have so much to give as we mature, so much wisdom born of hard-earned experience and loving kindness to share. So let's keep our good health and vitality and reap the profit of a life well-lived. The practices in this part of the book focus on just that. Yoga keeps us well-oiled as we age, and you'll find a few exercises that help prevent arthritis, as well as yoga that maintains good bone density and helps prevent osteoporosis. Just for the fun of it, and because we women love to look and feel beautiful, I've included yoga for your face and a special yoga set for enchanting beauty. Enjoy, and feel like the beautiful soul that you are!

BENDING CIRCLES

This exercise aids in the prevention of arthritis. It improves spinal flexibility and helps you feel young and energetic. If you have arthritis or bursitis in your shoulders or back, use slower, smaller movements.

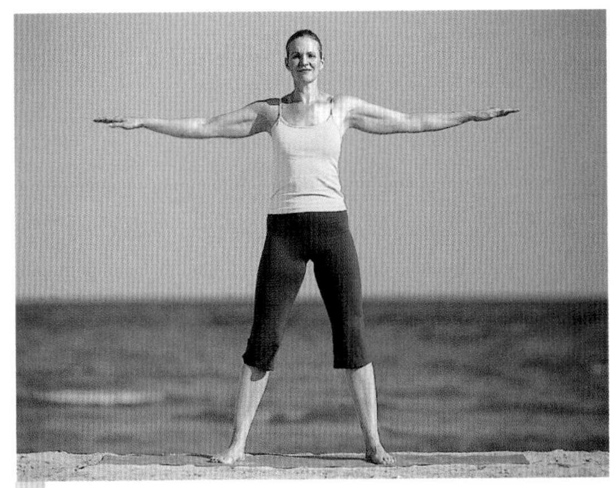

1 Stand with your feet shoulder-width apart, your spine straight, and your knees soft. Bring your arms straight out to the sides of your body.

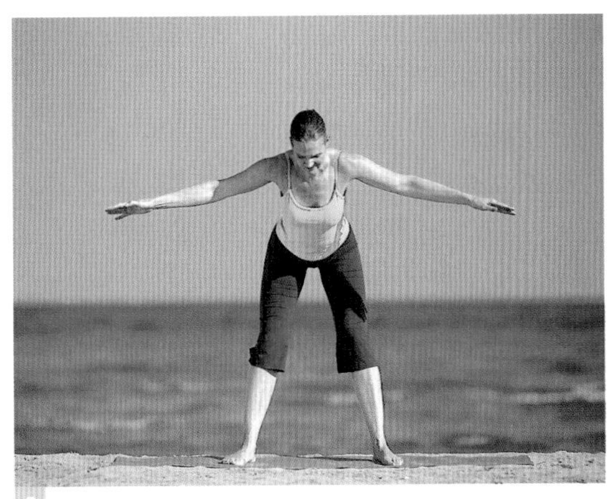

2 Counting out loud from 1 to 8, begin to bend forwards slowly from the waist while moving the arms in forward circles, about the size of a dinner plate.

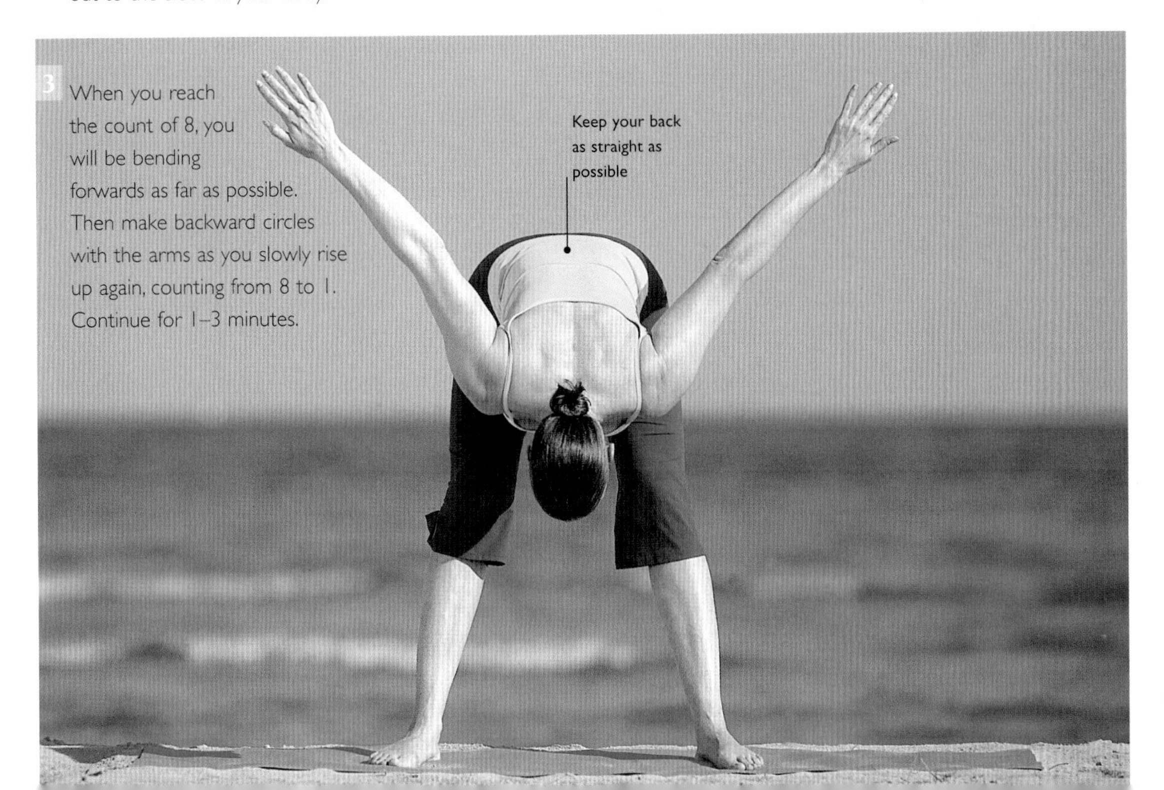

3 When you reach the count of 8, you will be bending forwards as far as possible. Then make backward circles with the arms as you slowly rise up again, counting from 8 to 1. Continue for 1–3 minutes.

LIONESS POSE

This pose works on firming your neck muscles, exercising your eye muscles, and opening your throat. The strong breathing that you practise in this exercise releases toxins from the body.

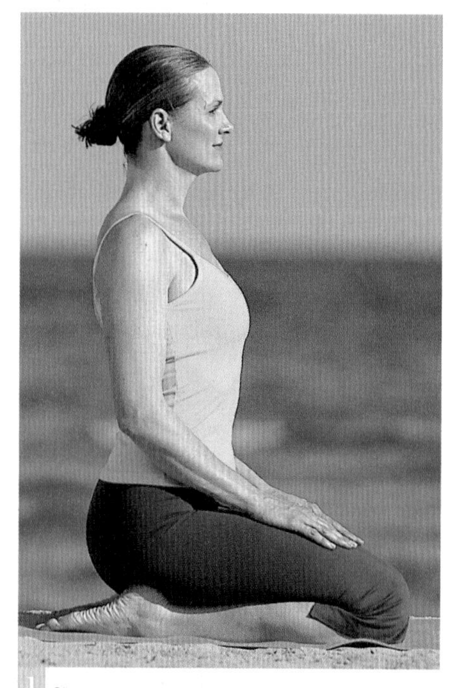

1 Sit on your knees in Rock pose *(p.20)*. Then place your hands on the ground in front of your knees, palms down.

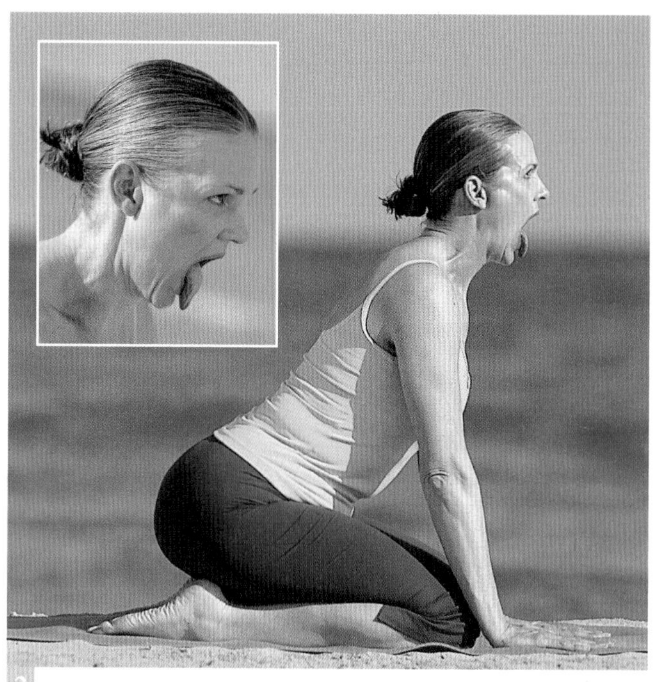

2 Draw your chin in towards your chest. Stretch out your tongue as far as possible. Open your eyes wide and breathe through your mouth. Make the sound of a lioness. Continue for 1 minute.

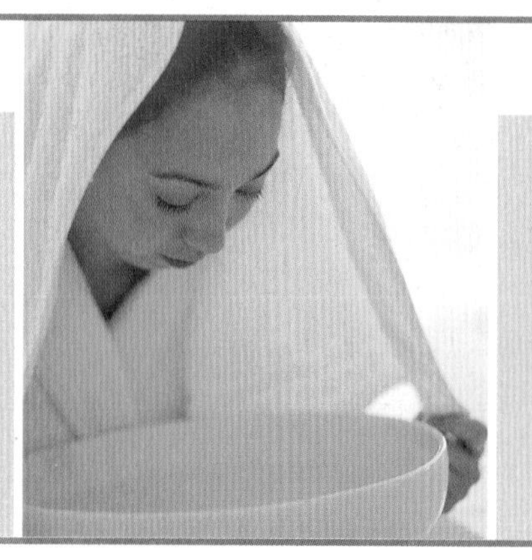

CHAMOMILE STEAM FACIAL

Your pores will open and a cleansing sweat will be created in a few minutes with this steam facial. Bring a saucepan of water to a boil, then remove from the heat. Add a handful of chamomile flowers, cover, and let steep for 10 minutes. Place a towel over your head and bring your face close enough to the steam that you can smell and feel the steam opening your pores, but without burning your skin or nostrils. Follow with a mask of plain home-made yogurt if you like.

QUEEN DANCER

Originally called King Dancer, Queen Dancer is a more appropriate name for this women's yoga book! It gives you a sense of elation and power, rejuvenates your spine and internal organs, and improves your sense of balance. A good sense of balance can help prevent falls, which can be a serious problem as we age, especially if bone density is weakened.

What is the relationship between yoga and healthy bone density? Bone production is stimulated when tension and resistance are applied to the tendons that attach to bones. Yoga, being weight-bearing, does just that.

If you need help reaching your bent leg loop a belt around your foot
Gaze straight ahead for focus and balance

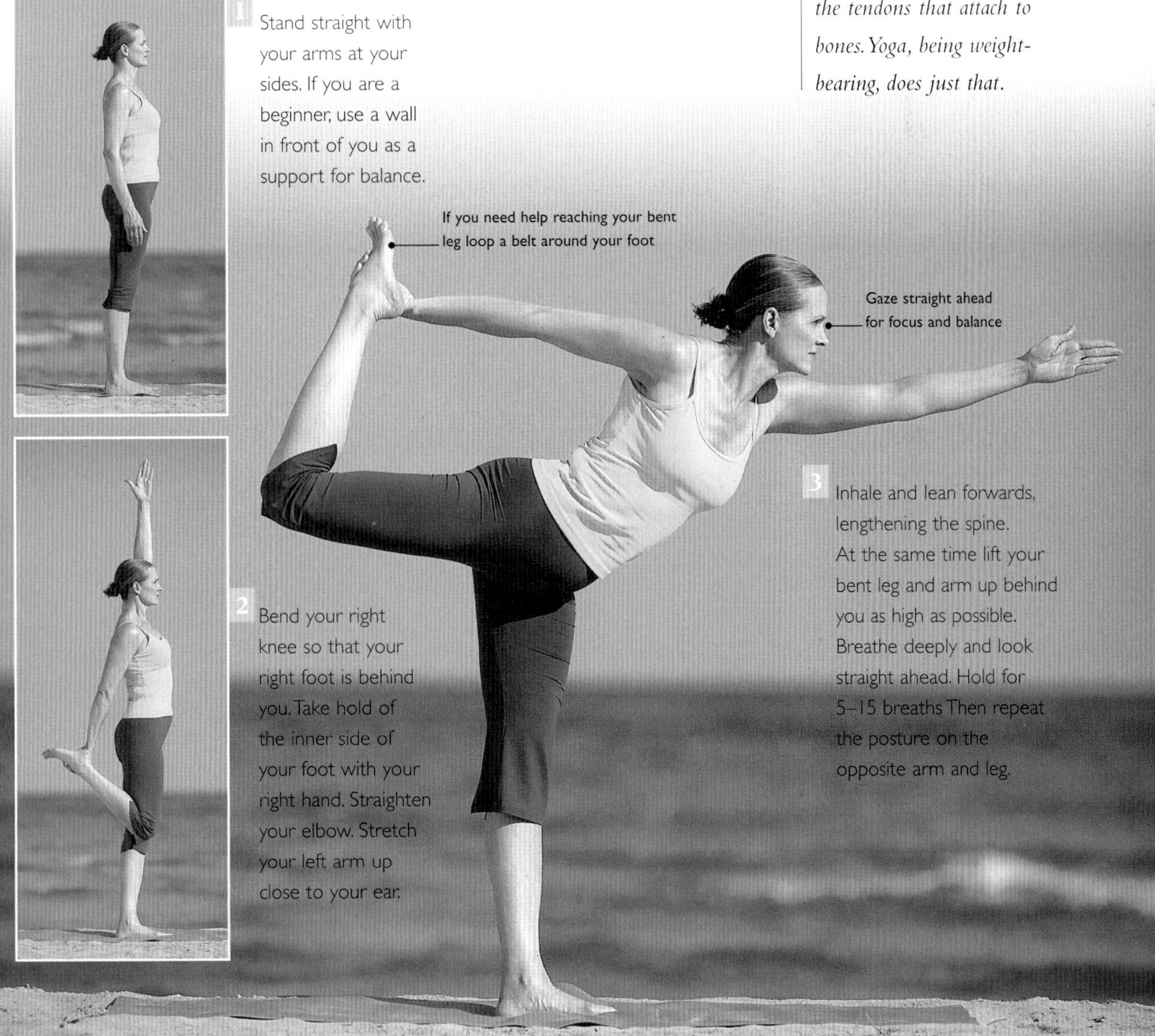

1 Stand straight with your arms at your sides. If you are a beginner, use a wall in front of you as a support for balance.

2 Bend your right knee so that your right foot is behind you. Take hold of the inner side of your foot with your right hand. Straighten your elbow. Stretch your left arm up close to your ear.

3 Inhale and lean forwards, lengthening the spine. At the same time lift your bent leg and arm up behind you as high as possible. Breathe deeply and look straight ahead. Hold for 5–15 breaths Then repeat the posture on the opposite arm and leg.

PLANK

This pose strengthens the arms and legs and builds upper body muscle mass, which is a factor in helping to increase bone density. Spend a few moments in Child's pose *(p.63)* afterwards to relax the lower spine.

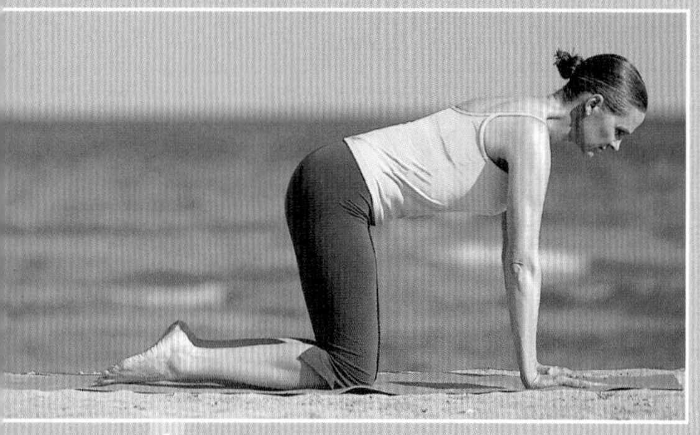

1 This pose is best done on a non-slip mat. Begin on your hands and knees.

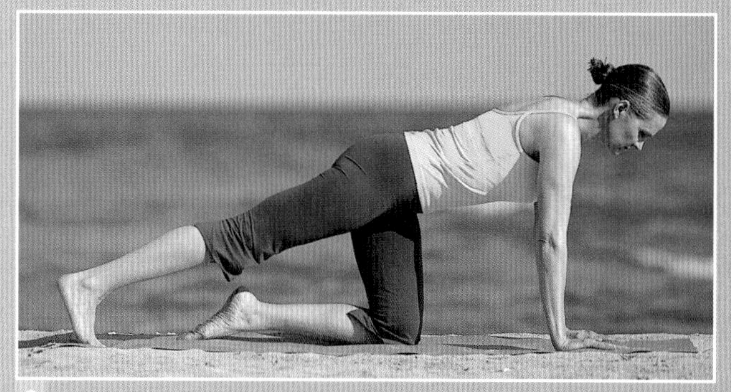

2 Extend your right leg back and place your toes only on the ground, then extend the left leg back. Balance your weight on your toes.

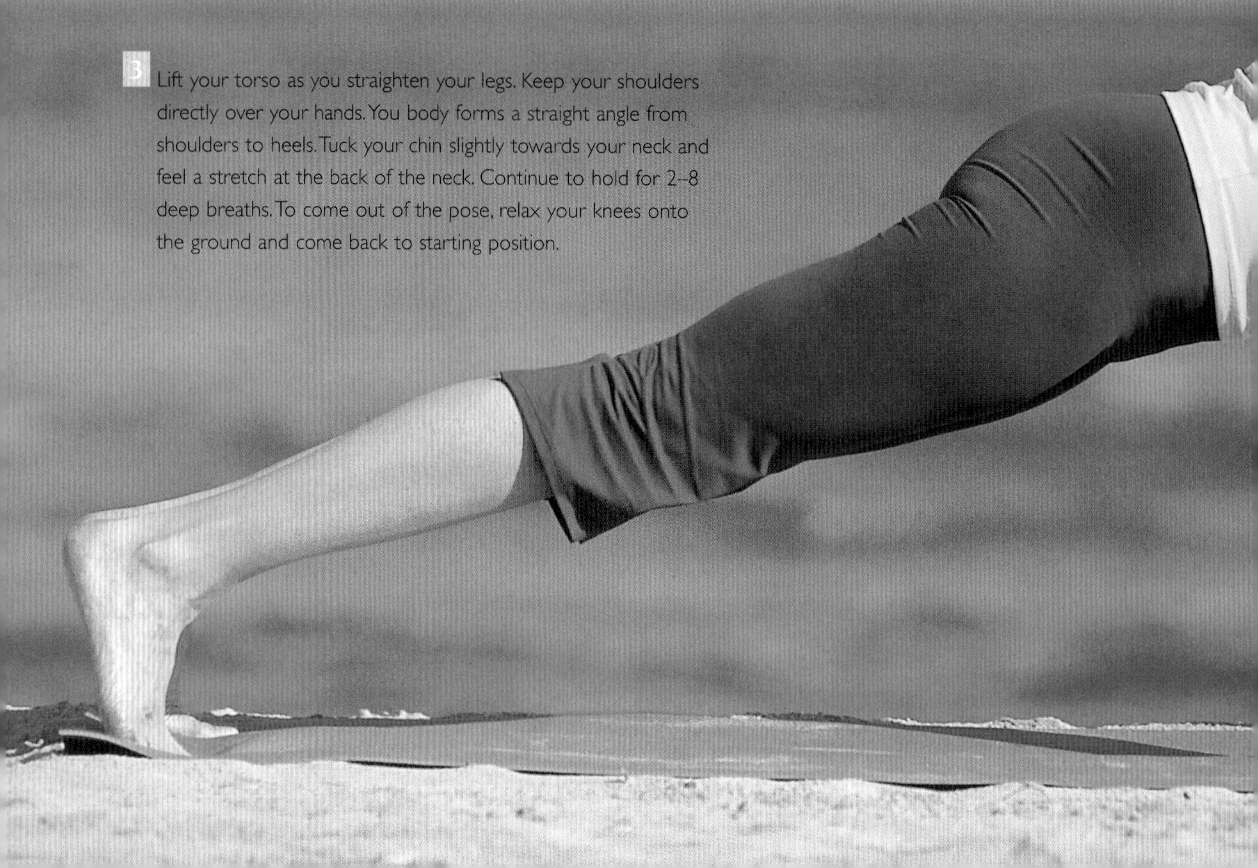

3 Lift your torso as you straighten your legs. Keep your shoulders directly over your hands. You body forms a straight angle from shoulders to heels. Tuck your chin slightly towards your neck and feel a stretch at the back of the neck. Continue to hold for 2–8 deep breaths. To come out of the pose, relax your knees onto the ground and come back to starting position.

MARY ANN'S STORY (USA)

I began yoga classes on my 57th birthday and have been practising for five years now. I found out I had severe osteoporosis of the spine and had a lot of lower back pain. My doctor told me that, should I fall, I was six times as likely to break my back as a normal person. Now I don't worry about falling as I feel I have gained balance through practising yoga. Kundalini Yoga was the perfect fit for my spine, and I love the breathing exercises which have empowered me so much. Some people say I do not look my age, but I tell them it is the yoga, breathing exercises, and the water I drink. I tend to be a worrier and a perfectionist, but the mental serenity I achieve from yoga is unbelievable. Each Christmas my husband purchases several months' worth of classes as my gift. It is the best thing he can give me: yoga is now and always will be a part of my life.

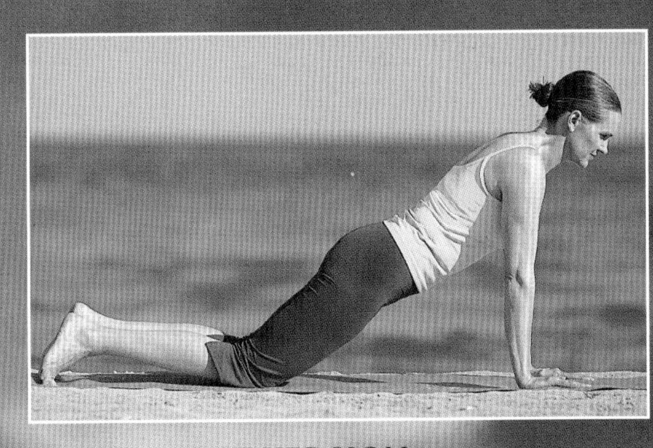

EASY-DOES-IT VERSION

Begin on your hands and knees. Lean forwards onto your arms and stretch out your torso so that your body is at a straight angle from knees to shoulders. Your shoulders are directly over your elbows, with your head facing the ground and your chin tucked in slightly. Continue to hold for 2–8 deep breaths.

TO BE ENCHANTINGLY BEAUTIFUL

This short set brings vibrant, radiant health and helps develop a meditative mind; it increases your beauty both physically and mentally. To become beautiful inside and out you need a flow of pranic energy to brighten your eyes and skin, and generate glowing health.

1 LION FLEX

This exercise increases flexibility in the spine, which is the true measure of youthfulness. Be aware of flexing each vertebra of your spine in a flowing movement.

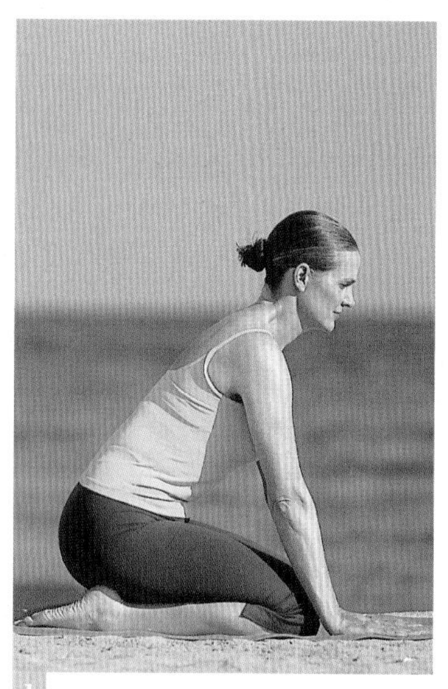

1 Sit on your heels with a straight spine. Place the palms of your hands on the ground just in front of the knees. Bring your neck vertebrae in line with your spine by lifting your head and tucking the chin in slightly.

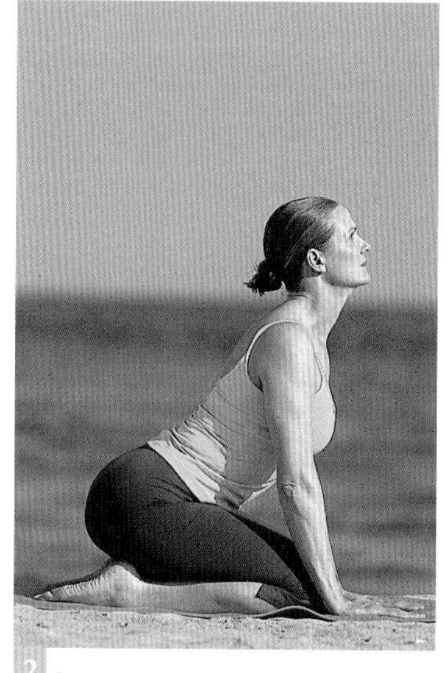

2 Begin flexing your spine to its maximum capacity, keeping the elbows straight as you flex: inhale and arch your spine, lifting your chest while keeping your head level.

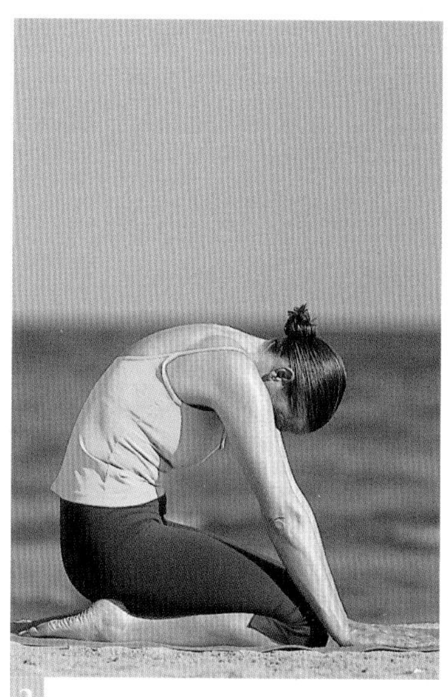

3 Exhale as you round your spine so that your chest curls inwards. Keep a constant rhythm as you repeat the pose. You may begin to sweat lightly on the forehead and spine. Continue for 2–3 minutes.

2 VENUS LOCK STRETCH

This exercise brings circulation to your face and cheeks. Try smiling while you breathe in this exercise; the best face lift you can get is to smile as often as possible. Besides, you cannot think a negative thought when you are smiling – try it and see!

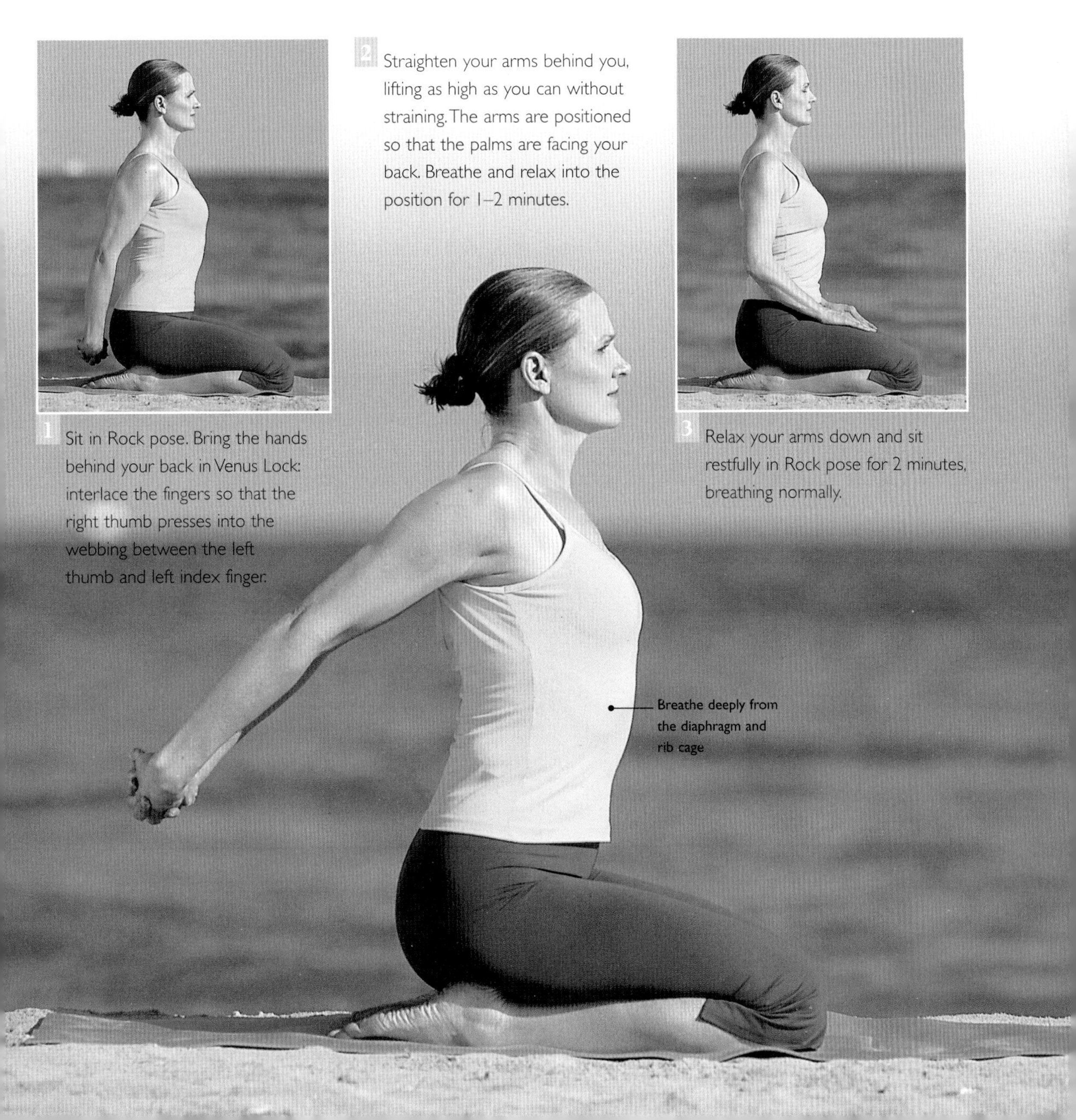

1 Sit in Rock pose. Bring the hands behind your back in Venus Lock: interlace the fingers so that the right thumb presses into the webbing between the left thumb and left index finger.

2 Straighten your arms behind you, lifting as high as you can without straining. The arms are positioned so that the palms are facing your back. Breathe and relax into the position for 1–2 minutes.

3 Relax your arms down and sit restfully in Rock pose for 2 minutes, breathing normally.

3 LIFT AND HOLD

This pose helps to relieve headaches. It also stretches and strengthens the sciatic nerves in the legs. There is a strong, automatic tendency to shake in this position, which strengthens the entire nervous system.

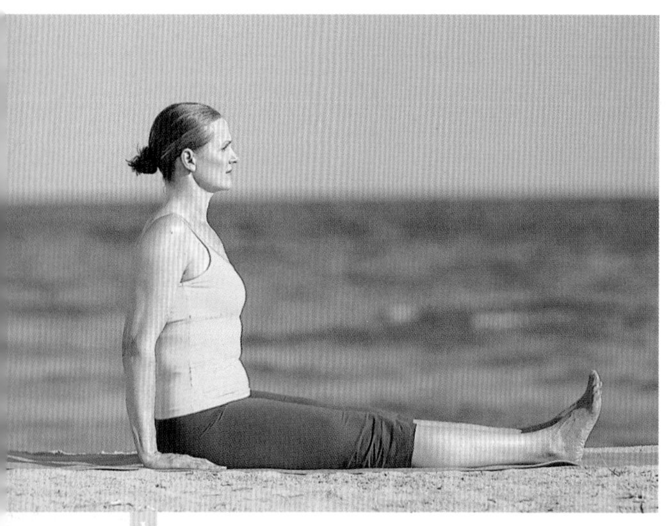

1 Sit with a straight spine and your legs outstretched in front of you, with your heels together. Your hands are flat on the ground beside your hips.

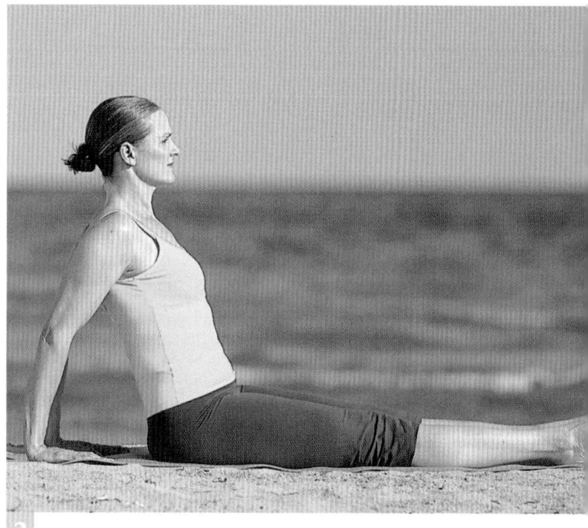

2 Place your hands slightly behind your hips and lean back, keeping your chest lifted. Point your toes.

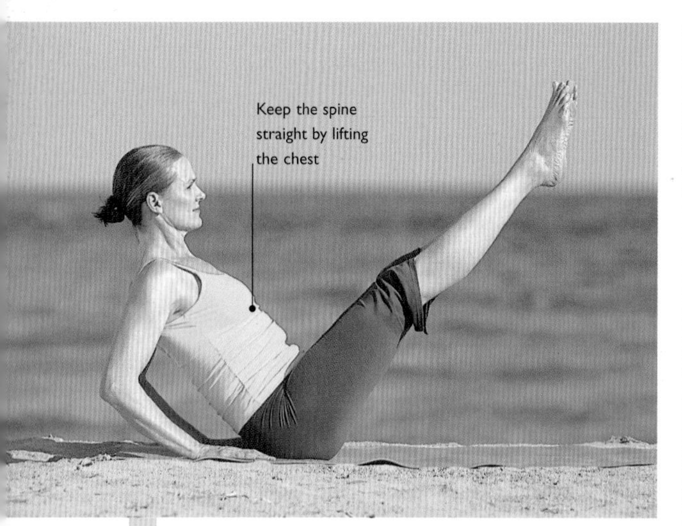

3 Bending your elbows, lean back as you inhale and raise your legs slowly to a 60° angle and hold. Keep your legs together and breathe deeply for 1–3 minutes.

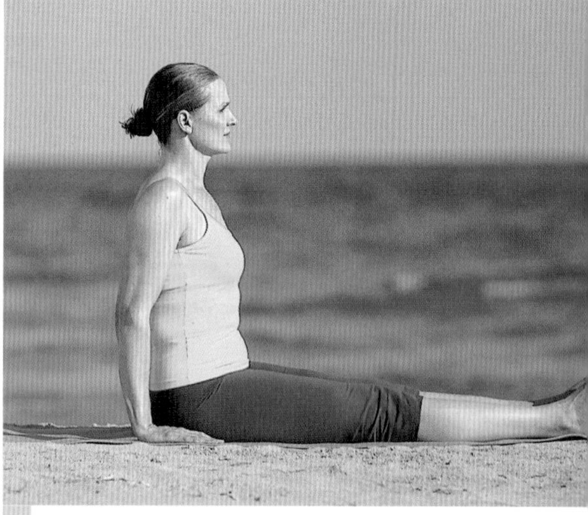

4 Come out of the pose by relaxing your legs down onto the ground. Relax and sit straight or rest in a Forward Bend for a few seconds.

4 FEET UP

Fifty powerful and continuous repetitions of Breath of Fire while in this pose cleanse and improve blood circulation. Feet Up cleans the lungs and stimulates the prana so that you are able to retain your youth and power.

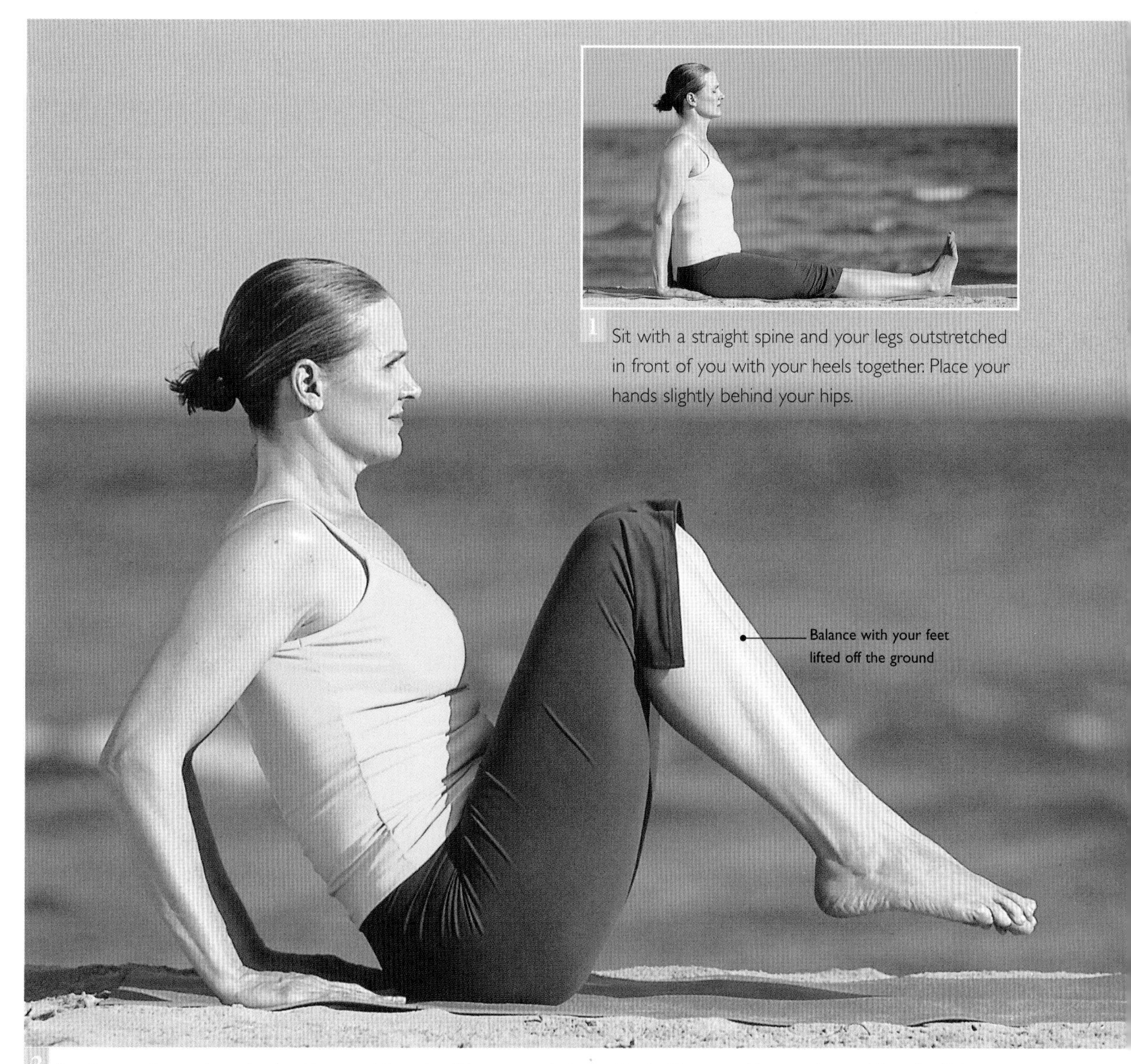

1 Sit with a straight spine and your legs outstretched in front of you with your heels together. Place your hands slightly behind your hips.

2 Bend your elbows. Lean back with a straight spine. Then bend your knees and bring them as close to your chest as possible. Hold your feet 15cm (6in) off the ground and balance. Begin 50 powerful repetitions of Breath of Fire. Inhale deeply, exhale, and relax your legs onto the ground. Rest in a Forward Bend for a few seconds if you wish.

5 FORWARD STRETCH

This exercise invigorates the liver and spleen. Pressing your toes with your fingers stimulates reflexology points that in turn stimulate brain activity. The top back area of the big toe stimulates the pituitary gland. Chanting cleans the lungs and creates such a stimulation to the pranic life force that you can retain your youth, power, and work potency.

As you hold this posture, chant the sound Hum. *It means "we", and it helps to take you out of your own smallness and feel a unity with all life. The "mmm" sound is continuous.*

Lengthen your spine and stretch it up fully
Keep your arms straight

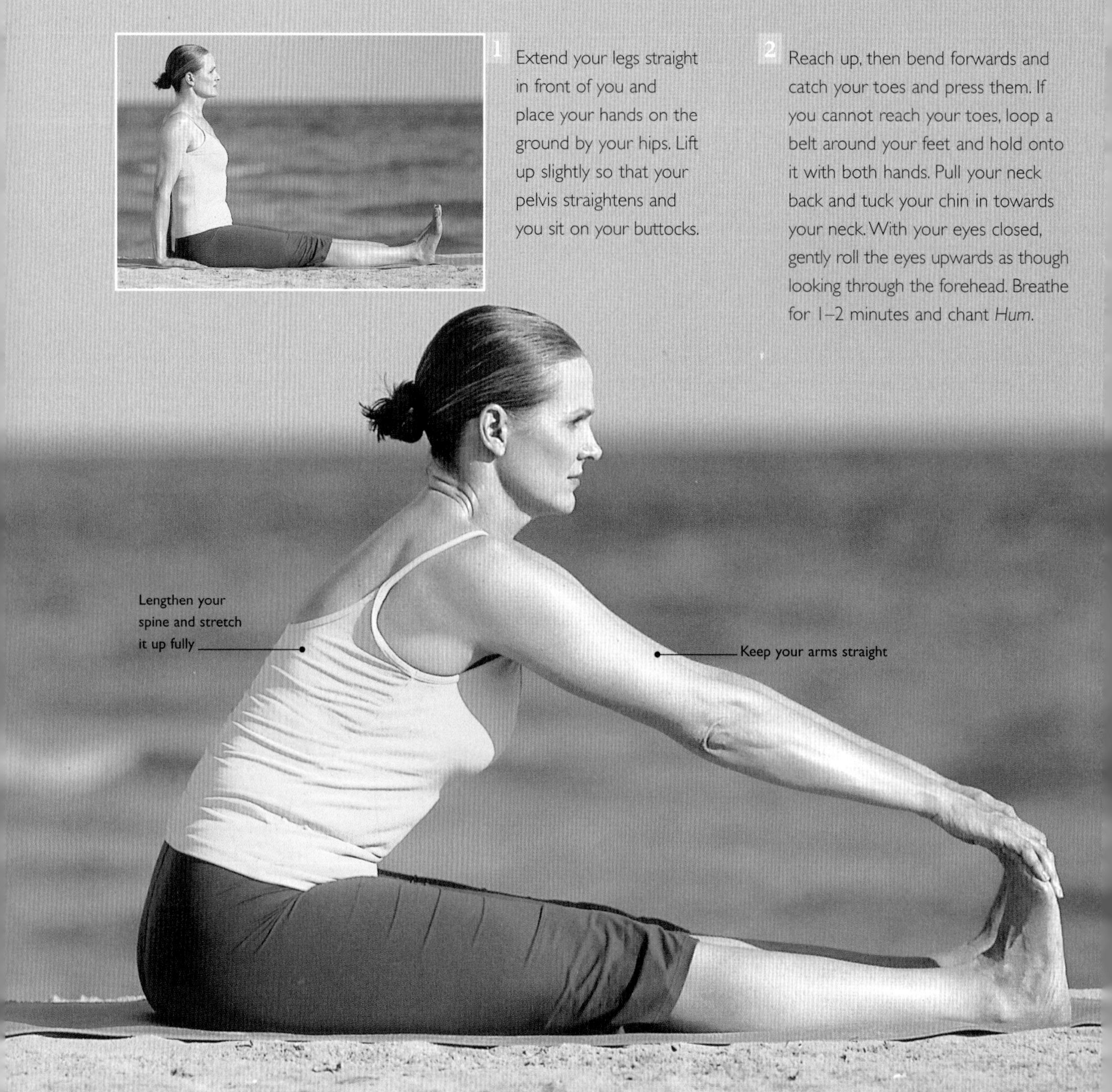

1 Extend your legs straight in front of you and place your hands on the ground by your hips. Lift up slightly so that your pelvis straightens and you sit on your buttocks.

2 Reach up, then bend forwards and catch your toes and press them. If you cannot reach your toes, loop a belt around your feet and hold onto it with both hands. Pull your neck back and tuck your chin in towards your neck. With your eyes closed, gently roll the eyes upwards as though looking through the forehead. Breathe for 1–2 minutes and chant *Hum*.

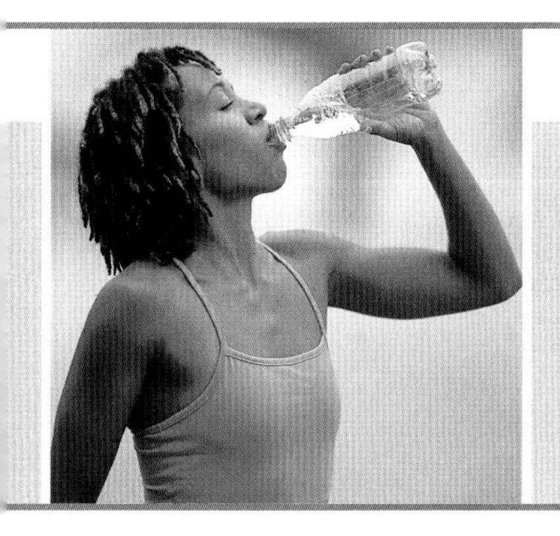

DRINK WATER

Sip pure water throughout the day to balance your brain, glands, and nervous systems. If you feel the urge to eat something, but you are not really hungry, drink water. Keeping hydrated can also help to neutralize food cravings. Drink plenty of water in between meals rather than with them since liquids dilute the digestive juices. Water is the best thirst quencher; any other beverage can only quench your thirst in proportion to the amount of water it contains.

TO MAKE YOUR FACE INNOCENTLY CHARMING

This is a beautiful meditation. It is said to have the ability to make a woman feel happy and extend her life. The mudra (hand position) and breath affect the brain chemistry in ways that allow you to feel cosy and relaxed, and your face reflects an innocent charm. This is a relaxing meditation, perfect to do before bedtime or to feel refreshed after work. Do not practise it if you have work to do. You may like to practise for 11 minutes, a complete meditation cycle of time.

1 *Sit comfortably in a meditative pose with your spine straight. Bring your hands in front of you so that the palms of the hands face each other. Curl the fingers of your left hand into a fist, then wrap the fingers of your right hand around the left with the heels of the hands touching. When you look down at your hands, your left index finger should be closest to you. Bring your thumbs together so the sides are touching, then rest them on the index finger of the left hand. They should not touch the right index finger at all. An air space is naturally created between the hands.*

2 *With the hands positioned 21–24cm (8–10in) from the face at mouth level, begin inhaling deeply through the nose and exhaling through the mouth, directing the air through the opening created between your thumbs. Exhale completely. Close your eyes and continue the breath meditation for however long you wish – even until you fall asleep.*

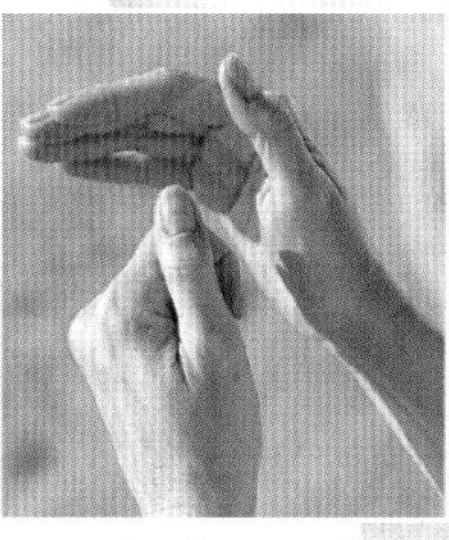

Wrap the fingers of the right hand around the left

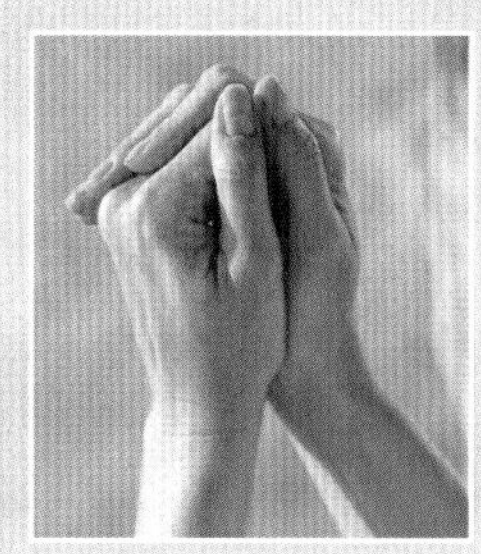

The thumbs rest on the left index finger

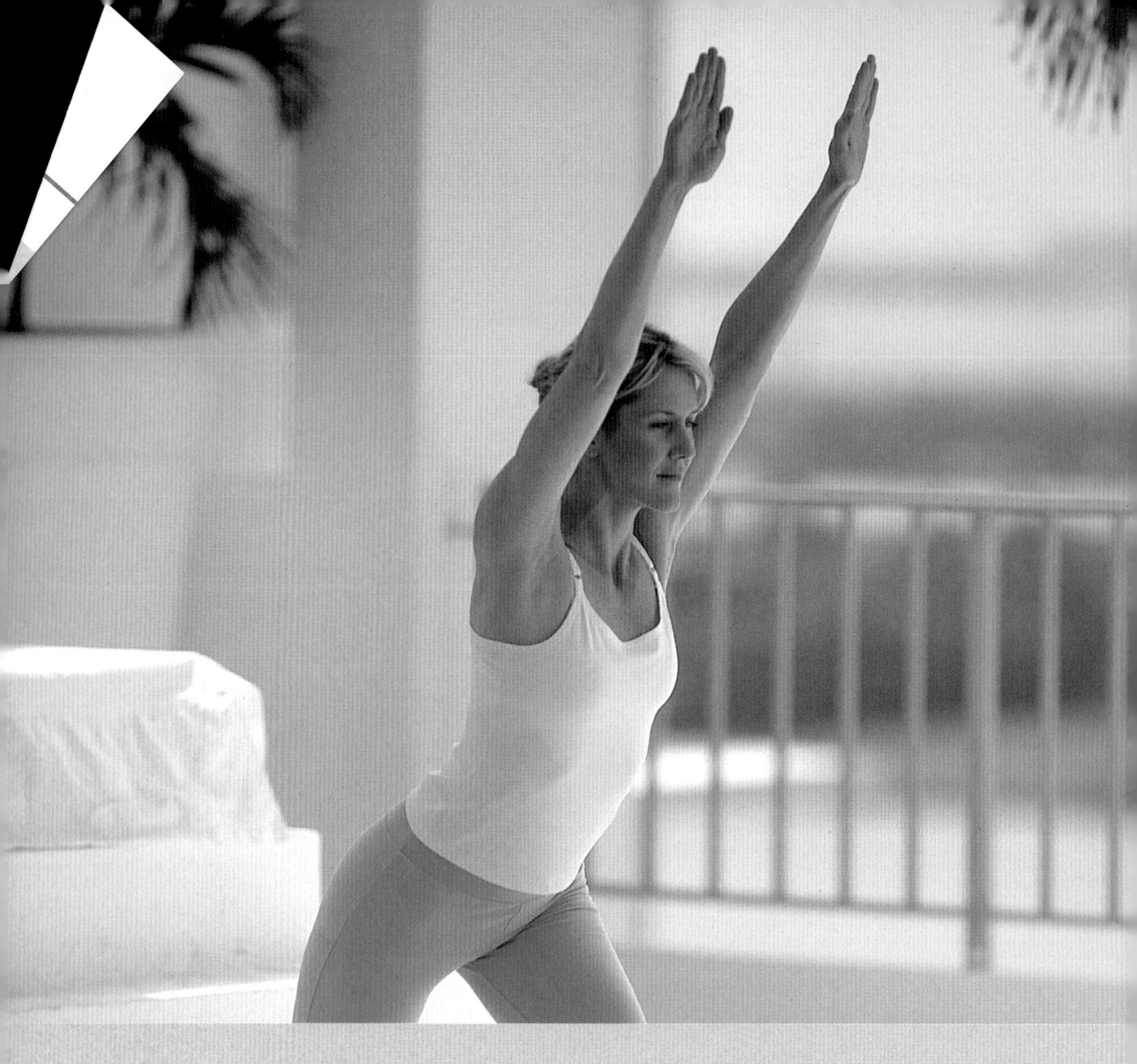

LIVING IN THE MOMENT

Right now is the only time you actually exist. The past exists only in memory, and the future only in your mind's projection. Being "present" to the present is truly living. What does it feel like to be present? Some describe it as feeling grounded, stable, expansive, and peaceful, deeply peaceful. There is no need for judgement, guilt, anger – or even patience – fortitude, and forgiveness, as they all stem from resistance to what "is". Being present is being with life as it is and allowing it, simply because it is what it is! In being present to the eternal "Now", you experience what in yoga is called Shunia, the zero point, where the neutral mind, the loving heart, and the expanded awareness exist as one.

THE WARRIOR SEQUENCE

The dance of breath, movement, and awareness is the signature of a vinyasa. In this powerful vinyasa, be mindful of the interplay of breath and movement. Pause the breath at the end of both the inhalation and exhalation. In that pause of one or two seconds, relate to the stillness inside, outside and all around.

Practise Full Warrior for a week or so, then add Extended Warrior, and so on, until you know the entire sequence.

1 FULL WARRIOR

The vertebrae of the mid-spine are flexed, and digestion is stimulated in this pose. Energy is also circulated throughout the middle and upper back.

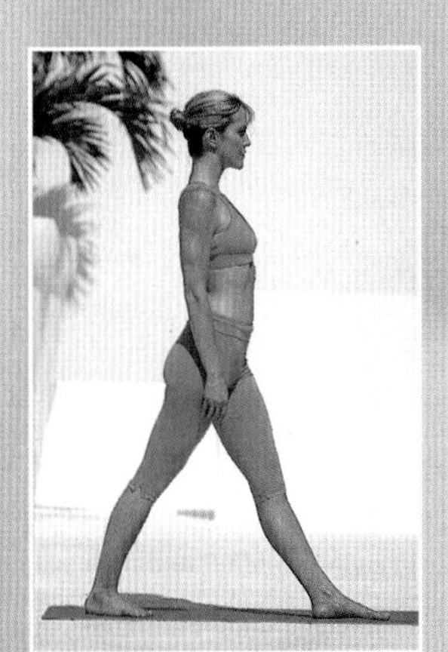

1 Stand with your left leg 60–120cm (2–4ft) forwards and your right foot behind you, turned out slightly. Your arms are by your sides. Your back leg is the grounding element in this pose: keep your right leg strong and maintain a lifting feeling in the left knee.

2 On a slow, deep inhalation, bend the left knee so that it is directly above your ankle. Lift your arms up close to your ears, palms facing forwards. As the movement and breath end, tilt the chin up slightly and focus on the horizon. Exhale and return to the starting position. Repeat 2–3 times, then change legs and repeat.

The whole movement is all done on one long, relaxed inhalation

Your chest is lifted over your thigh and the upper back is arched slightly

2 EXTENDED WARRIOR

This pose strengthens the spine and legs, tones the abdominal muscles and nervous system. Keep the mind focused and the eyes gazing forwards as you practise Extended Warrior.

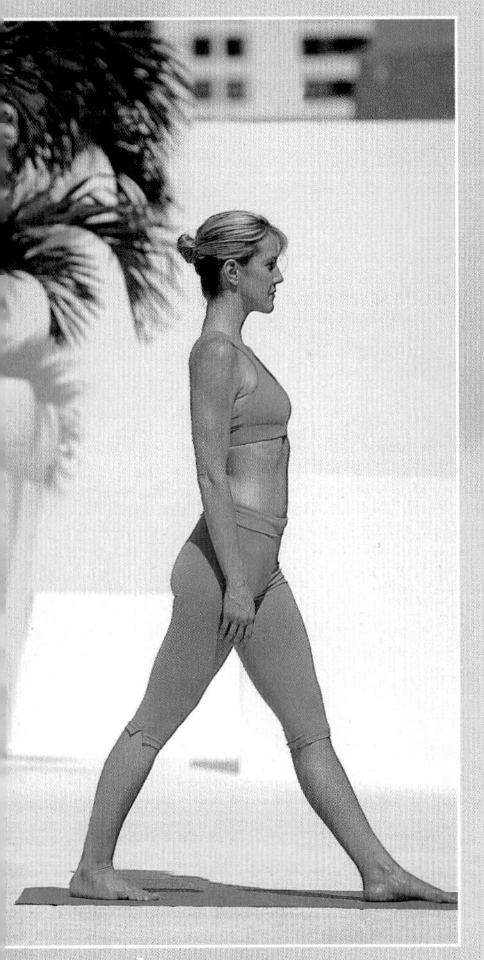

1 Stand with your left leg 60–120cm (2–4ft) forwards and your right foot behind you, turned out slightly. Your arms are by your sides.

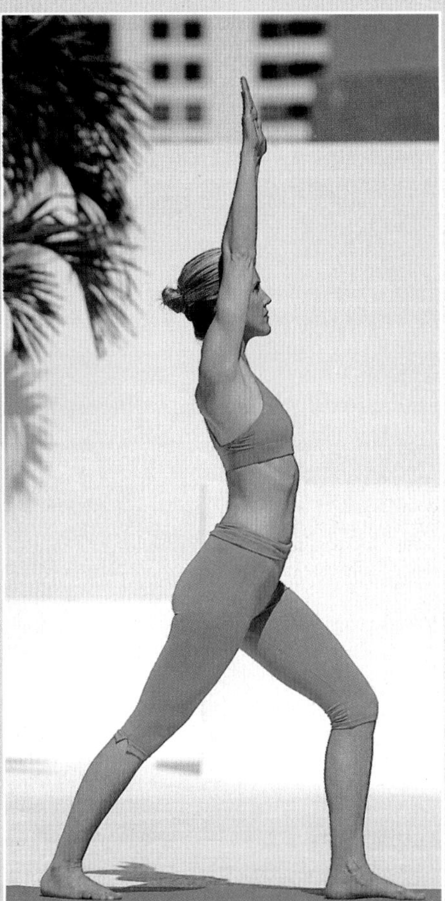

2 Inhale and come up into Full Warrior pose: bend the left knee so that it is directly above your ankle, and lift your arms up close to your ears, palms facing forwards.

Practise this sequence 2–3 times, then rest in the counterpose (p.220) before repeating the sequence again with the right foot in front.

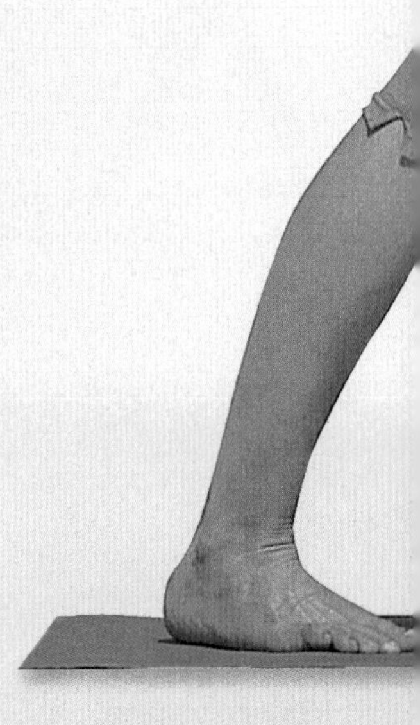

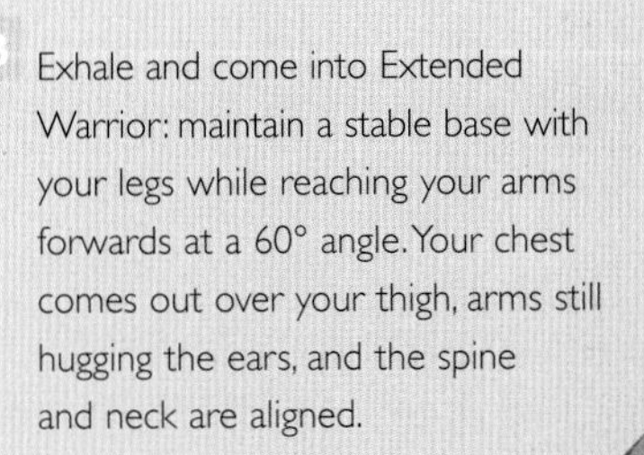

3 Exhale and come into Extended Warrior: maintain a stable base with your legs while reaching your arms forwards at a 60° angle. Your chest comes out over your thigh, arms still hugging the ears, and the spine and neck are aligned.

Your body forms a straight angle from the spine through the arms and hands

Maintain a stable base and lift the muscles around the knees

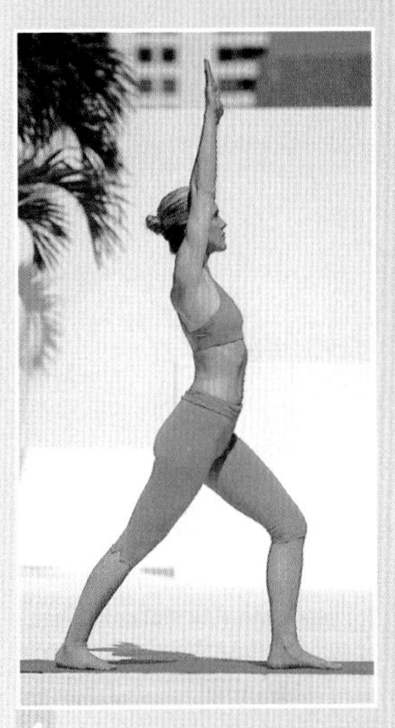

4 Inhale deeply and return to Full Warrior position as before.

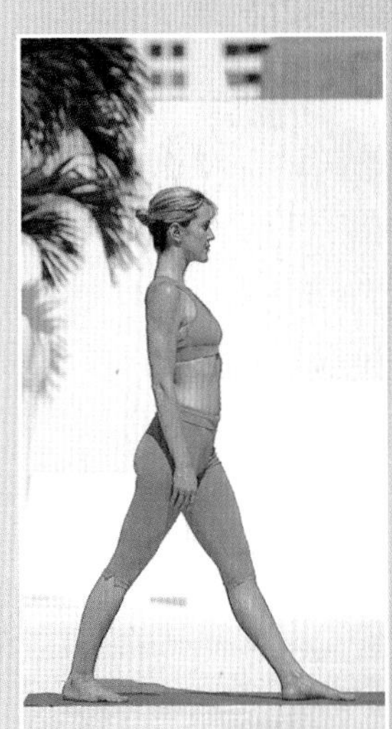

5 Exhale and bring the arms down, returning to the starting position.

3 WARRIOR BEND

This pose invigorates and refreshes the mind since it increases the blood supply to the brain, greatly enhancing concentration and mental capacity. Adding this forward bend into the Warrior sequence stretches and strengthens the lower and upper spine. If you have a weak back, bring your arms down towards the ground before you bend fully forwards. Rise up slowly if you begin to feel dizzy or off-balance.

Continue to practise all nine steps of Warrior Bend 2–3 times with the left foot in front, then rest in counterpose (p.220) *for 30 seconds to 1 minute, and repeat the sequence with the right foot in front.*

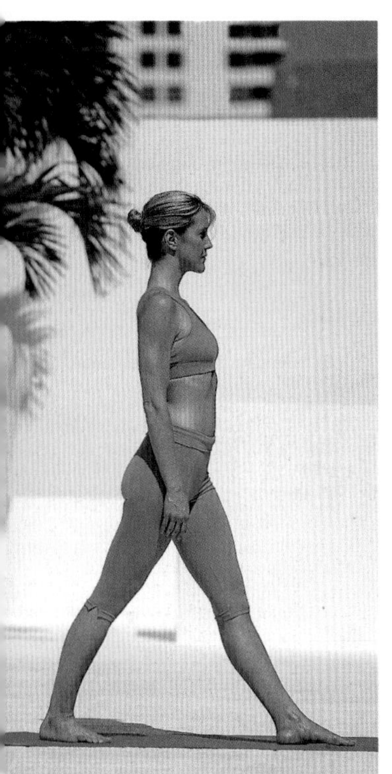

1 Stand with your left leg 60–120cm (2–4ft) forwards and your right foot behind you, turned out slightly. Your arms are by your sides.

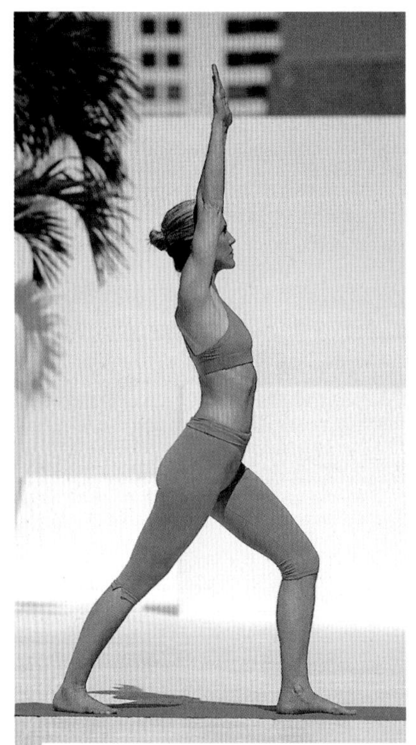

2 Inhale and come up into Full Warrior pose: bend the left knee so that it is directly above your ankle, and lift your arms up close to your ears, palms facing forwards.

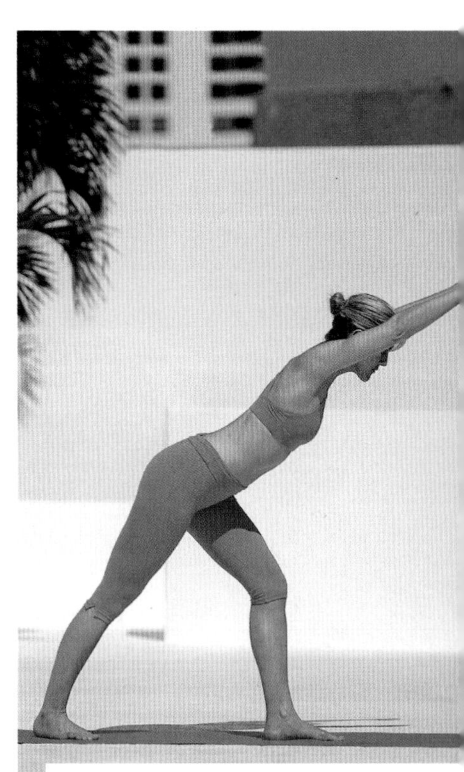

3 Exhale into Extended Warrior: reach your arms and upper body forwards so that your chest is over your thigh, your arms by your ears, and the spine and neck are aligned.

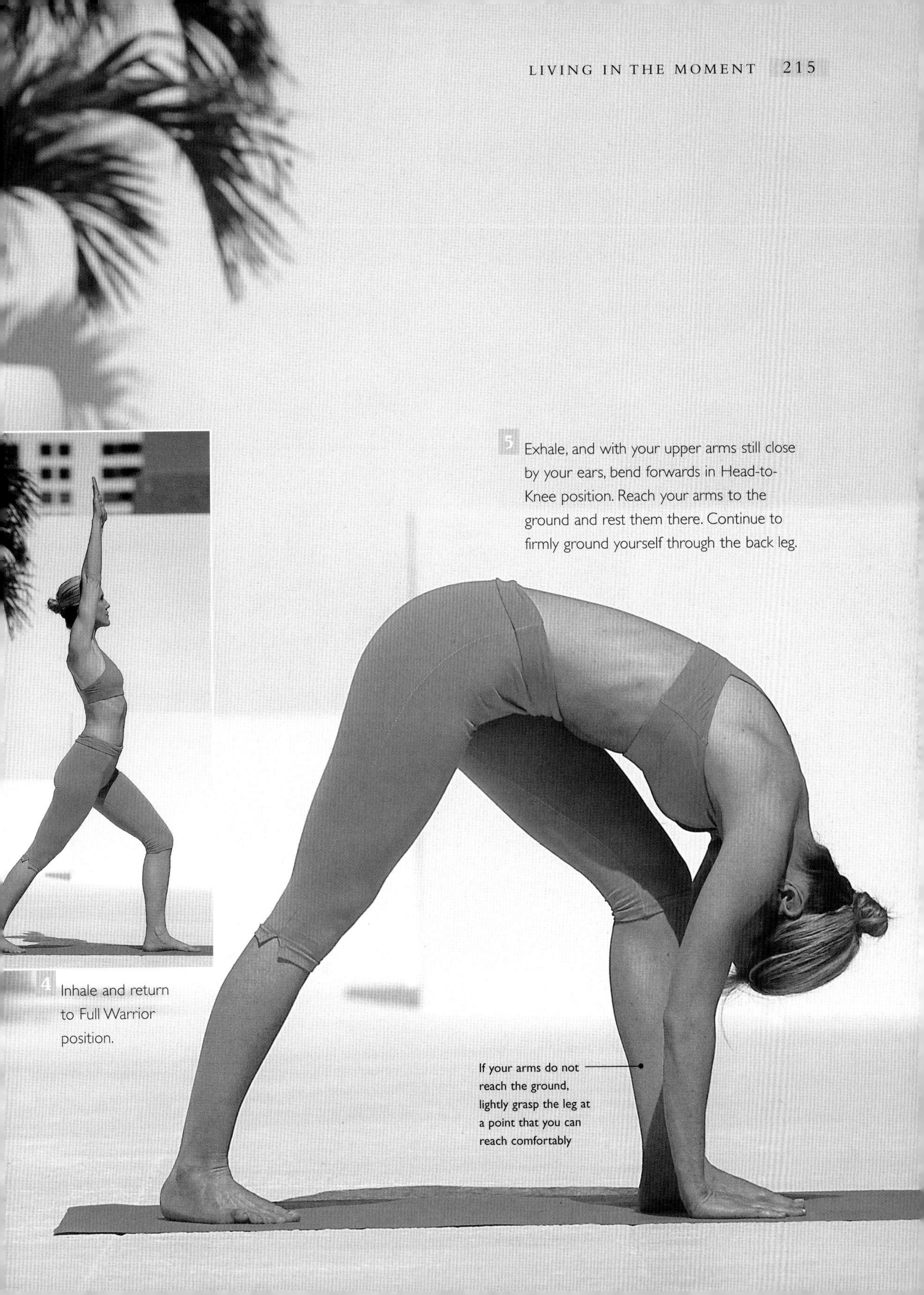

5 Exhale, and with your upper arms still close by your ears, bend forwards in Head-to-Knee position. Reach your arms to the ground and rest them there. Continue to firmly ground yourself through the back leg.

4 Inhale and return to Full Warrior position.

If your arms do not reach the ground, lightly grasp the leg at a point that you can reach comfortably

MARTHA'S STORY (USA)

One of the most profound and life-changing events in our lives has to be the moment we face the reality of our mother's death. My mother died of ovarian cancer, and I was blessed with the opportunity to spend several months with her as she struggled with the disease. I have had some training in the yogic healing practice of Sat Nam Rasayan, which teaches you to simply "be" with whatever situation presents to you, and consequently find healing and transformation in doing so. It was this knowledge that served me best during this difficult time.

I felt that my role, as her daughter, was to simply and gracefully "hold the sacred space" so that she could go through this transition with grace and dignity. The very simple yet profound act of listening, practising kindness, and being aware of the breath and its steady, rhythmic tide allowed me to stay and be present in the moment even during the sad and terrible moment of her death. I know it was a blessing to her, and it helped me to grieve and release her to the arms of the Infinite without remorse or guilt.

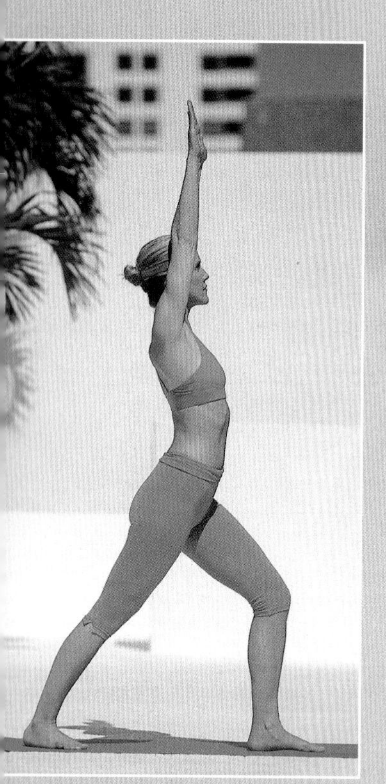

6 Inhale and return to Full Warrior position as before.

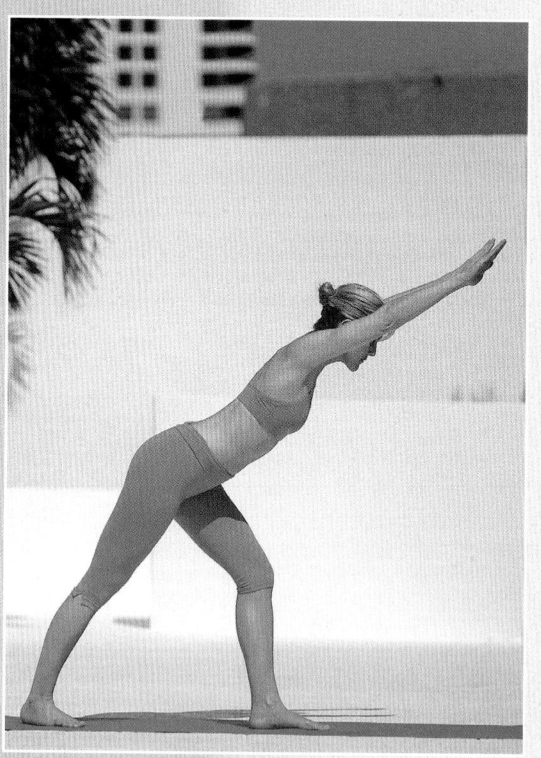

7 Exhale and return to Extended Warrior pose, maintaining a stable base with your legs while reaching your arms and upper body forwards.

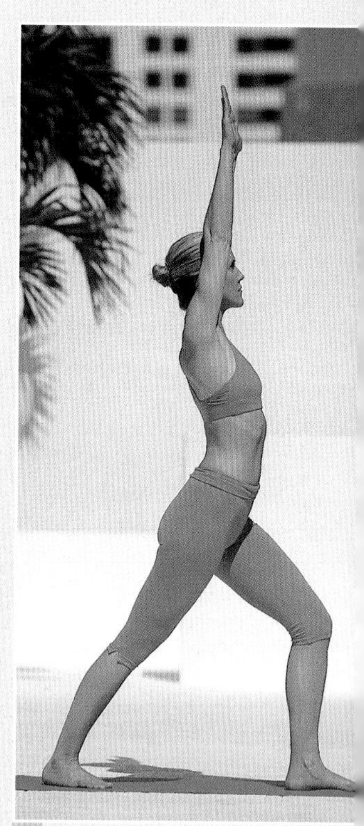

8 Inhale and return to Full Warrior position. Exhale and and return to the starting position. Repeat 2–3 times.

NADABRAHMA MEDITATION

Through this meditation, from Osho's book, Meditation (see p.224), *you learn to listen – to yourself, your partner, and everyone you meet. Ultimately you learn to listen to, and and be guided by, the soundless sound of the universe.*

1 *Sit in a relaxed position with your eyes closed and lips together, relaxed. Start humming loudly enough to be heard by others, and to create a vibration throughout your body. Visualize a hollow tube or empty vessel, filled only with the vibrations of the humming. A point will come when the humming continues by itself and you become the listener. There is no special breathing. Alter the pitch or move your body smoothly and slowly if you feel it. Continue for 30 minutes.*

2 *The second stage of the meditation is divided into two 7½ minute sections. For the first half, move the hands, palms up, in an outward circular motion. Starting at the navel, both hands move forwards, then divide to make two large circles mirroring each other on the left and right. The movement should be so slow that at times there will appear to be no movement at all. Feel that you are giving energy outwards to the universe.*

3 *After 7½ minutes, turn the hands so that the palms are down, and move them in the opposite direction. Now the hands come together towards the navel and divide outwards to the sides of the body. Feel that you are taking energy in. As in the previous movement, move extremely slowly. As in the first part of the meditation, don't inhibit any soft, slow movements of the rest of your body with these hand movements. Sit or lie absolutely quiet and still for 15 minutes.*

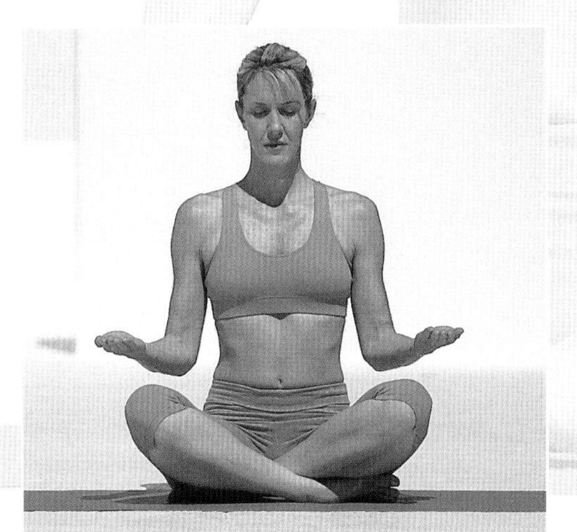

Giving motion: circle hands outwards, palms up

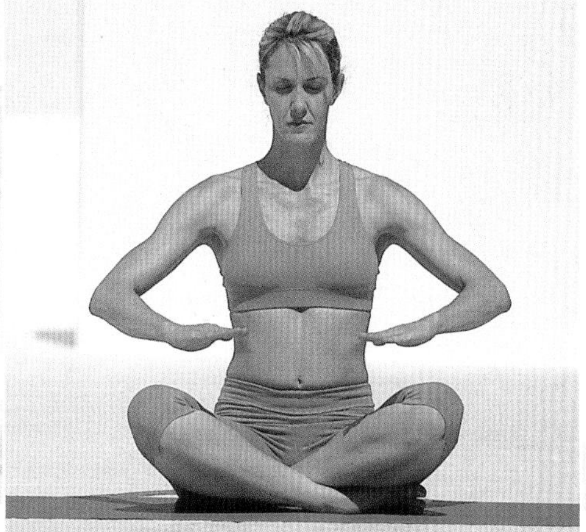

Receiving motion: circle hands inwards, palms down

4 WARRIOR BALANCE

This additional pose may be added to the vinyasa at the intermediate level. For extra balancing support, position yourself near a wall so that when you lean forwards your fingertips touch the wall.

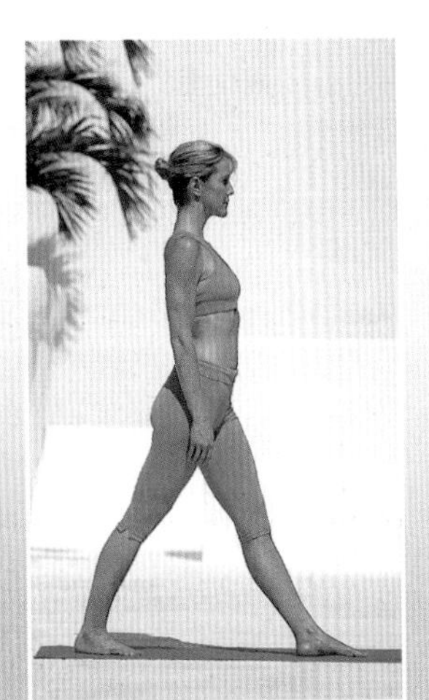

1 Stand with your left leg forwards, right foot behind and turned out slightly, and arms by your sides.

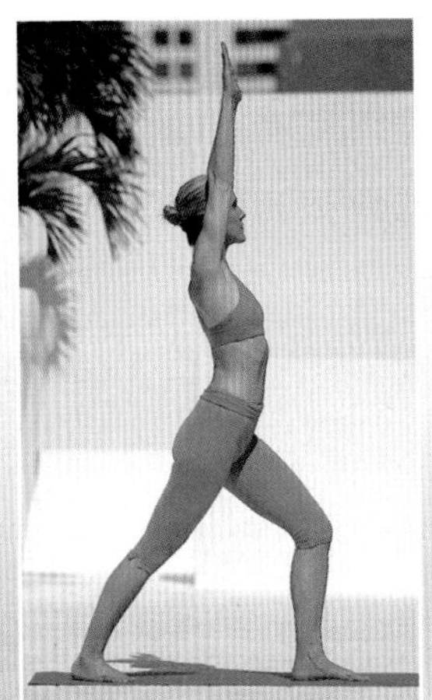

2 Inhale into Full Warrior pose as before.

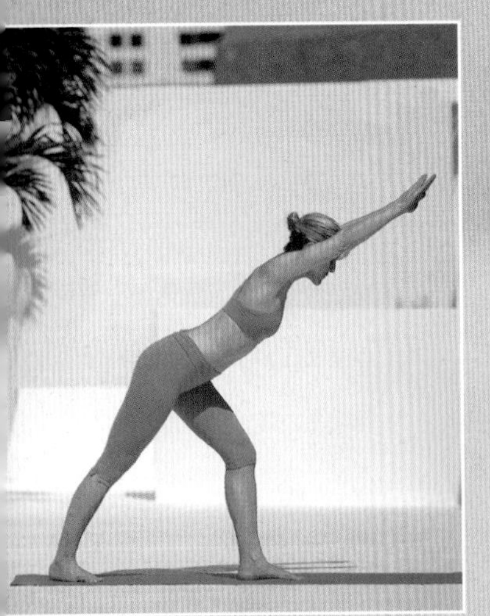

3 Exhale into Extended Warrior pose as before, maintaining a stable base with your legs.

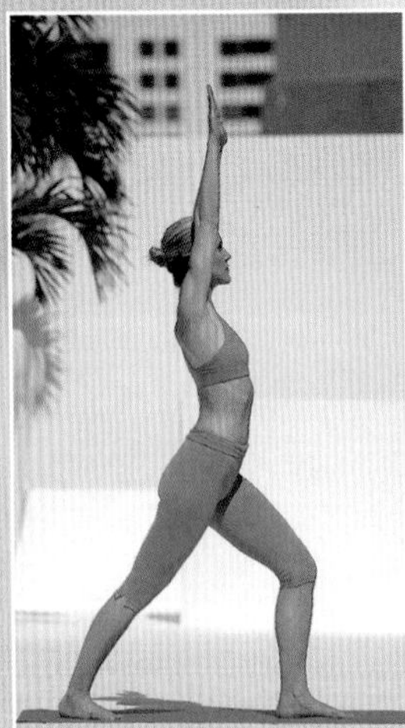

4 Inhale into Full Warrior pose as before.

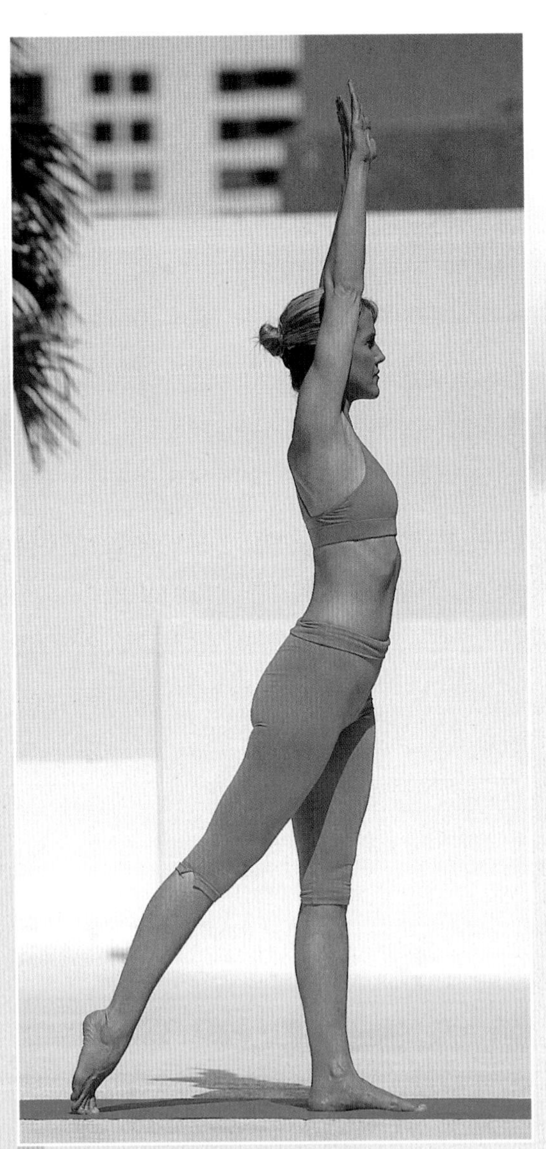

5 Exhale and lift the heel of your right foot up and lean forwards with the spine lengthened. Keep your arms up and reach out and up as you shift your weight to your left foot and lift your right foot off the ground.

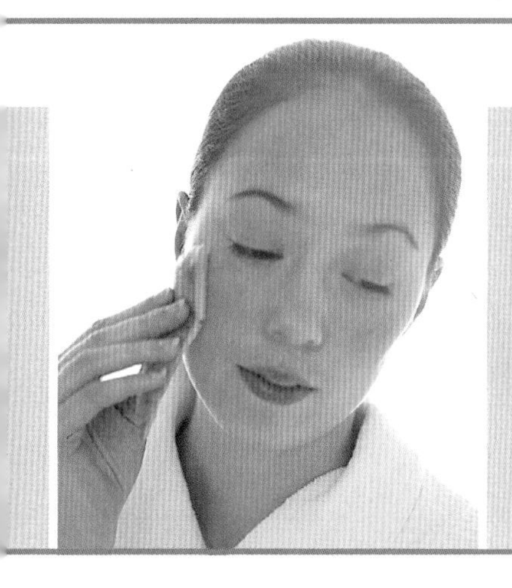

PAPAYA FACE MASK

Papaya is a heavenly fruit. It is soothing to the stomach and intestinal tract, and contains the digestive juice papain. It is rich in vitamins A, B, C, and D, which are all good for your skin and internal health. The inside skin of the papaya has been used as a beauty treatment since ancient times. For a beautiful complexion, cut up a papaya so that a very small layer of the flesh remains on the inside of the papaya skin. Rub this layer over your face until only the outside skin is left. Allow to dry, then rinse your face in warm water.

Arms are close to
the sides of the head
Leg is lifted to
hip height

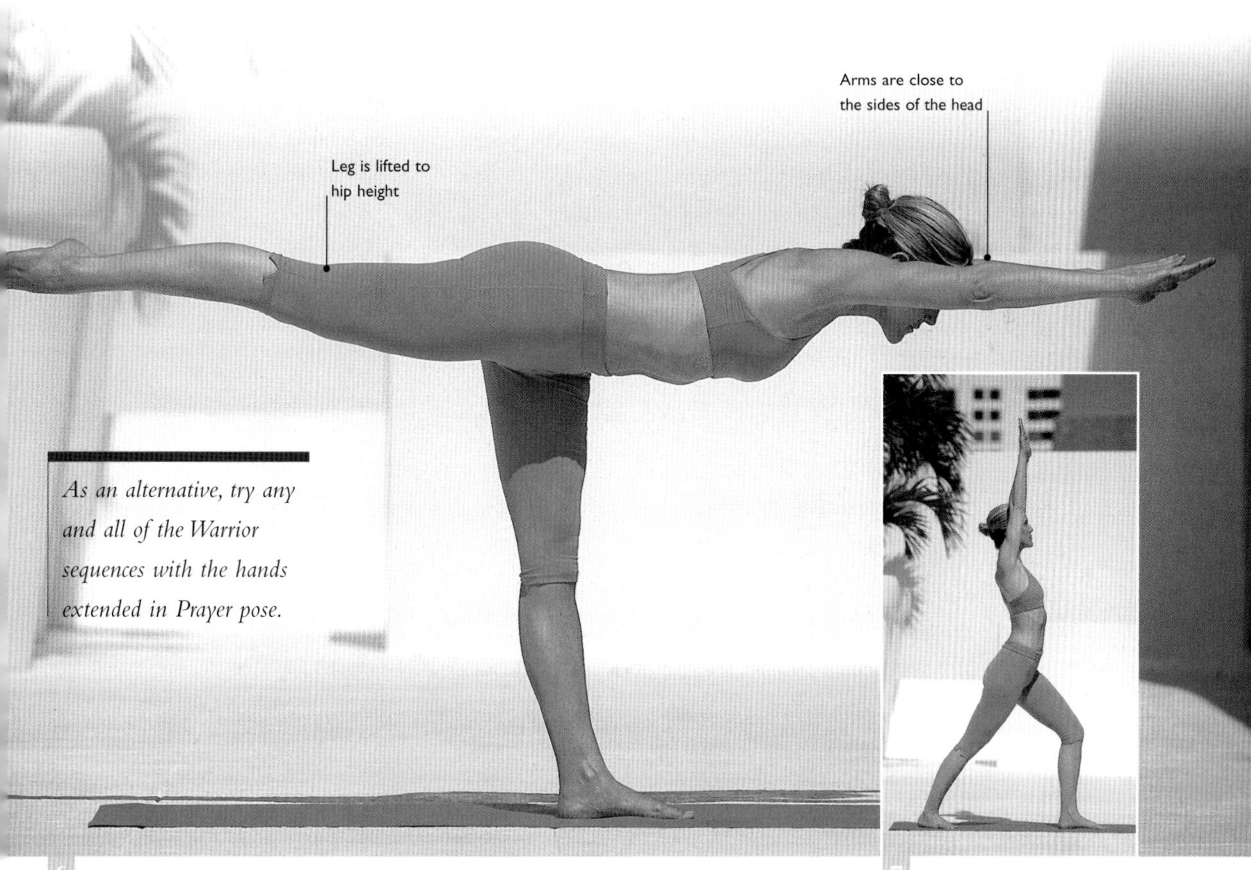

As an alternative, try any and all of the Warrior sequences with the hands extended in Prayer pose.

6 Lift your back leg so that your body forms a straight line from your hands to your toes. It may help to point the toes of your lifted leg. Gaze ahead as you feel the extension in your torso, arms, and leg.

7 Bend your left knee and lower your right leg. Inhale into Full Warrior pose.

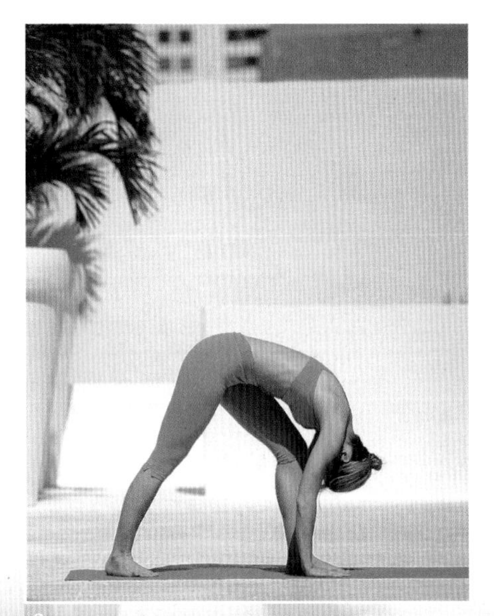

8 Exhale into Warrior Bend (*step 5, p.215*) as before, firmly grounding yourself through the back leg.

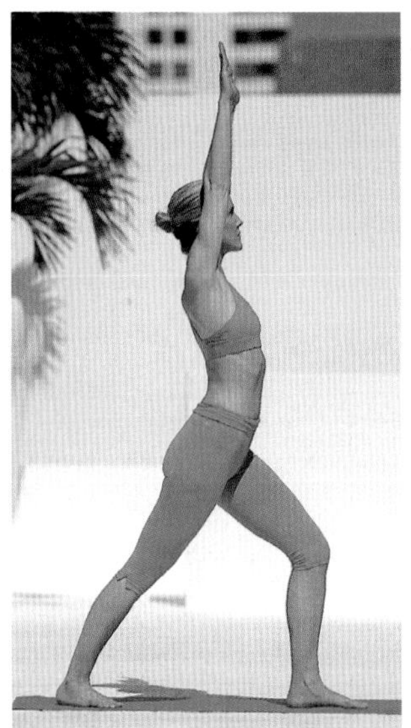

9 Inhale into Full Warrior pose as before.

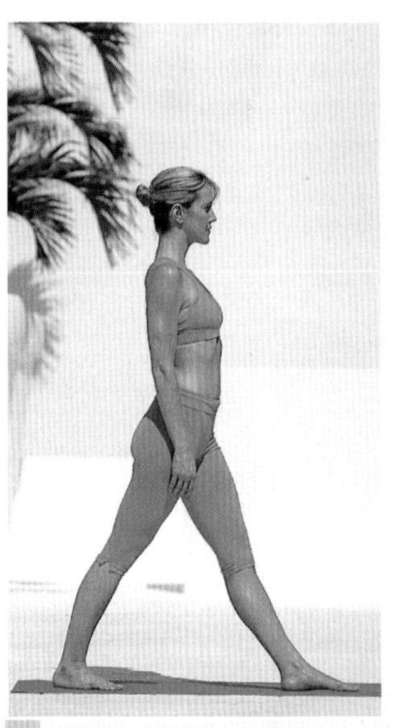

10 Exhale and come back to the starting position to end. Practise 2–3 rounds, then rest in the counterpose before repeating the sequence with the right leg forwards.

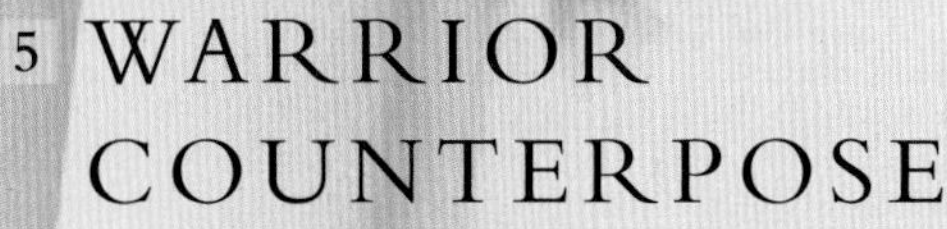

5 WARRIOR COUNTERPOSE

This allows your body to stretch and relax in the opposite direction from the Warrior sequence. Practise it after each round or at the end of the set.

With your legs straddled, pivot your feet so they are parallel to each other. Bend forwards and rest your hands on the ground, or just allow your arms to hang down. Relax in the forward bending position, yield to gravity, and let all tension go. Smile from the inside! Relax for 30 seconds to 2 minutes.

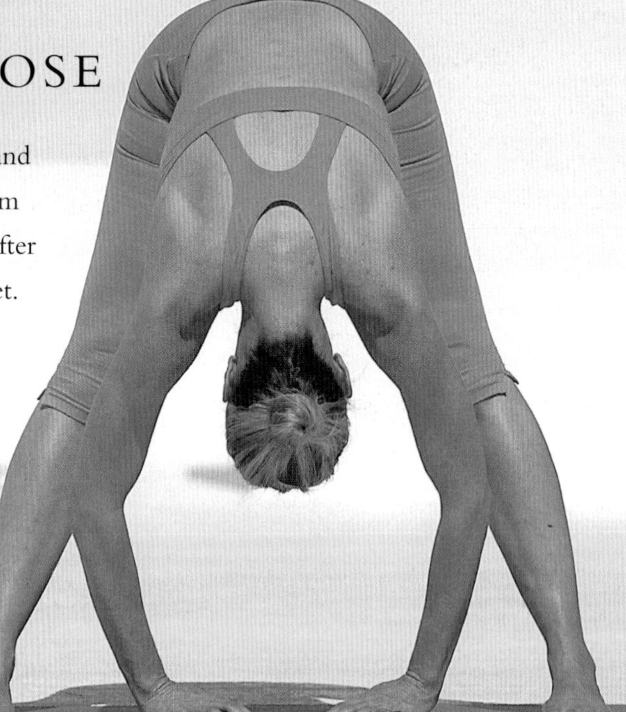

MOMENT TO MOMENT PRACTICE OF PEACE

This practice draws upon elements of present moment awareness as well as from the healing practice Sat Nam Rasayan (see Resources). *If you wish, you can record this meditation in your own voice and then play it back to practise. To deepen the effect, pauses have been added to allow the previous practice to subtly resonate in your awareness. Stay with the sensation until you feel it settle into a deep stillness, then move on to the next part.*

Observing and Allowing

Focus your awareness on your sensations. The feelings in your physical body, your breath, the sounds. Allow them all equally, without any special focus on any one of them. Let thoughts arise and watch them, as waves washing up on the shore of your awareness (pause).

Some feelings and thoughts that arise may be painful. Experiment with allowing the pain to be. Everything is allowed, nothing is judged. See that it cannot hurt you to let it be (pause).

After some few moments of observing and allowing the pain, a new element of acceptance is introduced and pain with total acceptance is no longer pain (pause).

Being in the Empty Space of Creation

Settle into your inner self. Experience a feeling of extending out in all directions. In observing these sensations, experience a deep space around you and inside you, a profound stillness and silence. Let a few seconds go by and realize that the "I" that seems to be you did not exist for a time. There is only beingness in this space. Experience this expanded awareness as an emptiness in which all potential of creation exists. Know that anything is possible in this creative emptiness, and that it exists all the time, whether you experience it or not (pause).

Adding Intention to your Awareness

Without effort, allow intention into the empty space of all possibilities. The intention may feel like a bubble rising from the water's depth to break on the surface. Insights that are related to the intention may come forwards into your consciousness. You may have a sense of what would heal a particular situation or person, or an insight into how to move forwards in your life. Remain neutral and non-resistant as intention and insight stabilize in your awareness (pause).

Living Life with Awareness

After a sitting practice, hold the intention of moving through your life with awareness of each moment. Bit by bit, find your way to the practice of peace until it becomes a way of life.

INDEX

RESOURCES

BOOKS

Easy Does It Yoga, Alice Christensen, Fireside Books, NY NY, 1999

Relax and Renew, Judith Lasater, PhD, PT, Rodmell Press, Berkeley CA, 1995

Easy Exercises for Pregnancy, Janet Balaskas, Macmillian, NY NY, 1997

Meditation: The First and Last Freedom, Osho, St. Martin's Press, NY NY, 1996

A Call to Women: The Healthy Breast Program & Workbook, Sat Dharam Kaur, ND, Quarry Press, Ontario, Canada, 2000

Anatomy of Miracles, Subagh Singh Khalsa (The Practice of Sat Nam Rasayan), Tuttle Publications, Boston MA, 1999

Baby and Mom (Video), Gurmukh Khalsa, Parade Videos, Peter Pan Ind., Newark NJ

Fly Like A Butterfly: Yoga for Children, Shakta Kaur Khalsa, Sterling Publishing Co., NY NY, 1998

Kundalini Yoga, Shakta Kaur Khalsa, DK Publishing, UK, 2001

Keep It Simple Series (KISS) Guide to Yoga, Shakta Kaur Khalsa, DK Publishing UK, 2001

Meditation as Medicine, Dharma Singh Khalsa, MD, Pocket Books, NY NY, 2001

Yoga for Your Life, Margaret and Martin Pierce, Sterling Publishing Co, NY NY, 1996

The Wisdom of Menopause, Christiane Northrup, M.D., Bantam Books, NY NY 2001

The Power of Now, Eckhart Tolle New World Library, Novato CA, 1999

Yoga Builds Bones, Jan Maddern, Harper Collins, UK, 2002

The Path of Practice: A Women's Book of Healing, Maya Tiwari, Ballantine Books, NY NY, 2000

Kundalini Yoga: The Flow of Eternal Power, Shakti Parwha K. Khalsa, Perigree, NY NY, 1998

Breathwalk, Yogi Bhajan, Ph.D. and Gurucharan S. Khalsa, Ph.D., Broadway Books, NY NY, 2000

Foods for Health and Healing, Yogi Bhajan, Ph. D., KRI, Espanola, NM, 1983

A Woman's Book of Yoga – Embracing Our Natural Life Cycles, Machelle Seibel, MD, and Hari Kaur Khalsa, Penguin Putnam (Avery) NY NY, 2002

WEBSITES

www.blessbless.com
Click on Women's Quote Express for inspiring quotes for women from the teachings of Yogi Bhajan.

www.SpiritVoyage.com
Providing powerfully uplifting music and mantra

www.grdcenter.com
Provides health education using yogic methods to people with chronic or life-threatening illness, such as HIV disease, cancer, and chronic pain.

www.Breathwalk.com
Information about Breathwalk, the walking meditation.

www.shaktakhalsa.com
Information about the author's books and writings on yoga and spiritual living.

www.kundaliniyoga.com
Kundalini Yoga as taught by Yogi Bhajan, White Tantric Yoga, and listings of trained Kundalini Yoga teachers worldwide.

www.yogafinder.com
Classes and teachers of all types of yoga.

www.yogainternational.com
Produced by the Himalayan Institute.

www.yogajournal.com
Articles about yoga, book reviews, information about yoga retreats, and much more.

www.yogitea.com
Healthy and tasty herbal teas.

www.yogamovement.com
Everything yoga-related.

www.transitionsforhealth.com
High-quality products, services and information to improve the health and lives of women.

www.momwell.com
Medically proven programmes in yoga and exercise for health, for expectant and new mothers.

www.bwy.org.uk
Learn about yoga or find a class in your area through The British Wheel of Yoga, a registered charity and leading member of the European Union of Yoga.

www.australian-institute-yoga.com.au
The Australian Institute of Yoga Therapy provides education, training and consultancy in yoga, ayurveda, general counselling and nutrition. Its services are available to groups, educational institutions and all individuals.

www.nzhealth.net.nz
Click on Business & Services Directory, then New Zealand Register of Complementary Health Professionals to find a qualified teacher in your area.

MUSIC CD

Women's Yoga Music CD compiled by Shakta Kaur Khalsa.

Available from Spirit Voyage Music. To hear a selection or to order, go to **www.SpiritVoyage.com**

ACKNOWLEDGMENTS

Author's acknowledgments
I am deeply grateful for the love and support of my teacher, Yogi Bhajan, my husband, Kartar Singh Khalsa, my son, Ram Das Singh Khalsa. My gratitude goes to the wonderful women whose insight, creativity, and plain hard work shaped this book; Gillian Roberts, Mary-Clare Jerram, Susannah Steel, Claire Legemah, Karen Sawyer, LaVonne Carlson; to the talented photographer, Russell Sadur, and his assistant, Nina Duncan; to Cindy Andrews for hair and make-up; to the superb models who gave their best to this book. My thanks to all who offered their expertise; Patricia Miller, Kay Hawkins, Dr. Nirmala Lamaye, Bonnie Berk, Gururam Kaur, and to all those women whose stories appear in this book. Special thanks go to Satya Kaur Khalsa for making KRI a joy to work with.

Publisher's acknowledgments
Thanks to Dawn Young and Anna Benjamin for design assistance, and Hilary Bird for the index.
All photographs © Dorling Kindersley
For further information visit www.dkimages.com
Photography: photographer Russell Sadur, assisted by Nina Duncan; photographic production and location services in Miami, Sharon Weems.
Models: Clinton Archambault, Gurmeet K. Cheng, Rudy Estripeant, Mia Rosen Glick, Sarah Ruby Glick, Catherine Goodrum, Anna Karina Gutierrez, Anastasia Levinson, Mary E. Schroeder, Spencer Singer, Kelly Smith-Beany, Cate Williams
Hair and makeup: Cindy Andrews
Hair and makeup for front jacket photograph: Toko
Stylist: Liz Hancock

Yoga mats kindly supplied by: Hugger Mugger Yoga Products
www.huggermugger.com & www.yoga.co.uk
email: yme@ednet.co.uk
Yoga props kindly supplied by: Yoga Matters
www.yogamatters.co.uk
email: enquiries@yogamatters.co.uk
Leisure clothing kindly supplied by: Toast
www.toastbypost.co.uk
email: contact@toastbypost.co.uk
Nadabrahama Meditation (*p.217*) reprinted with permission by Osho International (www.osho.com).
Pranayama to Expel Negativity and Disease (*p.163*) reprinted with permission from *A Year with the Master* by Atma Singh and Guruprem Kaur Khalsa (info@yogagems.net)